Drugs of Abuse
Their Genetic
and Other Chronic
Nonpsychiatric Hazards

The MIT Press

Cambridge, Massachusetts, and

London, England

Drugs of Abuse
Their Genetic
and Other Chronic
Nonpsychiatric Hazards

Based on a symposium
cosponsored by the Center for
Studies of Narcotic
and Drug Abuse, NIMH, and by
the Environmental Mutagen Society
San Francisco, October 29 and 30, 1969

edited by
Samuel S. Epstein

with associate editors

Joshua Lederberg

Marvin Legator

Eleanor E. Carroll, and

Jack D. Blaine

ISBN 0 262 05009 9 (hardcover)

Library of Congress catalog card number: 78–148969

Appendixes

Contributors and
Invited Participants

Seymour Abrahamson
Departments of Genetics and Zoology,
University of Wisconsin, Madison, Wisconsin.

Kimball C. Atwood
Department of Human Genetics and Develop-
ment, College of Physicians and Surgeons,
Columbia University, New York, N.Y.

Jack D. Blaine
Center for Studies of Narcotic and Drug
Abuse, National Institute of Mental Health,
Chevy Chase, Maryland.

Henry Brill
Pilgrim State Hospital, West Brentwood,
New York.

Bertram S. Brown
National Institute of Mental Health, Chevy
Chase, Maryland.

Eleanor E. Carroll
Center for Studies of Narcotic and Drug
Abuse, National Institute of Mental Health,
Chevy Chase, Maryland.

Maimon M. Cohen
Department of Pediatrics and Division of
Human Genetics, State University of New York,
Buffalo, New York.

Seymour I. Cohen
Bureau of Occupational Health and Environ-
mental Epidemiology, California State
Department of Public Health, Berkeley,
California.

James F. Crow
Departments of Genetics and Medical Genetics,
University of Wisconsin, Madison, Wisconsin.

Alan C. Davis
American Cancer Society, New York, N.Y.

Frederick J. de Serres
Biology Division, Oak Ridge National
Laboratory, Oak Ridge, Tennessee.

Samuel S. Epstein
Swetland Professor of Environmental Health
and Human Ecology, School of Medicine,
Case Western Reserve University, Cleveland,
Ohio.

Ernst Freese
Laboratory of Molecular Biology, National Institute of Neurological Diseases and Stroke, Bethesda, Maryland.

John R. Goldsmith
Bureau of Occupational Health and Environmental Epidemiology, California State Department of Public Health, Berkeley, California.

Lissy F. Jarvik
Department of Medical Genetics, New York State Psychiatric Institute, and Department of Psychiatry, College of Physicians and Surgeons, Columbia University, New York, N.Y.

Milton H. Joffe
Division of Narcotic Addiction and Drug Abuse, National Institute of Mental Health, Chevy Chase, Maryland.

Harold Kalter
Children's Hospital Research Foundation and Department of Pediatrics, University of Cincinnati College of Medicine, Cincinnati, Ohio.

Charles J. Kensler
Arthur D. Little, Inc., Cambridge, Massachusetts.

Joshua Lederberg
Department of Genetics, Stanford University School of Medicine, Stanford Medical Centre, Palo Alto, California.

Marvin S. Legator
Cell Biology Branch, Division of Nutrition, Food and Drug Administration, and George Washington University, Washington, D.C.

Gilbert J. Mannering
Department of Pharmacology, University of Minnesota, Minneapolis, Minnesota.

William R. Martin
NIMH Addiction Research Center, Lexington, Kentucky.

James A. Miller
McArdle Laboratory for Cancer Research, University of Wisconsin Medical Center, Madison, Wisconsin.

Paul S. Moorhead
Department of Medical Genetics, School of Medicine, University of Pennsylvania, Philadelphia, Pennsylvania.

Robert C. Petersen
Center for Studies of Narcotic and Drug Abuse, National Institute of Mental Health, Chevy Chase, Maryland.

Alexander T. Shulgin
1483 Shulgin Road, Lafayette, California.

James Willis
Consultant psychiatrist, Department of Psychological Medicine, Guy's Hospital and Bexley Hospital, London, England.

Virginia Zaratzian
Psychopharmacology Research Branch, National Institute of Mental Health, Chevy Chase, Maryland.

Foreword

There have now been two conferences held under the aegis of the National Institute of Mental Health principally concerned with the nonpsychiatric hazards of drugs of abuse. The first, held in the fall of 1967, at a time of considerable public alarm over possible genetic implications of LSD use, did much to place the problem in perspective and to encourage additional research. The second conference, two years later, has, we hope, contributed further awareness of what is still needed to assess adequately the possible mutagenic, teratogenic, and carcinogenic aspects of drugs of abuse. Drug abuse remains a refractory problem to which there are few simple solutions. Assessment of the physical and mental health implications of drug abuse, particularly from the standpoint of chronic use, is not easy. It is the task of the National Institute of Mental Health to develop the research support strategies to deal flexibly with the many facets of drug abuse. Publication of this volume is part of the long-term effort to foster a greater awareness of the present state of our scientific knowledge and to further the research effort upon which enlightened public policy must inevitably rest.

Bertram S. Brown, M.D.

Director
National Institute of Mental Health

Preface

The use of an ever widening range of drugs for nonmedical purposes has engendered some of the most contentious and perplexing controversies of our social policy. The possible biological hazards of such drugs as LSD, which presently derive from conjecture as much as from controlled experiments, have attracted interest disproportionate to more plausible concerns on direct and residual psychotropic effects. Nevertheless, both an understanding of these side effects and an assessment of their potential hazards are important for the design of reasonable policies.

Available information on potential biological hazards due to drugs of abuse is extremely limited. However, a confusing variety of experimental data has been reported for the biological effects of LSD. These in turn have stimulated a variety of research projects submitted for funding to the National Institute of Mental Health (NIMH). Some of these projects were inadequate in concept or design; others still left unanswerable questions on the significance of their possible findings; yet others were potentially duplicative. Nevertheless, the growing dimensions of drug abuse necessitate urgent development of reliable data on adverse biological effects, particularly the chronic hazards of mutation, cancer, and teratology, as well as on psychotropic effects.

At the suggestion of the National Advisory Mental Health Council, the NIMH in association with the Environmental Mutagen Society sponsored a conference in October 1969 whose aims were to evaluate existing information on potential chronic biological hazards of drugs of abuse, and to outline the most effective methodologies for developing necessary information on the subject [Epstein and Lederberg 1970]. It was hoped that the findings of the conference would assure that the limited resources of the NIMH could be most productively deployed. However, the findings of the conference rest on the scientific reputation of its members, and they should not be taken as an NIMH policy statement.

The conclusions of the conference are not easy to summarize, and they may well be judged unsatisfactory by defenders of categorical positions. This is partly a reflection of some limitations in the methodology available until recently for answering questions on chronic hazards to man. Promising new approaches based on well-established theoretical and empirical principles, particularly in mutagenicity testing, have recently emerged. Such approaches have not as yet been properly exploited in the study of drugs of abuse, let alone in the more general study of environmental chemical pollutants [Epstein and Lederberg 1970].

Even in an idealized laboratory setting, there are still many complicating problems in dealing with drugs of abuse, as compared with therapeutic or prophylactic drugs, apart from the wider perspective of environmental chemical pollutants. Psychotropic agents often exhibit different effects in different species, which may reflect differences in metabolism, although plausibly attributed to differences at higher levels of neural organization. The use of drugs of abuse, which has increased dramatically over the last decade, is generally restricted to young adults. The street drugs are rarely pure or uncontaminated, and even if they were, with the possible exception of cannabis, very few drugs claim the undivided attention of their users ; the drug habitué is likely to practice ultimate polypharmacy and to be relatively unaware of what and how much he has actually taken by diverse routes, including ingestion, inhalation, and injection. The habitué may well be relatively idiosyncratic in other life styles as well, and he may experience bouts of intercurrent infection and malnutrition that may have their own chronic effects on health, besides specifically interacting with the drugs. Drugs of abuse

thus present quite unusual toxicological problems.

A most pressing question for which the conference found no satisfactory solution, was how to establish *quantitative* standards for the putative human cost of a given exposure to a chemical inducing adverse effects such as mutagenicity in an experimental animal. What level of mutagenicity would have to be imputed to LSD or to other more acceptable drugs, or to synthetic chemicals such as food additives, to be relevant to social controls ? The well-authenticated chromosome-breaking activity of a cyclamate metabolite, cyclohexylamine, prompted no early administrative action, owing partly to present lack of consensual standards ; this fact is all the more surprising in view of the questionable utility of cyclamate for the population at large. It may be argued, however, that our existing methods are unlikely to detect and prove mutagenic effects in man unless they exceed a 10 percent increase in the spontaneous mutation rate. This is an effect that would be comparable to a doubling of the background level of natural radiation. *Any* mutagenic effect that is demonstrable with present *in vivo* methods in mammals should thus be ample cause for concern.

The insensitivity of mammalian systems for prediction of chronic toxicity in man, especially carcinogenicity, teratogenicity, and mutagenicity, is now well recognized. Such insensitivity is a function of the restricted numbers of animals tested, commonly under 50 per dose of compound, in contrast with the millions of humans at presumptive risk. Let us assume that a new compound, such as a food additive or pesticide, produces cancer, birth defects, or hereditary genetic effects at the alarming rate of 1 per 10,000 humans ; let us assume further that the sensitivity of man and the test animal is of a similar order. Then test groups of 10,000 animals would be required to demonstrate a single adverse effect; for statistical significance, groups of approximately 30,000 animals would thus be required. Of course, in in any particular instance, man may be more or less sensitive than the test animal to the toxic effects of the compound in question. Thus, testing at the low levels of presumptive human exposure would preclude the possibility of detecting any but the grossest possible adverse effect.

For these reasons, it is routine practice to test up to maximally tolerated doses, in an effort to reduce the gross insensitivity of animal systems. Such overloading is the only practical method for detecting carcinogenic, teratogenic, and mutagenic effects, especially those due to agents with relatively low biological potency. In testing for carcinogenicity, commencing exposure of animals during early infancy is also helpful in enhancing sensitivity. Calculation of human risk by extrapolation from animal assays, with or without overload, is necessarily complex. In the absence of very specific information that overload induces abnormal metabolic pathways—due to saturation of enzyme receptor sites or to abnormal feedback—data based on overload responses are clearly legitimate and should be used for regulatory purposes and for the quantitative prediction of human risk. There are other cogent reasons, including problems of interaction and synergism, for the view that there is no acceptable method for predicting safe levels of carcinogens, teratogens, or mutagens, based on arbitrary fractions of no-effect doses in animal tests, with their built-in insensitivity as a function of small sample size [Epstein 1970]. Indeed, such considerations form the basis of the Delaney amendment, with reference to establishment of zero tolerances for food additives found to be carcinogenic by feeding at any level; this concept could well be extended to both teratogens and mutagens.

The conference emphasized that the restriction of the discussion to the evaluation of drugs of abuse alone, without consideration of other chemical pollutants of the environment such as pesticides and food additives, is an artificial restriction. Factual data on drugs of abuse are grossly inadequate; there is, furthermore, no rationale to single these drugs out as worse potential hazards than many environmental pollutants and common therapeutic or prophylactic drugs, such as tranquilizers, whose *abuse* is less widely recognized and labeled as such. The same methodology would apply to the evaluation of environmental pollutants, which would be somewhat less complicated by the secondary factors associated with drugs like LSD.

The conference's deliberations emphasized the need for more systematic and programmatic evaluation than is currently required of potential chronic hazards of drugs and other environmental pollutants, including food additives, pesticides, and fuel additives [Epstein 1970]. The conference discussed a wide range of specific toxicological procedures that are currently available, some of which could well bear improvement. The importance of the effect of a drug on *metabolism* was underscored; this effect can provoke suspicions about unusual kinds of hazard, and it is necessary for correlating human with animal responses, especially if results in different animal species prove discordant. Individual differences within human populations, be they of genetic or environmental origin, must be expected; drugs will interact with one another in the process of metabolism, and therefore also in side effects; the fetus cannot be expected to show the same metabolic patterns as the adult; infection and malnutrition may also complicate individual responses.

The impact of a chemically induced cancer falls so heavily on the afflicted patient that the cost of environmental cancer is likely to be perceived in very personal terms. The costs of mutations are mortgages against the future. The responsible citizen, when he functions in his social role, should give the same weight of passionate concern for his helpless posterity that he gives to his own health in one of the soundest, if not always best honored, of human motives, self-preservation.

J. Lederberg
S. S. Epstein

References

Epstein, S. S., and J. Lederberg (1970). *Science* 168:507.

Epstein, S. S. (1970). *Nature* 228:816.

Drugs of Abuse
Their Genetic
and Other Chronic
Nonpsychiatric Hazards

I. General Considerations

1 Chemistry and Sources

A. T. Shulgin

The purpose of this chapter is to assemble in a single convenient location the chemical and botanical definitions of those materials which may contribute to the drug abuse problem.

Many questions that concern these materials are now being answered, both socially as well as pharmacologically, but to a large measure these are questions that should have been asked years ago, before specific problems arose. A much larger number of questions can be anticipated now concerning drug problems of the future, and current research plans should be molded to provide needed answers as soon as possible. The instruments and skills required are available (see Sections II and III), and the only requirements that must be met are that the questions be honestly asked, and the subsequent research be supported without prejudice. It is hoped that this chapter will provide a compendium of factual information that might provide a reference foundation for future research.

1. Atlas of Drugs

Many of the drugs grouped under the general headings actually constitute mixtures of many different chemicals. The possibility always exists that some component other than the generally accepted "active principle" of a drug mixture may contribute to its hazard potential or to its undesirable side effects. For this reason, each drug presentation is expanded upon from the viewpoints both of congeneric contaminants and of synthetic by-products.

Those materials that are substantially of synthetic origin may generally be expected to be relatively pure. The contaminants that may be present will reflect the synthetic routes that have been employed. This debris, although both chemically and forensically meaningful, is rarely related pharmacologically to the synthetic end product. An exception to this must be made in those instances, such as the manufacture of LSD, where the end drug is produced from starting materials that are themselves of high biological activity—in this case, the natural ergot alkaloids. In any event all components in a given chemical pathway should be considered from the point of view of potential hazard. Unfortunately, far too often these concomitant chemicals have been isolated in quantities barely sufficient for structural studies, and most biological properties remain unknown.

This presentation of drugs has been arranged in a descending order of priority. The first discussed are those that constitute immediate social problems, and which certainly require the major attention of medical scientists. Within this first group, marijuana and LSD stand apart in their apparent capabilities for social disruption through subtle disturbances of the conventional mores. Their use has on occasion led, within the user, to a change in personal ethics regarding law and society; this change is certainly dissimilar to the generally disruptive or withdrawal-like behavior of the other abuse drugs mentioned. However, virtually all of the drugs to be discussed have upon one occasion or another led to some similiar emotional evolution.

The second group to be discussed contains those materials that are of limited availability, but that have not yet achieved a position of general abuse.

The least attention should be directed to the third group, which contains materials that are quite difficult to obtain. An extension of this is a group of odd botanical extracts and of several chemicals of totally synthetic origin, that can be classified as fads of the moment, or even as fraudulent put-ons. One cannot predict the future of such substances, and very little research work along these lines can be currently justified.

A frequently overlooked category of chemicals should at least be noted here. These are the excipients that are used in the preparation of illegal drugs or other intentional contaminants, not related to the manner of preparation, that might be introduced for the purpose of interference with analysis. These are often materials that are accepted as being pharmacologically inert in small dosages, such as ascorbic acid and lactose. Frequently, however, less well-studied chemicals, such as plant essential oils, or materials of known pharmacological efficacy, such as strychnine, are employed.

Each of the entries within these several classifications must be considered only as a representative example that stands for an entire group of drugs. Continuous reference must be made to Table 1, wherein each group is illustrated more completely. Each group is separated in the table under the single entry name that is used in the following text.

2. Drugs of Immediate Social Impact

2.1. Marijuana

All of the marijuana that is available on the street, and thus all of the marijuana that constitutes a drug problem, is of botanical origin. The material may be presented as a leafy substance, marijuana itself, or it may be encountered as hashish, which is properly the resinous exuate of the plant, but which is a name often applied to the concentrated extract of the plant. None of these forms involve any synthetic considerations and thus there are no aspects of purification; all together they constitute broad mixtures of related chemicals.

There are four principal groups of interrelated chemicals present in the resin of the plant. The first of these, the aromatic fraction, contains a single chemical, cannabinol [Wood et al. 1899; Adams et al. 1940b]. This compound appears to be the end product that results from both long-term storage and from animal metabolism of the various tetrahydro derivatives. These latter represent the second group of the cannabinoids, and are currently

Table 1. Chemical Classification of Drugs of Abuse

Molecular Structure	Chemical Names / Common Names	References (b) Biological (i) Isolation (s) Synthesis
Marijuana Group		
[structure: CH₃, HO, (CH₂)₄CH₃, H₃C CH₃, O]	6,6,9-trimethyl-3-pentyl-6H-dibenzo-(b,d)-pyran-1-ol. cannabinol	(b) Loewe 1950 (i) Wood et al., 1899 (s) Adams, Baker, et al, 1940b
[structure: CH₃, HO, (CH₂)₄CH₃, H₃C CH₃, C–O]	6a, 7, 8, 10a-tetrahydro-6,6,9-trimethyl-3-pentyl-6a,10a-trans-6H-dibenzo-(b, d)-pyran-1-ol. Δ^1-tetrahydrocannabinol Δ^1-THC Δ^9-tetrahydrocannabinol Δ^9-THC	(b)(i) Gaoni and Mechoulam 1964a; Bicher et al, 1966, Isbell, Gorodetsky, et al, 1967; Hollister, Richards, et al, 1968; Mechoulam and Bicher 1968 (s) Mechoulam and Gaoni, 1965a; Fahrenholtz et al 1966; Mechoulam, Braun, et al, 1967
[structure: CH₃, HO, (CH₂)₄CH₃, H₃C CH₃, C–O]	6a,7,10,10a-tetrahydro-6,6,9-trimethyl-3-pentyl-6a,10a-trans-6H-dibenzo-(b,d)-pyran-1-ol. $\Delta^{1(6)}$-tetrahydrocannabinol $\Delta^{1(6)}$-THC Δ^8-tetrahydrocannabinol Δ^8-THC	(b) Bicher et al, 1966; Mechoulam and Bicher 1968 (i) Hively et al, 1966 (s) Fahrenholtz et al, 1966; Taylor et al, 1966
[structure: CH₃, HO, (CH₂)₄CH₃, H₃C CH₃, O]	7,8,9,10-tetrahydro-6,6,9-trimethyl-3-pentyl-6H-dibenzo-(b,d)-pyran-1-ol. Δ^3-tetrahydrocannabinol Δ^3-THC	(b) Loewe 1950 (i) Not natural (s) Adams and Baker 1940; Adams, Smith, et al, 1941b; Ghosh et al, 1941
[structure: CH₃, HO, (CH₂)₅CH₃, H₃C CH₃, O]	3-hexyl-7,8,9,10-tetrahydro-6,6,9-trimethyl-6H-dibenzo-(b,d)-pyran-1-ol. Parahexyl Pyrahexyl (Abbott) Synhexyl (Roche)	(b) Loewe 1950; Hollister, Richards, et al, 1968 (i) Not natural (s) Adams, Loewes, et al, 1941a
[structure: CH₃, HO, CH(CH₂)₆CH₃, CH₃, H₃C CH₃, O]	7,8,9,10-tetrahydro-6,6,9-trimethyl-3-(1-methyloctyl)-6H-dibenzo-(b,d)-pyran-1-ol. methyloctylpyran MOP	(b) Dagirmanjian and Boyd 1962 (i) Not natural (s) Adams, Aycock, et al, 1948a

Table 1. Chemical Classification of Drugs of Abuse (continued)

Molecular Structure	Chemical Names Common Names	References (b) Biological (i) Isolation (s) Synthesis
	7,8,9,10-tetrahydro-6,6, 9-trimethyl-3-(1,2- dimethylheptyl)-6H- dibenzo-(b,d)-pyran-1-ol. dimethylheptylpyran DMHP SKF-5390 RA-122	(b) Loewe 1950; Dagirmanjian and Boyd 1962; Haertzen et al, 1963 (i) Not natural. (s) Adams, MacKenzie, et al, 1948b
	2-(p-mentha-1,8-dien-3- yl)-5-pentylresorcinol cannabidiol	(b) Jacob and Todd 1940; Loewe 1946 (i) Jacob and Todd 1940; Adams, Hunt, et al, 1940 (s) Mechoulam and Gaoni 1965a; Korte, Dlugosch, et al, 1966; Petrzilka et al, 1967
	2-(p-mentha-1,8-dien-3- yl)-5-pentylresorcinol- 4-carboxylic acid cannabidiolic acid	(b) Schultz and Haffner 1958; Kabelik et al, 1960 (i) Krejči et al, 1958; Mechoulam and Gaoni 1965b
	6a,7,8,10a-tetrahydro- 6,6,9-trimethyl-3-pentyl- 6H-dibenzo-(b,d)-pyran- 1-ol-2-carboxylic acid Δ^1-THC acid	(i) Korte, Haag, et al, 1965
	$\Delta^{4(8)}$-isotetrahydro- cannabinol	(s) Gaoni and Mechoulam 1966

LSD Group

	(d)-Lysergic acid, diethyl- amide N,N-diethyl lysergamide lysergide Delysid (Sandoz) LSD, LSD-25, "acid"	(b) Stoll 1947; Cohen 1960 (i) Not natural (s) Stoll and Hofmann 1943

Molecular Structure	Chemical Names Common Names	References (b) Biological (i) Isolation (s) Synthesis
	(d)-Isolysergic acid di-ethylamide Iso-LSD	(b) Hofmann 1958 (i) Not natural
	2-bromo-d-lysergic acid diethylamide bromlysergide BOL-148	(b) Stoll and Hofmann 1943; Jarvik et al, 1955 (i) Not natural
	N¹-methyl-d-lysergic acid diethylamide MLD-41	(b) Rothlin 1957; Cerletti 1959 (i) Not natural
	N¹-acetyl-d-lysergic acid diethylamide ALD-52	(b) Rothlin 1957; Cerletti 1959; Isbell, Miner, et al, 1959 (i) Not natural
	d-lysergic acid ethyl-amide LAE-32	(b) Stoll and Hofmann 1943; Cerletti 1959 (i) Not natural

Table 1. Chemical Classification of Drugs of Abuse (continued)

Molecular Structure	Chemical Names Common Names	References (b) Biological (i) Isolation (s) Synthesis
	d-lysergic acid morpholide LSM-777	(b) Cerletti 1959 (i) Not natural
	N^1-methyl-d-lysergic acid butanolamide Sansert (Sandoz) UML-491 methysergide	(b) PDR
	d-lysergic acid amide d-lysergamide ergine LA-111	(b) Solms 1956; Hofmann 1963 (i) Hofmann and Tscherter 1960; Hofmann 1963; Hylin and Watson 1965; Abou-Chaar and Digenis 1966; Der Marderosian and Youngken 1966
	d-iso-lysergic acid amide isoergine erginine	(b) Hofmann 1963 (i) Hofmann and Tscherter 1960; Hofmann 1963; Hylin and Watson 1965; Abou-Chaar and Digenis 1966; Der Marderosian and Youngken 1966
	d-lysergic acid, methyl-carbinolamide d-lysergic acid, (1-hydroxyethyl)-amide	(b) Glässer 1961 (i) This is a major product in ergot culture media

Molecular Structure	Chemical Names / Common Names	References (b) Biological (i) Isolation (s) Synthesis
	elymoclavine	(b) Yui and Takeo 1958; Isbell and Gorodetzky, 1966 (i) Hofmann 1963; Der Marderosian and Youngken 1966
	lysergol	(b) Yui and Takeo 1958 (i) Hofmann 1963; Abou-Chaar and Digenis 1966
	chanoclavine	(i) Hofmann and Tscherter 1960; Hofmann 1963; Genest 1965 Abou-Chaar and Digenis 1966; Der Marderosian and Youngken 1966
	ergonovine ergometrine ergobasine	(b) USP (i) Taber et al, 1963; Hofmann 1964; Der Marderosian and Youngken 1966
	ergometrinine ergobasinine	(i) Hofmann 1963; Abou-Chaar and Digenis 1966
	penniclavine	(i) Der Marderosian and Youngken 1966

Table 1. Chemical Classification of Drugs of Abuse (continued)

Molecular Structure	Chemical Names / Common Names	References (b) Biological (i) Isolation (s) Synthesis

Amphetamine Group

Molecular Structure	Chemical Names Common Names	References
Structure: benzene-CH₂CH(CH₃)NH₂	phenylisopropylamine α-methylphenethylamine amphetamine benzedrine (+) dexedrine dextroamphetamine	(b) PDR (i) Not natural (s) Jones and Wallis 1926
Structure: benzene-CH₂CH(CH₃)NHCH₃	desoxyephedrine N-methylphenylisopropyl-amine N,α-dimethylphenethyl-amine methamphetamine methedrine desoxyn	(b) PDR (i) Not natural (s) Ogata 1919; Emde 1929
Structure: morpholine ring	3-phenyl-2-methyl-morpholine phenmetrazine Preludin (Geigy)	(b) PDR (i) Not natural (s) Clarke 1962
Structure: piperidine ring	α-phenyl-2-piperidine-acetic acid, methyl ester methylphenidate Ritalin (Ciba)	(b) PDR (i) Not natural (s) Panizzon 1944
Structure: COCH(CH₃)N(CH₂CH₃)₂	2-diethylaminopropio-phenone diethylpropion Tenuate (Merrell) Tepanil (National)	(b) PDR (i) not natural (s) Hyde et al, 1928
Structure: tropane ring cocaine	2-β-carbomethoxy-3-β-benzotropane cocaine	(b) USP (i) Squibb 1885 (s) Willstätter et al, 1923; Findlay 1954

Barbiturates

Molecular Structure	Chemical Names Common Names	References
Structure: barbiturate ring with phenyl and CH₂CH₃	5-ethyl-5-phenylbarbituric acid phenobarbital phenobarbitone Luminal (Winthrop)	(b) All these materials are listed in the PDR, with pharmacological descriptions (i) All are synthetic chemicals not found in nature (s) Chamberlain et al 1935; Tagmann et al, 1952
Structure: barbiturate ring with CH(CH₂)₂CH₃ CH₃ and CH₂CH₃	5-ethyl-5-(1-methylbutyl barbituric acid pentobarbital Nembutal (Abbott)	

Molecular Structure	Chemical Names / Common Names	References (b) Biological (i) Isolation (s) Synthesis

	5-allyl-5-(1-methylbutyl) barbituric acid secobarbital Seconal (Lilly)	
	5-ethyl-5-isoamylbarbi- turic acid amobarbital Amytal (Lilly)	
	2-ethyl-2-phenylglutari- mide glutethimide Doriden (Ciba)	

Heroin Family

	diacetylmorphine heroin	(i) Not natural (s) Wright 1874
	morphine	(b) USP (i) Sertürner, 1805; Achor and Geiling, 1954;
	morphine, 3-methyl ether codeine	(b) USP (i) Freund et al, 1921; Schlöpf, 1927; Rodionow, 1929

Table 1. Chemical Classification of Drugs of Abuse (continued)

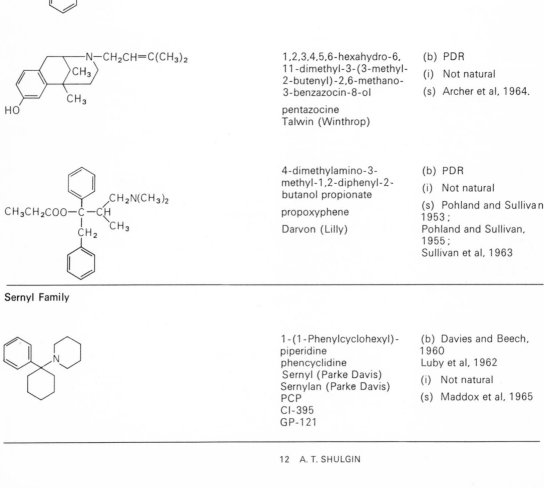

Molecular Structure	Chemical Names Common Names	References (b) Biological (i) Isolation (s) Synthesis
	dihydromorphinone hydromorphone dilaudid	(b) PDR (i) Not natural (s) Rapoport et al, 1950
	N-methyl-4-phenyl-4-carbethoxypiperidine ethyl 1-methyl-4-phenyl-isonipecotate meperidine Demerol (Winthrop)	(b) PDR (i) Not natural (s) Eisleb and Schaumann 1939
	6-Dimethylamino-4,4-diphenyl-3-heptanone methadone Dolophine (Lilly)	(b) PDR (i) Not natural (s) Schultz et al, 1947; Larson et al, 1948
	1,2,3,4,5,6-hexahydro-6,11-dimethyl-3-(3-methyl-2-butenyl)-2,6-methano-3-benzazocin-8-ol pentazocine Talwin (Winthrop)	(b) PDR (i) Not natural (s) Archer et al, 1964.
	4-dimethylamino-3-methyl-1,2-diphenyl-2-butanol propionate propoxyphene Darvon (Lilly)	(b) PDR (i) Not natural (s) Pohland and Sullivan 1953; Pohland and Sullivan, 1955; Sullivan et al, 1963

Sernyl Family

| | 1-(1-Phenylcyclohexyl)-piperidine phencyclidine Sernyl (Parke Davis) Sernylan (Parke Davis) PCP CI-395 GP-121 | (b) Davies and Beech, 1960 Luby et al, 1962 (i) Not natural (s) Maddox et al, 1965 |

Molecular Structure	Chemical Names / Common Names	References (b) Biological (i) Isolation (s) Synthesis
CH₃CH₂–NCH₂CH₂OC(=O)–C–OH (diphenyl)	β-diethylaminoethyl-benzylate benactyzine deprol	(b) Bultasova et al, 1960 (i) Not natural (s) Horenstein and Pählicke, 1938; Blicke and Maxwell 1942
	N-ethyl-3-piperidyl-benzylate JB-318 (Lakeside)	(b) Biel, Nuhfer, et al, 1962 (i) Not natural
	N-ethyl-2-pyrrolidylmethyl phenylcyclopentyl-glycolate; and N-ethyl-3-piperidyl-glycolate: Ratio, 7:3 ditran JB-329 (Lakeside)	(b) Abood and Meduna 1958 (i) Not natural (s) Biel, Sprengler, et al, 1955; Biel, Abood, et al, 1961
	N-methyl-3-piperidyl-benzylate LBJ JB-336 (Lakeside)	(i) Not natural (s) Abood, Ostfeld, et al, 1959; Biel, Nuhfer, et al, 1962

STP and Phenethylamines

	2,5-dimethoxy-4-methyl-phenylisopropylamine 2,5-dimethoxy-4,a-dimethylphenethylamine DOM STP	(b) Snyder et al, 1967; Hollister, Macnicol, et al, 1969 (i) Not natural (s) Shulgin, unpublished data

Table 1. Chemical Classification of Drugs of Abuse (continued)

Molecular Structure	Chemical Names Common Names	References (b) Biological (i) Isolatlon (s) Synthesis
	3,4,5-trimethoxyphen-ethylamine mescaline	(b) Heffter, 1897; Beringer 1927 (i) Heffter 1896 (s) Späth 1919
	anhalonidine 6,7-dimethoxy-1-methyl-1,2,3,4-tetrahydroiso-quinolin-8-ol	(b) Heffter 1897 (i) Heffter 1896 (s) Späth 1922
	anhalonine 6-methoxy-1-methyl-7 8-methylenedioxy-1,2,3,4-tetrahydroisoquinoline	(b) Heffter 1897 (i) Lewin 1894 (s) Späth and Kesztler 1935
	lophophorine 6-methoxy-1,2-dimethyl-7,8-methylenedioxy-1,2,3,4-tetrahydroisoquinoline	(b) Heffter 1897; Henry 1939 (i) Heffter 1898 (s) Späth and Gangl 1923
	peyotine pellotine 6.7-dimethoxy-1,2-di-methyl-1,2,3,4-tetra-hydroisoquinoline-8-ol	(b) Jolly 1896; Heffter 1897; Hutchings 1897 (i) Heffter 1894 (s) Späth 1922
	3,4,5-trimethoxyphenyl-isopropylamine 3,4,5-trimethoxy-α-methylphenethylamine TMA	(b) Hey 1947; Shulgin, Bunnell, et al, 1961 (i) Not natural (s) Hey 1947; Shulgin 1966
	3-methoxy-4,5-methylene-dioxyphenylisopropyl-amine MMDA	(b) Fairchild 1963; Shulgin 1964 (i) Not natural (s) Alles 1962; Naranjo, Sargent, et al, 1970

Molecular Structure	Chemical Names Common Names	References (b) Biological (i) Isolation (s) Synthesis
	3,4-methylenedioxyphenyl-isopropylamine MDA	(b) Alles 1959; Naranjo, Shulgin, et al, 1967 (i) Not natural

Datura Group

	(d1) atropine (1) hyoscyamine	(b) PDR (i) Kircher 1905; Schmidt and Kircher 1906 (s) Robinson, 1917; Evans and Griffin, 1963
	(d1) atroscine (1) scopolamine hyoscine	

Tryptamines

	N,N-dimethyltryptamine DMT	(b) Sai-Halasz et al, 1958 (i) Fish et al, 1955 (s) Speeter and Anthony 1954
	N,N-diethyltryptamine DET	(b) Szara et al, 1966 (i) Not natural (s) Barlow and Kahn 1959
	5-methoxy-N,N-dimethyl-tryptamine $5\text{-}OCH_3DMT$	(b) Gessner and Page 1962 (i) Holmstedt 1965 (s) Benington et al 1958; Gessner and Page 1962
	3-(dimethylaminoethyl)-indol-4-yl phosphate psilocybin	(b) Malitz et al, 1960 (i) Hofmann et al, 1958b (s) Hofmann et al, 1958a

Table 1. Chemical Classification of Drugs of Abuse (continued)

Molecular Structure	Chemical Names Common Names	References (b) Biological (i) Isolation (s) Synthesis
	3-(dimethylaminoethyl)-indol-4-ol psilocin	(b) see psilocybin above (i) Hofmann and Troxler 1959 (s) see psilocybin above
	ibogaine ibogine	(b) Schneider and Sigg 1957; Steinmetz 1961; Naranjo 1969 (i) Dybowsky and Landrin 1901

Harmala Group

	7-methoxy-1-methyl-carboline 7-methoxyharman harmine	
	3,4-dihydro-7-methoxy-1-methylcarboline 3,4-dihydro-7-methoxy-harman harmaline	(b) Pennes and Hoch 1957; Naranjo 1969 (i) Hochstein and Paradies 1957; Bernauer 1964 (s) Manske et al 1927; Späth and Lederer 1930
	1,2,3,4-tetrahydro-7-methoxy-1-methyl-carboline 1,2,3,4-tetrahydro-7-methoxyharman tetrahydroharmine leptoflorine	

presumed to be the active components of marijuana. Two of these, the Δ^1-3,4-*trans*-tetrahydrocannabinol and the $\Delta^{1(6)}$-3,4-*trans*-tetrahydrocannabinol, are both found in the natural cannabis resin [Wollner et al. 1942; DeRopp 1960; Hively et al. 1966). The structures have been established by Gaoni and Mechoulam [1964a and b], and there have been several total syntheses recently described (see Table 1). The various numbering systems in this family of chemicals have been described and compared [Mechoulam and Gaoni 1967; Shulgin 1969]; the system based upon the terpene ring is used in this report. Most of the interest in the biological activity of the cannabis components has centered on this second group, the tetrahydrocannabinoids, and most of the biologically active, synthetically produced analogs are closely related compounds. As mentioned above, the Δ^1- and the $\Delta^{1(6)}$- isomers are the naturally occurring ones; the former is much the more plentiful and is widely accepted as being largely responsible for the central activity of marijuana. A third tetrahydrocannabinol isomer, Δ^3-tetrahydrocannabinol, has been known for some thirty years. It is biologically active; it has been synthesized both by discrete chemical steps [Adams and Baker 1940] as well as by the condensation of natural products [Adams, Smith, et al. 1941b; Ghosh et al. 1941]; but it does not appear to occur in nature.

Although less active than the naturally occurring THC, the Δ^3-THC is much more easily obtained synthetically and has served as a reference point in a large number of structure-activity relationship studies. Three of these are described in the table; the first, parahexyl, since it had achieved considerable clinical application; and the other two, methyloctylpyran and dimethylheptylpyran, because of their exceptional potency in human subjects.

A third group of chemicals that can be obtained from the marijuana plant *Cannabis sativa* contains those that, although themselves not pharmacologically active, can be converted to active compounds either chemically or physically. The two-ring resorcinol cannabidiol is probably a biosynthetic precursor of the tetrahydrocannabinols [Mechoulam and Gaoni 1967] and is a frequent laboratory intermediate in their syntheses (see table). Similarly, of the several carboxylic acids that are found in the cannabinoid fraction of marijuana extracts, cannabidiolic acid and Δ^1-tetrahydrocannabinolic acid are entered in the table as they, too, are precursors to the active tetrahydrocannabinols and possibly may be converted to them through the pyrolysis associated with smoking. Recently the second possible positional isomer of Δ^1-THC acid has been isolated and characterized [Mechoulam, personal communication]. It is readily converted to the Δ^1-THC acid described in the table.

The fourth group of chemicals associated with the cannabis extracts contains a large number of structural oddities. There are currently no suggestions that they in any way contribute to the pharmacological description of the plant. There are two additional carboxylic acids, cannabinolic acid [Mechoulam and Gaoni 1965b] and cannabigerolic acid [Mechoulam and Gaoni 1965b], the latter yielding upon decarboxylation the open chain cannabinoid, cannabigerol [Gaoni and Mechoulam 1964b]. Cannabichromene [Claussen et al. 1966], cannabicyclol [Crombie and Ponsford 1968], cannabidivarin [Vollner et al. 1969], and the ester tetrahydrocannabitriolyl cannabidiolcarboxylate [von Spulak et al. 1968] all constitute minor components of the plant extract.

These minor components can serve a potentially valuable role in the study of drug abuse problems. Although tetrahydrocannabinol is not at present a drug problem, it might conceivably become one, and it is through the analysis of the impurities that accompany it that indications of its origins might be revealed. If it comes from natural sources, it is certainly likely that some of these chemically similar compounds will be present as impurities. If, on the other hand, the tetrahydrocannabinol is completely synthetic, these biosynthetically related materials cannot accompany it, and the more likely contaminant would be iso-tetrahydrocannabinol. This is a completely synthetic by-product that is not known in nature. It is entered in the table as it might be encountered if synthetic THC ever becomes a drug problem.

2.2. LSD

Properly, LSD is the name of a single chemical individual, but in fact it has been used to embrace both synthetic mixtures and biological extracts as well. This discussion will consider these substances in three sections: first, the chemical itself and the contaminants that might be present as impurities; second, synthetic chemical individuals that are LSD-like in their central action in man; and last, the composition and description of botanical extracts that have been used as LSD.

LSD is a semisynthetic alkaloid, prepared by the action of diethylamine on lysergic acid. The latter, a mandatory intermediate, is invariably obtained from natural sources, from amides produced biosynthetically by the ergot fungus *Claviceps purpurea*. The intermediate lysergic acid is easily isomerized to a mixture of epimers, lysergic acid, and iso-lysergic acid, and the latter can give rise to an inactive form of LSD, vis., iso-LSD. The starting ergot amides such as ergonovine and ergotoxine, more particularly the isomeric acids which will arise from the fermentation production of lysergic acid amides, and the iso-LSD all may be expected to occur as contaminants of the drug LSD.

There is a large number of synthetic allies of LSD that have been synthesized and evaluated in clinical trials. Some of these analogs (such as the N^1-acetyl and N^1-methyl counterparts, ALD-52 and MLD-41) have proved to be as potent as LSD itself [Rothlin 1957]. Other analogs that have involved the amide area of the molecule have in general proved to decrease the potency of the LSD molecule. The N-ethyl, the N,N-pyrrolidyl, and the morpholinyl amides (LAE-32, LSM-777) approach LSD in potency [Giarman 1967]; other amides, such as the methyl, dimethyl, propyl, and butyl, appear to decrease in potency. The optical enantiomorphs, and the isomeric diastereoisomers of LSD (vis., l-LSD, d-iso-LSD and l-iso-LSD) have been also assayed in human subjects and have been found inactive [Hofmann 1958; Murphree et al. 1960]. Those chemical entities that are active have been included in the table. Yet another individual should be mentioned, Sansert (Sandoz) or UML-491. This amide has found value in the prophylactic treatment of migraine headache, yet it has been used as an LSD substitute; it can be estimated that about 20 mg is equivalent to one one-hundredth this weight of LSD from the viewpoint of its central activity.

The third group of chemicals that must be considered under the LSD classification contains those alkaloids that have been identified in the various morning glory plant extracts, and that appear collectively to imitate LSD in their pharmacological descriptions. Some of the alkaloids found in these seeds are carbanolamides, amides of hydroxyethylamine, which would readily hydrolyze to the corresponding lysergide [Arcamone et al. 1960]. Others are fully stable, and may certainly contribute to the reported activity of the plant extract. Most of these Convovulaceae have been described under the general name Ololiuqui, and many related plants have been analyzed chemically. The several identified components are listed in the table, along with the plant name associated with its identification. An excellent recent review of these Ipomoeae has appeared [Der Marderosian 1967] which helps in the botanical classification of these plants. In the table, references are listed according to botanical name.

2.3. Amphetamine

The name amphetamine properly applies to the single chemical phenylisopropylamine, although it has socially come to embrace the N-methyl homolog, methamphetamine.

A number of pharmacologically related materials, occasional drugs of abuse, are best considered here, and they are generally listed in the table as amphetamines. There is also a large number of chemically related materials that pharmacologically more closely resemble mescaline and MDA; they are considered later.

The majority of the amphetamines, as described in this section, are derived from commercial sources, such as dexedrine or benzedrine, and should be relatively free from impurities. Illicit material is prepared from phenylacetone, or from norephedrine by reduction, and these starting materials may be present as impurities.

A large number of synthetic drugs should be considered here under the amphetamine classification, for they are, indeed, sympathomimetic stimulants and they all have at some time or other been socially abused. The structures and direct references are listed in Table 1. In most instances these materials are, as mentioned for amphetamine itself, diverted into illicit usage from legitimate sources, and they may be expected to be correspondingly pure. The structures of these amphetamine-like compounds are drawn in a manner that emphasizes the phenethylamine nucleus common to all of them (see table).

Several of the drugs listed can exist as isomerically distinct chemicals. Amphetamine itself is found as the racemate, as benzedrine, or as the dextrorotatory isomer, dexedrine.

The levorotatory isomer is the active ingredient in at least one drug, levamfetamine, or Cydril (Tutag). Methedrine is the DL-racemate if synthesized from phenylacetone and methylamine; it is optically active (dextro-) when synthesized through the reduction of natural ephedrine. None of the stimulants listed in the table is found in nature. Ephedrine itself is a natural alkaloid, the active ingredient of the plant *Ephedra distachia*. The plant *Catha edulis*, or khat, contains norpseudoephedrine and is used extensively in Ethiopia and some Arab states. These plants have a very limited range of abuse, and they are not listed here. Cocaine is also a natural plant product.

2.4. Barbiturates

This group of well-established drugs is extremely widely used among young people today, and in measure of gross abuse it might well constitute the most serious single problem. Their use is that of a psychological escape, and they are recognized as being depressants.

The structures of those currently most misused are given. All are presented as the un-ionized form, although most are found as the water-soluble sodium salts. The chemistry associated with these materials is uninteresting; all are prepared by essentially the same reaction (fusion of an appropriately substituted malonate with urea) and as most examples found on the street are originally from commercial sources, few impurities are to be expected. None is found in nature.

Slang names that have been associated with these drugs usually reflect the appearance of the commercial capsule. Thus phenobarbital is called "purple hearts," pentobarbital and secobarbital are "yellows" and "reds," amobarbital is "blue heaven," and the mixture Tuinal (secobarbital and amobarbital) is called "rainbow" (a red and blue capsule).

Glutethimide is provided in the table as an example of a group of sedatives that, although technically not barbiturates, are properly classified with them, as they have led to similar abuse problems and appear to lead to the same style of drug dependence. A common slang name of glutethimide tablets reflects the origin rather than the appearance; they are called "Cibas"!

2.5. Heroin

Under this general heading have been gathered drugs that are chemical modifications or derivatives of the naturally occurring opiates as well as pharmacologically similar drugs that are completely synthetic. With the exception of heroin, all of the listed materials have accepted medical uses, and are listed either in the U S. Pharmacopoeia or the Physicians' Desk Reference. In Table 1, under the heading of biological reference, this will be noted as USP or PDR, and no literature source will be cited.

Care should be taken not to confuse pentazocine (Talwin [Winthrop]) with the closely related phenazocine (Prinadol [SKF]) or cyclazocine (Sterling). These latter two drugs are substituted with an N-phenethyl and an N-cyclopropylmethyl group in place of the N-methylbutenyl group in pentazocine. The hallucinogenic abuse potential of pentazocine has already been noted in the published medical literature [Keup 1968; De Nosaquo 1969].

Propoxyphene represents an interesting isomer problem. The two diastereoisomeric forms are known. It is the dextro-isomer (d-) of the less soluble racemic pair (α-) that is marketed by Lilly as Darvon.

2.6. Sernyl

Sernyl is representative of a large group of parasympatholytic drugs that are pharmacologically but not chemically related to the Datura alkaloids. The synthetics, mostly benzylate esters, are listed here, as they are widely abused at the present time, and their use seems to be increasing. The actual alkaloids, for example atropine, are less commonly found and are listed under section 3.

The lead drug, Sernyl or phencyclidine, is largely manufactured in clandestine laboratories, as it is a very simple synthesis. The requisite starting materials are all commercially available (e.g. cyclohexanone, piperidine, bromobenzene) and illustrate contaminants that might be expected [Maddox et al. 1965]. As these three chemicals are all amenable to easy chemical modification, it is clearly possible that chemical variants of phencyclidine might be expected. Ketamine (C.I. 581; 2-(o-chlorophenyl)-2-(methylamino)-cyclohexanone) has been evaluated as a clinical substitute for phencyclidine, but it is not likely to become a drug problem as it is only a tenth as active, and it is more difficult to synthesize.

A more serious problem occurs with the benzylate ester family of drugs. Benactyzine is one of the oldest of these, and is of relatively low potency (approximately 1 mg per Kg). Many of the more recently developed analogs are literally hundreds of times more potent, and although they are not commercially available, they can be prepared directly from organic chemicals that are available. Several of these "JB" compounds are listed in Table 1.

2.7. STP

This chemical is a close structural analog of mescaline. Due to the fact that it is both highly potent and easy to synthesize, it has had a regular and continuous appearance in the areas of drug abuse. It is usually found alone, diluted with inert excipients and binders, although it is occasionally observed admixed with LSD. It is probable that this drug is manufactured from 2,5-dimethoxy-4-methyl-β-nitrophenylpropene, and this yellow, neutral compound will be a likely contaminant. The chemical reduction product, DOM or STP, does not occur in nature, and it is not available commercially, although the necessary starting materials for its synthesis are easily available through chemical supply houses. It is listed in Table 1 along with mescaline, the peyote alkaloids, and the other substituted amphetamines, with which it is closely related both chemically and pharmacologically.

3. Drugs that Represent Potential Problems

3.1. Mescaline

Mescaline is placed in the classification of drugs with a low priority for research attention, for two reasons. First, although many drugs are sold in the illegal market as mescaline, very few of them are indeed this chemical. Second, the drug has been the subject of hundreds of research studies, and there is a large body of information already at hand concerning it.

The listings in Table 1 are arranged to present first the better known alkaloids that accompany mescaline in its native form, peyote, followed by a listing of some of the synthetic relatives of mescaline that are subject to abuse.

Peyote is the common name given to the New World cactus *Anhalonium lewinii,* the principal botanical source of mescaline. Rouhier [1927] has given several descriptions of the human pharmacology of the total plant materials, and the individual pharmacological properties of the separated components are referenced in Table 1.

Three alkoxylated phenylisopropylamines (amphetamines) are also listed. Although these bases are not found in nature, evidence has been found [Oswald et al. 1969] that suggests that they might arise from essential oils such as elemicin, myristicin, and safrol, known constituents of plants such as nutmeg [Shulgin, et al. 1967].

3.2. Datura

There are many plants of the family Solanaceae that have been employed in widely separated social groups as intoxicants. Although these are broadly defined botanically [Schultes 1969], there are consistently present two alkaloids, atropine and scopolamine. The optically active form of atropine is the levo-

form, called hyoscyamine, whereas scopolamine (synonym : hyoscine) is easily racemized to the racemic form, atroscine.

A number of minor aklaloids have been isolated from atropine-containing plants, but in general they have not been studied pharmacologically, and they are not entered in the table. The demethylated homolog of atropine is noratropine, the intramolecular ether of the nonaromatic fragment of scopolamine is known as oscine or scopoline, and an aliphatic (tiglate) ester of this triol is known as meteloidine. Bristol et al. [1969] has published an excellent correlation between botanic identity and alkaloid content.

3.3. DMT

The indolic base dimethyltryptamine (DMT) is a chemical that can be obtained either from chemical synthesis or from botanical sources. All of the illicit instances of its appearance derive from laboratory synthesis, as the snuffs which contain it are difficult to obtain and even more difficult to resolve into components. Both DMT and a number of its unnatural (synthetic) homologs have come into usage over the last few years as a result of the discovery of simple and direct syntheses. A three-step synthesis from indole and oxalyl chloride, with the generation of an appropriate amide and subsequent hydrogenation, has made available a variety of N,N-dialkyltryptamines. Both the dimethyl and the diethyl compounds (DMT and DET) are commercially available ; the dipropyl and di-isopropyl amines are known in the areas of drug abuse.

A principal contaminant to be found in the synthesis of DMT, and presumably in the syntheses of the various homologs, is the result of incomplete reduction, the dialkylindolylethanolamine. The hydroxylated contaminants appear to be difficult to remove.

A closely related base, found in many botanical extracts along with DMT, is the 5-methoxy analog, 5-methoxy-N,N-dimethyltryptamine. The human pharmacology of the total plant substance has been described by Wassén and Holmstedt [1963]; leading references to the descriptions of the specific chemical are found in Table 1. This chemical is also commercially available.

4. Rare Drugs

4.1. Psilocybin

At the lowest end of the priority scale are gathered those chemicals that are certainly pharmacologically effective but which are to a large measure unobtainable. In this category fall psilocybin and psilocin. Both chemicals can be obtained from botanical sources as well as through synthetic procedures, and neither is available commercially. The collection of these bases from natural sources, mushrooms related to *Psilocybe mexicana,* is difficult, for these sources are scarce and hard to identify. The synthesis of these chemicals is a many-stepped process which lies beyond the ability of the average attic chemist. Even though they are widely claimed to be available, these chemicals are not problems, nor will they soon become so.

The monomethyl homolog of psilocybin has recently been isolated from a related mushroom, *Psilocybe baeocystis* [Leung and Paul 1967]. It has not been explored pharmacologically.

4.2. Ibogaine

Here again is a problem that is defined substantially by the writing of laws. Recently ibogaine has been specifically defined as a dangerous drug, yet this material is completely impractical to synthesize. It may be obtained, along with its structural isomer tabernanthine, from the bark of the African plant *Tabernanthe iboga.* The abuse of this chemical depends upon the occasional availability of the plant extract; the separated and purified alkaloid is offered commercially, as a research chemical, but it cannot be considered a serious problem, within present economics.

The isomeric tabernanthine is active only as a peripheral anaesthetic. It appears to be devoid of central activity.

4.3. Harmala

Here again is an area of drug study that is not a problem due to the difficult availability of the alkaloids involved. The plant source, vines found in the genus Banisteriopsis, has been the subject of several reports [see Efron 1967]. The three principal alkaloids apparently responsible for biological activity are grouped together at the end of the table on p. 16. These bases, and especially the isomeric but equally active 6-methoxyharman counterparts, are considered potentially valuable tools in the study of mental health, as they can theoretically arise in the course of human metabolic chemistry (McIsaac et al. 1961). These carboline alkaloids have all recently become commercially available.

5. Other Botanicals and Synthetics

There is a limitless number of materials of unpredictable identity that will drift in and out of the area of drug abuse. People will forever smoke the spice cabinet and proceed through the over-the-counter drugs alphabetically. Recent examples such as catnip, nutmeg, and scotch broom will always be part of the youthful adventure. Further, any suggestion of scientific documentation in the literature will certainly be pursued. These are problems that must be anticipated, and that are discussed briefly here.

6. Present Technology and Research Needs

The devices and skills that are available to the analytical chemist today are almost beyond belief. Instruments are at hand that will reveal subtle molecular structure by infrared spectroscopy and atomic arrangements by nuclear magnetic resonance spectrometers. High resolution separations are easily made by gas-liquid, liquid-liquid, and partition chromatography, and both molecular weight and fragmental structures can be determined on microgram quantities by mass spectroscopy. There is no technical reason why any questionable material could not be broken down and identified as to its chemical components within minutes, in a properly equipped laboratory.

But consider the present problem from its social considerations. There is at present little communication between those with social needs and those with scientific facilities. The naive child on the street wonders if he has good "acid," and the only available facility for this determination is the law enforcement establishment. There are few honest answers available to the people who constitute the drug-abuse problem. As an outgrowth of this condition, much valuable information, detail, and fact concerning drug usage is either inaccurate or even totally unavailable to researchers and students in this area. The drug problem as it is presently evolving bids well to embrace an ever increasing number of chemicals, and there appears to be an ever increasing information gap between the person who uses drugs and the person who describes their use.

There is no question but that all efforts must be made to study those materials that are now being explored socially, in every possible aspect. Marijuana, LSD, and peyote all represent complex mixtures of chemicals, and the many components of these mixtures must be separated and individually studied. Further, these studies must be from the point of view of searches for factual information, not from the argument of legal or punitive definition.

Problems that may arise in the near future must be anticipated. There are currently many hints that analogs of DMT and STP, as well as structural variations of THC, may be soon presented to the enthusiastic drug market. These inventions must be anticipated, and defensive information, if not constructive and useful information, must be at hand to answer future questions. These questions must be answered honestly without the reservations or moralizing that would suggest prejudice on the part of the scientific researcher.

7. Table of Chemical Classification of Drugs of Abuse

In this table of drugs of abuse, structures are given for those drugs that are synthetic, and for the components of those drugs that are of biological origin. Principal chemical names are listed, along with references to the most important scientific sources.

References

Abood, L. G., and L. Meduna (1958). *J. Nerv. Ment. Dis.* 127:546.

——, A. Ostfeld, and J. H. Biel (1959). *Arch. Int. Pharmacodyn.* 120:186.

Abou-Chaar, C. I., and G. A. Digenis (1966). *Nature* 212:618.

Achor, L. B., and E. M. K. Geiling (1954). *Anal. Chem.* 26:1061.

Adams, R., B. F. Aycock, and S. Loewe (1948a). *J. Amer. Chem. Soc.* 70:622.

——, and B. R. Baker (1940a). *J. Amer. Chem. Soc.* 62:2405.

——, B. R. Baker, and R. B. Wearn (1940b). *J. Amer. Chem. Soc.* 62:2204.

——, M. Hunt, and J. H. Clark (1940c). *J. Amer. Chem. Soc.* 62:196.

——, S. Loewe, C. Jelinek, and H. Wolff (1941a). *J. Amer. Chem. Soc.* 63:1971.

——, S. MacKenzie, and S. Loewe (1948b). *J. Amer. Chem. Soc.* 70:664.

——, C. M. Smith, and S. Loewe (1941b). *J. Amer. Chem. Soc.* 63:1973.

Alles, G. A. (1959). In *Neuropharmacology*, Abramson, ed., New York: Macy.

—— (1962). Personal communication to M. D. Fairchild (1963), q.v.

Arcamone, F., C. Bonino, E. B. Chain, A. Ferretti, P. Pennella, A. Tolono, and L. Vero (1960). *Nature* 187:238.

Archer, S., N. F. Albertson, L. S. Harris, A. K. Pierson, and J. G. Bird (1964). *J. Med. Chem.* 7:123.

Barlow, R. B., and I. Khan (1959). *Brit. J. Pharmacol.* 14:99.

Benington, F., R. D. Morin, and L. C. Clark (1958). *J. Org. Chem.* 23:1977.

Beringer, K. (1927). *Der Meskalinrauch seine Geschichte und Erscheinungsweise.* Berlin: J. Springer.

Bernauer, K. (1964). *Helvi. Chim. Acta* 47:1075.

Bicher, H. I., J. Krupnik, and S. Eliash (1966). *Proc. Int. Cong. Pharm. Brazil,* p. 114 (see Mechoulam and Gaoni 1967).

Biel, J. H., L. G. Abood, W. K. Hoya, H. A. Leiser, P. A. Nuhfer, and E. Kluchesky (1961). *J. Org. Chem.* 26:4096.

―――, P. A. Nuhfer, W. K. Hoya, H. A. Leiser, and L. G. Abood (1962). *Ann. N.Y. Acad. Sci.* 96:251.

―――, E. P. Sprengeler, H. A. Leiser, J. Horner, A. Drukker, and H. L. Friedman (1955). *J. Amer. Chem. Soc.* 77:2250.

Blicke, F. F., and C. E. Maxwell (1942). *J. Amer. Chem. Soc.* 64:428.

Boszormenyi, Z., P. Der, and T. Nagy (1959). *J. Ment. Sci.* 105:171.

Bristol, M. L., W. C. Evans, and J. F. Lampard (1969). *Lloydia* 32:123.

Bultasova, H., E. Grof, E. Horackova, E. Kuhn, K. Rysenek, V. Vitek, and M. Vojtechovsky (1960). *Ideggyogy Szemle* 13:225.

Cerletti A. (1959). In *Neuropharmacology,* Bradley, et al., eds., New York: Elsevier. p. 117.

Chamberlain, J. S., J. J. Chap, J. E. Doyle, and L. B. Spaulding (1935). *J. Amer. Chem. Soc.* 57:352.

Clarke, F. H. (1962). *J. Org. Chem.* 27:3251.

Claussen, U., F. v. Spulak, and F. Korte (1966). *Tetrahedron* 22:1477.

Cohen, S. (1960). *J. Nerv. Ment. Dis.* 139:30.

Crombie, L., and R. Ponsford (1968). *Tetrahedron Letters* p. 5771.

Dagirmanjian, R., and E. S. Boyd (1962). *J. Pharmacol. Exp. Ther.* 135:26.

Davies, B. M., and H. R. Beech (1960). *J. Ment. Sci.* 106:912.

De Nosaquo, N. (1969). *J.A.M.A.* 210:502.

Der Marderosian, A. (1967). *Lloydia* 30:23.

―――, and H. W. Youngken (1966). *Lloydia* 29:35.

De Ropp, R. S. (1960). *J. Amer. Pharm. Ass.* 49:756.

Dybowsky and Laudrin (1901). *Compt. rend.* 133:748.

Efron, D. H. (1967). Ed. *Ethnopharmologic Search for Psychoactive Drugs.* PHSP No. 1647.

Eisleb, O., and O. Schaumaan (1939). *Deut. Med. Wochschr.* 65:967.

Emde, H. (1929). *Helv. Chim. Acta* 12:365.

Evans, W. C., and Griffin (1963). *J. Chem. Soc.* p. 4348.

Fahrenholtz, K. E., M. Lurie, and R. W. Kierstead (1966). *J. Amer. Chem. Soc.* 88:2079.

Fairchild, M. D. (1963). Thesis, Ph.D. Pharmacology, UCLA.

Findlay, S. P. (1954). *J. Amer. Chem. Soc.* 76:2855.

Fish, M. S., N. M. Johnson, and E.C. Horning (1955). *J. Amer. Chem. Soc.* 77:5892.

Freund, M., W. W. Melber, and E. Schlesinger (1921). *J. Prakt. Chem.* 101:1.

Gaoni, Y., and R. Mechoulam (1964a). *J. Amer. Chem. Soc.* 86:1646.

―――, (1964b). *Proc. Chem. Soc.* 82.

――― (1966). *J. Amer. Chem. Soc.* 88:5673.

Genest, K. (1965) *J. Chromatog.* 19:531.

Gessner, P. K., and I. H. Page (1962). *Amer. J. Physiol.* 203:167.

Ghosh, R., A. R. Todd, and D. C. Wright (1941). *J. Chem. Soc.* p. 137.

Giarman, N. J. (1967). *LSD, Man and Society.* Wesleyan, p. 143.

Glässer, A. (1961). *Nature* 189:313.

Heffter, A. (1894). *Arch. Exp. Path. Pharmak.* 34:65.

――― (1896). *Ber.* 29:216.

――― (1897). *Arch. Exp. Path. Pharmak.* 40:385.

――― (1898). *Ber.* 31:1196.

Henry, T. A. (1939). *The Plant Alkaloids.* Philadelphia: Blakison.

Hey, P. (1947). *Quart. J. Pharm. Pharmacol.* 20:129.

Hively, R. L., W. A. Mosher, and F. W. Hoffman (1966). *J. Amer. Chem. Soc.* 88:1832.

Hochstein, F. A., and A. M. Paradies (1957). *J. Amer. Chem. Soc.* 79:5735.

Hofmann, A. (1958). In Rinkel and Denber, eds., *Chemical Concepts of Psychosis,* New York:

———, (1963). *Bot. Mus. Leafl. Harvard.* 20:194.

——— (1964). *Psychedelic Review* 1:302.

———, A. Frey, H. Ott, T. Petrzilka, and F. Troxler (1958a). *Experientia* 14:397.

———, R. Heim, A. Brack, and H. Kobel (1958b). *Experientia* 14:107.

———, and F. Troxler (1959). *Experientia* 15:101.

———, and H. Tscherter (1960). *Experientia* 16:414.

Hollister, L. E., M. F. Macnicol, and H. K. Gillespie (1969). *Psychopharmacologia* 14:62.

———, R. K. Richards, and H. K. Gillespie (1968). *Clin. Pharm. Ther.* 9:783.

Holmstedt, B. (1965). *Arch. Int. Pharmacodyn.* 156:285.

Horenstein, H., and H. Pählicke (1938). *Ber.* 71:1654.

Hutchings (1897). *St. Lawrance State Hospital Bull.* No. 1.

Hyde, J. F., E. Browning, and R. Adams (1928). *J. Amer. Chem. Soc.* 50:2287.

Hylin, J. W., and D. P. Watson (1965). *Science* 148:449.

Isbell, H., and C. W. Gorodetzky (1966). *Psychopharmacologia* 8:331.

———, C. W. Gorodetzky, D. Jasinski, U. Claussen, F. v. Spulak, and F. Korte (1967). *Psychopharmacologia* 11:184.

———, E. J. Miner, and C. R. Logan (1959). *Psychopharmacologia* 1:20.

Jacob, A., and A. R. Todd (1940). *J. Chem. Soc.* p. 649.

Jarvik, M. E., H. A. Abramson, and M. W. Hirsch (1955). *J. Abnorm. Soc. Psychol.* 51:657.

Jolly, (1896). *Deutsch. Med. Wochenschr.*

Jones and Wallis (1926). *J. Amer. Chem. Soc.* 48:180.

Kabelik, J., Z. Krejči, and F. Šantavý (1960). *Bull. Narcotics* 12:5.

Keup, W. (1968). *Dis. Nerv. Syst.* 29:599.

Kircher, A. (1905). *Arch. Pharm.* 243:309.

Korte, F., E. Dlugosch, and U. Claussen (1966). *Ann.* 693:165.

———, M. Haag, and U. Claussen (1965). *Angew. Chem.* (Int.) 4:872.

Krejči, Z., M. Horák, and F. Šantavý (1959). *Pharmazie* 14:349.

Larson, A. A., B. F. Tullar, B. Elpern, and J. S. Buck (1948). *J. Amer. Chem. Soc.* 70:4194.

Laurie, P. (1967). *Drugs.* Middlesex, England: Penguin Books.

Leete, E. (1959). *J. Amer. Chem. Soc.* 81:3948.

Leung, A. Y., and A. G. Paul (1967). *J. Pharm. Sci.* 56:146.

Lewin, L. (1894). *Arch. Exp. Path. Pharm.* 34:374.

Loewe, S. (1946). *J. Pharmacol. Exp. Therap.* 88:154.

——— (1950). *Arch. Exp. Path. Pharm.* 211:175.

Luby, E. D., J. S. Gottlieb, B. D. Cohen, G. Rosenbaum, and E. F. Domino (1962). *Amer. J. Psychiat.* 119:61.

McIsaac, W. M., P. A. Khairallah, and I. H. Page (1961). *Science* 134:674.

Maddox, V. H., E. F. Godefroi, and R. F. Parcell (1965). *J. Med. Chem.* 8:230.

Malitz, S., H. Esecover, B. Wilkens, and P. H. Hoch (1960). *Compr. Psychiat.* 1:8.

Manske, R. H. F., W. H. Perkins, and R. Robinson (1927). *J. Chem. Soc.,* p. 1.

Mechoulam, R., and H. I. Bicher (1968). *Arch. Int. Pharm. Ther.* 172:24.

———, P. Braun, and Y. Gaoni (1967). *J. Amer. Chem. Soc.* 89:4552.

———, and Y. Gaoni (1965a). *J. Amer. Chem. Soc.* 87:3273.

———, and Y. Gaoni (1965b). *Tetrahedron* 21:1223.

———, and Y. Gaoni (1967). *Fort. Chem. Org. Natur.* 25:175.

Naranjo, C. (1969). *Clin. Tox.* 2:209.

———, T. Sargent, and A. T. Shulgin (1970). *J. Psychopharm.* (in press).

———, A. T. Shulgin, and T. Sargent (1967). *Med. Pharm. Exp.* 17:357.

Ogata (1919). *J. Pharm. Soc. Japan* 451:751.

Oswald, E. O., L. Fishbein, and B. J. Corbett (1969). *J. Chromatog.* 45:437.

Panizzon, L. (1944). *Helv. Chim. Acta* 27:1748.

Paris, R. R., F. Percheron, J. Manil, and R. Goutarel (1957). *Bull. Soc. Chim.* p. 780.

Pennes, H. H., and Hoch, P. H. (1957). *Amer. J. Psychiat.* 113:887.

Petrzilka, T., W. Haefliger, C. Sikemeier, G. Ohloff, and A. Eschenmoser (1967). *Helv. Chim. Acta* 50:719.

Pohland, A., and H. R. Sullivan (1953). *J. Amer. Chem. Soc.* 75:4458.

———, and H. R. Sullivan (1955). *J. Amer. Chem. Soc.* 77:3400.

Rapoport, H., R. Naumann, E. R. Bissell, and R. M. Bonner (1950). *J. Org. Chem.* 15:1103.

Robinson, R. (1917). *J. Chem. Soc.* 111:762.

Rodionow, W. M. (1929). *Bull. Soc. Chim.* 45:119.

Rothlin, E. (1957). *J. Pharm. Pharmacol.* 9:569.

Rouhier, A. (1927). *La plante qui fait les yeux emerveilles, le peyote.* Paris: G. Dain.

Sai-Halasz, A., G. Brunacker, and S. Szara (1958). *Psychiat. Neurol.* 135:285.

Schlöpf, C. (1927). *Ann.* 452:211.

Schmidt, E., and A. Kircher (1906). *Arch. Pharm.* 244:66.

Schneider, J. A., and E. B. Sigg (1957). *Ann. N.Y. Acad. Sci.* 66:765.

Schultes, R. E. (1969). *Science* 163:245.

Schultz, E. M., C. M. Robb, and J. M. Sprague (1942). *J. Amer. Chem. Soc.* 69:2454.

Schultz, O. E., and G. Haffner (1958). *Arch. Pharm.* 291:391.

Sertürner, F. W. (1805). See Krömeke, *Fr. Wilh. Sertürner, der Entdecker des Morphiums*, Jena: Fischer, 1925.

Shulgin, A. T. (1964). *Nature* 201:1120.

——— (1966). *J. Med. Chem.* 9:445.

——— (1969). *Psychedelic Drugs* 2:15.

———, S. Bunnell, and T. Sargent (1961). *Nature* 189:1011.

———, T. Sargent, and C. Naranjo (1967). In Efron, ed., *Ethnopharmacologic Search for Psychoactive Drugs*, PHSP No. 1645. p. 202.

Snyder, S. H., L. Faillace, and L. E. Hollister (1967). *Science* 158:669.

Solms, H. (1956). *J. Clin. Exp. Psychopath. Quart. Rev. Psychiat. Neurol.* 17:429.

Späth, E. (1919). *Monatsh.* 40:129.

——— (1922). *Monatsh.* 43:477.

———, and Gangl (1923). *Monatsh.* 44:103.

———, and F. Kesztler (1935). *Ber.* 68:1663.

———, and E. Lederer (1930). *Ber.* 63B:120.

Speeter, M. E., and W. C. Anthony (1954). *J. Amer. Chem. Soc.* 76:6208.

von Spulak, F., U. Claussen, H. W. Fehlhaper, and F. Korte (1968). *Tetrahedron* 24:5379.

Squibb (1885). *Pharm. J.* 15:775; 796.

Steinmetz, E. F. (1961). *Quart. J. Crude Drug Res.* 1:30.

Stoll, A. (1947). *Proc. 108th Meet. Swiss Soc. Psychiat.* 22, 23 Nov.

———, and A. Hofmann (1943). *Helv. Chim. Acta* 26:944.

Sullivan, H. R., I. R. Beck, and A. Pohland (1963). *J. Org. Chem.* 28:2381.

Steinmetz, E. F. (1961). *Quart. J. Crude Drug Res.* 1:30.

Szara, S., L. H. Rockland, D. Rosenthan, and J. H. Handlon (1966). *Arch. Gen. Psychiat.* 15:320.

Taber, W. A., L. C. Vining, and R. A. Heacock (1963). *Phytochem.* 2:65.

Tagmann, E., E. Sury, and K. Hoffmann (1952). *Helv. Chim. Acta* 35:1541.

Taylor, E. C., K. Lenard, and Y. Shvo (1966). *J. Amer. Chem. Soc.* 88:367.

Vollner, L., D. Bieniek, and F. Korte (1969). *Tetrahedron Letters*, p. 145.

Wassén, S. H., and B. Holmstedt (1963). *Ethnos* 28:5.

Willstätter, R., O. Wolfes, and H. Mäder (1923). *Ann.* 434:111.

Wollner, H. J., J. R. Matchett, J. Levine, and S. Loewe (1942). *J. Amer. Chem. Soc.* 64:26.

Wood, T. B., W. T. N. Spivey, and T. H. Easterfield (1899). *J. Chem. Soc.* 75:20.

Wright, C. R. (1874). *J. Chem. Soc.* 27:1031.

Yui, T., and Y. Takeo (1958). *Japan. J. Pharmacol.* 7:157

2 Epidemiology

S. I. Cohen and
J. R. Goldsmith

This chapter is concerned with acute and chronic health effects of various drugs used without medical sanction, including considerations of mutagenesis, teratogenesis, carcinogenesis, and other nonpsychiatric reactions. In the epidemiologic approach, it is necessary to characterize the groups of people who are using drugs as well as the types and quantities of drugs being used. Only then does it become possible to make pertinent observations about the occurrence of unfavorable drug effects.

By the very nature of the health indices available, the information first obtained may not be specific to a given drug or even to a specific population. Indices such as the mean birth rate among population groups, the mean age of the newborn in weeks of gestation, the ratio of newborn males to females, the presence of congenital malformations, diseases of early infancy, the nature, timing, and magnitude of fetal mortality, the occurrence of certain neoplasia, and the cause-specific death rate among designated groups are some examples of potential indicators which might be utilized.

It is also necessary to define populations with regard to their differences in exposure to drugs of abuse. If, for example, it is known that use of a new type of drug has recently become frequent in a community, then one would like to see whether this temporal change is reflected over a suitable interval in certain health indices when one compares such a community with others likely to have had less use of this drug. This "temporo-spatial" strategy has been developed and applied to a substantial extent in studies of air pollution health effects, and it may give useful results with data when a considerable number of confounding variables are present.

There are also specific effects which can be followed in carefully selected smaller populations. Examples include abnormal chromosomal patterns in newborns, the relative magnitude of rare conditions such as carcinoma of the liver or buccal cavity, leukemia rates, and the frequency of metabolic abnormalities. The focus on specific events will depend in large part upon the previous laboratory or clinical demonstration of the possibility that such an effect may be related to drug use. In this sense, epidemiology must never be too far removed from laboratory research.

Accumulated experience makes it abundantly clear that long-term unfavorable reactions to a given agent may substantially depend upon the combined presence of other agents or upon unusual susceptibility such as the existence of inborn metabolic defects. Any practical epidemiologic program for determining the effects of exposures to drugs of abuse must therefore deal with such variables as occupational exposures, cigarette smoking, community air pollution exposures, radiation exposures, and exposures to household agents. In short, the study of drugs of abuse needs to be closely interwoven with the epidemiologic study of a large number of other factors.

Economies of scale emerge when this is undertaken which make the entire effort immensely worthwhile. However, there have not yet developed the new types of research organizations which are required for this type of joint effort to evaluate the effects of man's technical and scientific resourcefulness upon man. In various places, excellent population rosters are available for many types of epidemiological analysis; also available are techniques for record linkage [U.S. National Committee on Vital and Health Statistics 1968]. What is needed is a determined effort to include drug abuse epidemiology with the other uses of these data sets. These efforts should be multinational, since several of these unusual sets are in other countries such as Sweden [Cederlof et al. 1965] and Japan [Yanese 1962].

The experience with alcohol, tobacco, and air pollution provides perspectives in the evaluation of long-term consequences of drug use. While the initial reactions to many of these agents were widely known, long-term consequences—cirrhosis, lung cancer, and emphysema, and the interaction of one agent with another—were not understood until recently. It is reasonable to assume that the same hiatus of information may be true for drugs of abuse. It would be unfortunate, however, if we must wait as many decades for evidence of long-term drug abuse effects as we did between the first widespread increase in cigarette tobacco use and the recognition and acceptance of its relationship to cancer of the lung.

It is important, therefore, that we know which populations to study and that we use appropriate methods for carrying out observations so that we can respond to the earliest possible indicators of unfavorable long-term effects. Unfortunately, current drug abuse research proposals do not indicate any trend toward studies of this type. Of over 125 projects funded in 1969 and 1970 by the National Institute of Mental Health, only three propose to deal in any fashion with longitudinal methods of study.

Further compounding this problem is the illegality, by current statutes, of most drug abuse activities. Identification of individuals for the purpose of long-term follow-up becomes tenuous when this information may be subject to subpoena by law enforcement agencies. Suggestions that certain agencies or organizations may not be subject to this problem have not completely resolved the ethical doubts that many researchers have about potential self-incrimination by study subjects. Several studies which plan to follow populations of drug abusers longitudinally will utilize code assignments known only to the individual himself. It will be possible in this way to link subjects over time without the necessity for specific identification of individuals. Approaches which guarantee anonymity are not only ethically important, but they also ensure more honest information about personal drug abuse practices.

1. Frequency of Drug Use and Abuse

1.1. Reliability of Data

The number of persons addicted to opium derivatives in the United States today is estimated to range between 60,000 to 150,000 individuals. This contrasts with the approximately 1.5 million persons said to be addicted to narcotics in the United States in the early 1900s. These figures, however, are only crude estimates.

Estimates of nonnarcotic drug abuse are even more difficult to substantiate. The Federal Food and Drug Administration, in a now frequently cited statement, has estimated that 9 billion doses of amphetamines and 854,000 pounds of barbiturates were produced annually in the United States in 1962, with about half finding their way into illicit channels of distribution [Sadusk 1966]. The development of adequate statistics regarding drug usage is difficult because, as we have previously noted, possession of many of these substances is illegal and users are often unwilling to disclose this information to researchers. This fact is of even more importance when comparisons of drug abuse patterns are made between countries having different drug abuse laws.

An additional problem is that available data are often subject to different interpretations. This is reflected in a follow-up study of juvenile drug offenders recently carried out in California [Polonsky et al. 1967]. Investigators found that of 866 youths arrested for marijuana offenses between 1960 and 1965, 12 percent of the arrestees subsequently were rearrested for involvement with opiates. This statistic is currently being used by some spokesmen to indicate the high percentage of opiate use following initial marijuana use, and by others to indicate that only a small percentage of individuals who are arrested for marijuana offenses go on to opiate use. Because this situation has occurred quite frequently, it is not surprising that many individuals have developed a negative attitude about what is called "statistics." Nevertheless, rosters of persons in contact with law enforcement or health agencies, because of drug use, can be potentially valuable from an epidemiologic viewpoint [Menachem et al. 1968].

1.2. Drug Use in Normal Populations

In 1965, 167 million prescriptions were written for stimulants, sedatives, and tranquilizers. This information, obtained in a national prescription audit, indicates that approximately 590 million dollars were spent for these drugs.

Several studies have attempted to determine what patterns of drug abuse exists among groups not considered to be unusual in any way. Roney and Nall [1967] investigated medication practices in 86 San Francisco households and found that there were a total of 2,539 medications available, representing an average of 30 medications per household. Approximately 20 percent of the total were prescription drugs. Of the total medications, 14 percent were analgesic or central nervous system-active drugs.

A study of Health Insurance Plan members carried out in New York indicated that 21 psychotropic drug prescriptions were written per 100 members each year [Shapiro and Baron 1961]. There was twice as much psychotropic drug use among females, and this finding persisted among all age groups. Psychotropic drug use was also noted to be higher in the elderly.

Manheimer et al. [1968] have reported that approximately 50 percent of a representative sample of California adults, 21 years of age or older, have at one time or another used

Table 1. Proportion of Adults in California and in Selected Subgroups Reporting Frequent Use of One or More of Three Drug Types—Stimulants, Sedatives, and Tranquilizers

	Stimulants %	Sedatives %	Tranquilizers %	Any of the Three %	Base for Percents
All Adults	6	7	10	17	1,026
Sex					
Male	4	5	6	12	527
Female	8	8	14	22	499
Age					
21–29	8	3	7	13	210
30–39	10	4	12	21	197
40–49	6	7	11	17	230
50–59	4	8	11	18	161
60+	2	11	8	16	228
Marital Status					
Married	6	6	10	16	813
Single	7	7	3	14	73
Widowed	4	14	10	20	80
Separated-divorced	8	10	18	27	60
Race					
White	6	7	9	17	909
Negro	5	10	15	19	78
Other	5	5	13	15	39
Education					
Grade school graduate	4	8	10	16	315
High school graduate	5	6	9	16	287
Some college	9	6	9	19	255
College graduate or more	7	6	11	17	169
Family Income[1]					
3,000	5	10	10	19	122
3–5,000	6	5	8	14	118
5–7,000	6	8	9	18	171
7–10,000	6	5	11	16	227
10–15,000	7	5	8	16	238
15,000 or more	5	8	11	20	134
Respondent's Occupation					
Professional, technician, etc.	8	6	8	17	192
Clerical	8	10	9	18	79
Sales	9	9	10	22	67
Skilled craftsmen	5	4	2	9	97
Service and semi-skilled	3	1	9	12	98
Laborers	0	0	3	3	37
Males not in labor force	1	11	8	16	118
Females not in labor force	7	7	14	21	338

[1] Omitted from this table were 16 persons for whom income data were not ascertained.
Source: *California's Health* 26 : 8 (February 1969), p. 6.

psychotherapeutic drugs. Of the 1,026 individuals surveyed, 30 percent had used one of these drugs in the past year and 17 percent were using them frequently. Women were again noted to use psychotherapeutic drugs twice as often as men. Data in Table 1 indicate that drug use is greatest among those who are divorced, better educated, and belong to higher income groups. It is lowest among skilled, semiskilled, or unskilled workers. The type of drugs used differs by age. In men, stimulants are most frequently used during the thirties, tranquilizers during the forties and fifties, and sedatives at age sixty and above. In women, stimulants are most frequently used during the thirties and forties, tranquilizers during the thirties with another peak at age fifty, and sedatives are most commonly used at age sixty and above.

1.3. Drug Use Among College Students

During 1967, a drug use survey was conducted by the Gallup poll organization [Dickenson 1967] on 426 college campuses. Personal interviews with students indicated that 6 percent had tried marijuana and 1 percent had tried LSD. Of these students, 51 percent stated that they did not know any drug users at all. A similar Gallup poll [1969] taken two years later indicates how remarkable the upward trend in student drug use has been. At this time 20 percent had used marijuana and 4 percent LSD (an apparent 300–400 percent increase !).

During 1967, a study was carried out by the Student Health Service at two eastern universities, utilizing a mailed questionnaire [Imperi et al. 1968]. At both campuses, 20 percent of the students stated that they had used hallucinogens at one time or another. At one of the schools, 7 percent of the students had used LSD, while at the other, 2 percent had done so. Approximately 70 percent of the students who tried drugs had taken them in the past year. Of those who said they had never used drugs, over 70

percent had acquaintances who had used drugs. Interestingly, 25 percent of nonusers considered using hallucinogens at some future time.

A number of similar studies have become available since 1967 (Table 2). These show some consistency with marijuana use ranging from 10 to 33 percent and an indication of a trend toward increased usage. LSD usage has been considerably lower.

1.4. Drug Use Among California High School Students

Since 1967, surveys have been conducted in several California counties to determine the extent of drug use among high school students (Table 3). A study at a northern California high school [Sir Francis Drake High School, 1968] indicated that 26 percent of students were using various drugs at the time of the study. Of these students, 39 percent stated that they had tried marijuana, methamphetamine, or LSD at one time or another. Marijuana users smoked it on the average of six times per month. Students indicated that LSD was the most difficult drug to obtain, then methamphetamine, with marijuana being obtained most easily. Surveys on the east coast [Miller 1969] have usually indicated less student drug involvement.

Of students in a San Francisco high school [Rhodes 1968], 20 percent used marijuana frequently, while another 11 percent had used it once or twice. Thirty-six percent of students indicated that they knew someone at school who could get marijuana for them. When asked to give some opinion about the relative dangers of marijuana, heroin, amphetamines, and LSD, the students indicated that marijuana was the least dangerous of these drugs.

A similar study [Lambert and Price 1967] was conducted in one Alameda County school district. Thirty-eight percent of male and 24 percent of female junior and senior high school students admitted to having taken

Table 2. College Students Reporting Use of Drugs (percent)

Survey	Year of Study	Number Surveyed	Mari-juana	LSD	Amphe-tamine	Barbi-turate	Opi-ates	Comments
Gallup polls Nationwide-College Campuses [Dickenson 1967, Gallup 1969]	1967 1969		6 20	1 4				
Yale University [Imperi et al.]	1967	367	18	2				20% had used "hallucinogens"
Wesleyan [Imperi et al.]	1967	251	20	7				20% had used "hallucinogens"
California State College at Long Beach [Demos and Shainline]	1967	540		6				11% had taken LSD, marijuana, mescaline
California Institute of Technology [Eells]	1967	1,290	20	9				
"A West Coast University" [Suchman]	1967	600	20	2				21% had taken some illicit drug
A San Mateo County, Calif. Junior College [Devonshire]	1967	700	23	7				10% has taken "hallucinogens"
Brooklyn College [Pearlman]	1965	1,245						6% had taken some illicit drug
Five Western Colleges [Blum] School I II III IV V	1967	300 270 201 250 293	21 11 21 33 10	6 2 7 9 2	25 11 26 32 13	31 18 29 25 21	1 1 2 1 1	LSD in this survey refers to all hallucinogens

Table 3. California High School Students Reporting Use of Drugs (percent)

Survey	Year of Study	Number Surveyed	Mari-juana	LSD	Amphe-tamine	Barbi-turate	Opi-ates	Glue	Al-cohol	To-bacco	Comments
A Marin County High School (Sir Francis Drake High School)	1968	1,356									26% were currently using and 29% had used marijuana, LSD, or methamphetamine
A San Francisco High School [Rhodes]	1968	232	31								
A Castro Valley High School [Lambert and Price]	1967	1,272	29	12	20	14	4	7	65	36	
Fresno City Unified School District [Thomas]	1967	21,185	7	3	5	5		13			18% had used drugs
Conejo Valley High School Study [Brown]	1968	2,300	21								14% currently using marijuana
California High Schools [Cohen and Deane]	1969	Male 2,169 Female 2,073	23 18	8 6	18 15	11 10	5 4	21 17	47 37	30 29	Conducted in selected schools in Los Angeles, San Francisco, Alameda, and San Diego counties (LSD here refers to all hallucinogens)

drugs not prescribed by a physician. Thirty-five percent of males and 22 percent of females had taken marijuana, the majority for three or more times. Fifteen percent of males and 9 percent of females had taken LSD. Approximately 5 percent of males and 3 percent of females stated that they had used "hard narcotics" such as heroin. A majority of these drugs was said to have been used in the student's homes. The usual age when drugs were first taken was between fifteen and sixteen years of age for both males and females. The most common source of these drugs was classmates, and the usual reason given for taking drugs was "for experimentation."

Studies have also been carried out in less urbanized areas of California [Thomas 1967]. Of twenty-one thousand students surveyed, 18 percent indicated that they had used one of more drugs. Of these students, 5 percent had taken barbiturates, 5 percent amphetamines, 3 percent LSD, and 8 percent had tried marijuana. Students who were involved in extracurricular activities and students with higher grades were less likely to use drugs as continuously or as frequently as other students.

Brown [1968] has obtained drug use data in a survey of 2,300 high school students in a recently urbanized area near Los Angeles. Twenty-one percent of students replied that they had used marijuana at some time in the past and usually planned to continue its use. Users indicate that they will continue marijuana use primarily because of its pleasurable effects. Those who do not use marijuana give reasons such as "don't need it" and "fear bad effects or addiction" for being nonusers. No information on other drug use was obtained. A study more comprehensive in scope was conducted in the City of Berkeley by Fort [1968]. A breakdown of drug use in grades seven through twelve and by sex is presented in Table 4.

A recent study in San Mateo County [Blackford 1969] is of particular importance because surveys of student drug use were conducted in both 1968 and 1969 (Table 5). With this information it has become possible to obtain on a large scale some concept of recent trends in drug use. The 1968 survey included the responses of 18,774 high school students and the 1969 survey of 23,649 students. Included in 1969 were 2,234 seventh-grade and eighth-grade students. The results indicate that girls have consistently lower rates of drug usage than boys, drug use increases with increasing grade level, and with the exception of tobacco, all drugs were used with greater frequency in 1969 than they were in 1968. This last finding is particularly of interest, since the general impression has been that LSD use had diminished as students have become aware of its potentially adverse effects upon chromosomes. Also noteworthy is the finding of an increase in alcohol consumption between 1968 and 1969, particularly when one argument offered by students for use of other drugs is that "they are less harmful than alcohol."

The California Department of Education and the Department of Public Health are cooperating in a statewide study [Cohen and Deane 1969] to obtain more information about the attitudes, opinions, knowledge, and behavior of students relative to drug abuse. Preliminary drug use data has been summarized in Table 3. This information, in combination with pertinent demographic variables may make more relevant educational approaches available as well as point toward more appropriate preventive approaches.

Some preliminary impressions from the data are as follows: Use of drugs increases with age in both males and females. Students whose fathers are currently unemployed are more likely to be users, or to have been users, of drugs. Students who are not living with both parents also are more likely to be users

Table 4. Percent High School Drug Use in Berkeley, California

Sex	Grade	Marijuana	LSD[1]	Amphe-tamine	Barbiturate	Opiates	Glue	Alcohol
	1968							
Male	7	18	6	4	5	3	15	67
	8	27	11	8	—	3	12	81
	10	38	8	12	13	3	11	83
	12	41	6	15	10	5	8	71
Female	7	12	4	5	4	3	7	70
	8	18	3	7	—	3	7	77
	10	43	6	12	13	3	6	81
	12	41	7	15	15	8	11	87

[1] Refers to all hallucinogens.

Table 5. Percent High School Drug Use in San Mateo County, California

Sex	Grade	Marijuana	LSD	Amphetamines	Alcohol	Tobacco
	1968					
Male	9	27	8	12	61	57
	10	32	11	16	64	54
	11	37	15	18	71	57
	12	45	17	20	76	58
Female	9	23	7	13	52	52
	10	28	8	16	60	55
	11	32	9	17	67	57
	12	32	9	16	71	55
	1969					
Male	7	11	3	5	52	44
	8	24	9	12	60	51
	9	35	11	15	66	51
	10	42	17	19	75	50
	11	46	19	22	79	55
	12	50	23	26	82	58
Female	7	11	2	6	38	40
	8	22	6	10	51	50
	9	32	11	20	63	56
	10	36	13	20	67	56
	11	38	13	22	71	55
	12	38	11	20	76	58

Source: Compiled from an article by Lillian Blackford, *California's Health* 27 (November 1969), p. 3.

of drugs. Students who indicate that they have a close relationship with their parents are less likely to be users of drugs. Those whose grades are below average or failing use drugs more frequently than students receiving passing grades. Those who intend to receive a college education or go into the armed forces are less likely to be users of drugs than those who intend to get a job. Those who plan to pursue a four-year college course are much more likely to be nonusers of drugs. Tabulation of various after school activities indicate that as the number of after-school activities increase, use of drugs falls. Nonsmokers are much less likely to be users of drugs than smokers. This observation is also true of those who drink alcohol, with drug use increasing as alcohol consumption increases. Individuals who drink alcohol to get "high" are more likely to use other drugs than those who use alcohol for social reasons. The most frequent reasons given for using drugs are curiosity and "because drugs make you feel good." Those who indicate that their motives for drug use are curiosity are less likely to persist in its use. A study is currently underway in Toronto, Canada, in an attempt to obtain similar information [Jackson 1969].

1.5. Drug Use in Special Populations

Robins and Murphy [1967] have described drug use patterns in 240 individuals representing a sample of Negro males born in St. Louis who had attended elementary school for six years or more and who had an I.Q. score of at least 85. This study is important because it provides a sample which is unselected for prior drug use, and it does not exclude cases which have been institutionalized for addiction or other reasons. Information was obtained by personal interviews as well as by a review of available school records.

One out of ten individuals in this sample had been addicted to heroin; 14 percent of these addicts had used heroin in the past year. Heroin addicts and ex-heroin addicts frequently were using a variety of drugs at follow-up. Of the total sample, 50 percent had at one time used some drug illegally. Virtually every one who used any drug used marijuana as well. Half of the marijuana users never used any other drug, and one-third of marijuana users stated that they did not continue use for more than one year. The younger the age when marijuana use began, the more likely was the user to become addicted to heroin. Sixteen percent of the sample used amphetamines, and 15 percent used barbiturates at one time or another. The combination of an absent father in the household, delinquency, and dropping out of high school characterized the group of boys that was most vulnerable to heroin addiction.

Adolescent marijuana users were further studied with regard to long-term outcome [Robins, Darvish, et al. 1969]. They were less likely than nonusers to graduate from high school, reported increased infidelity on their part and had an increased number of illegitimate children, more frequently required financial aid, had adult records for nondrug offenses, drank heavily, and were more likely to report violent behavior. If they had used other drugs as adolescents, the above problems were even further compounded. Controlling for dropping out of school, juvenile delinquency, and early drinking patterns did not eliminate the outcome differences between drug users and nonusers.

A study carried out in the Haight-Ashbury hippie subculture of San Francisco by Smith [1969] during the summer of 1967 indicated that drugs were used by almost everyone interviewed. Over 95 percent of the individuals had used marijuana. Multiple drug use in this subculture was common, and a single individual often used various combinations of hallucinogens, stimulants, and depressants.

There appeared to be a recent shift in drug use from hallucinogens to intravenous methamphetamine. Studies are currently underway to determine the extent and pattern of amphetamine use.

Brown, Craemer, et al. [1968] have reported on drug use in male alcoholics at Napa State Hospital and find patterns of multiple drug abuse among these individuals. Of 129 alcoholics studied, 91 percent had used sedatives and tranquilizers at least once during their lifetime, and 75 percent had used one of these drugs in the previous 12 months. Frequently these drugs were obtained for the treatment of their alcoholism; however, they were obviously misused on many occasions.

Investigations of patients admitted for drug abuse problems to Bellevue Psychiatric Hospital indicated that individuals were commonly schizophrenic before taking drugs [Hekimian and Gershon 1968]. Of this population, 37 percent required extended hospitalization. Heroin users were usually older than nonusers, and 50 percent of this population were thought to have "sociopathetic" personalities prior to their addiction.

Goldberg [1968] has comprehensively reviewed drug abuse problems in Sweden. He notes that a number of surveys currently underway include studies of hospital patients, those arrested for criminal offenses, alcoholic patients, automobile drivers, and adolescents. Hospital patients were found commonly to abuse sedatives and tranquilizers. These individuals rarely had any criminal background. There were approximately 1,000 patients in Sweden during 1966 with narcotic problems being treated in psychiatric clinics or mental hospitals. Of those arrested for illegal activity associated with drug abuse, the most commonly used drugs were volatile solvents by those between 10 and 19 years of age; stimulants by those 20 to 29; stimulants and hypnotics by those 30 to 39; and hypnotics above 40 years of age. This is similar to the

patterns of drug use found by Manheimer et al. [1968] in the California study of normal adults.

Surveys were also carried out by Goldberg [1960] to determine the prevalence of drug abuse among high school students, of whom 95 percent had never used drugs. Two percent had previously used drugs but stopped, and 1.5 percent were currently using drugs. Seventy-five percent of drug users had used hypnotics or tranquilizers. A similar study in a larger city (Stockholm) indicated that 22 percent of boys and 16 percent of girls had taken drugs on one or more occasions. A majority of these users (81 percent) had smoked cannabis and 26 percent had used stimulant drugs. In Sweden the most commonly abused stimulant drugs are phenmetrazine (Preludin) and methylphenidate (Ritalin). Opiates were used by 6 percent of those taking drugs, 5 percent had taken LSD, and 9 percent had used other drugs such as hypnotics or tranquilizers.

It is quite apparent from the studies cited that drug abuse epidemiology is in an early stage of development and the majority of information available deals primarily with extent as well as trends in drug use by students. These studies do indicate, however, that there is a wide range of drug abuse behavior, and provide opportunities for follow-up studies, which we feel should receive very high priority.

2. Adverse Drug Reactions

Drugs which are being abused differ from drugs used for therapeutic purposes in that they are illicitly obtained, they may not contain the expected ingredients, and they frequently are manufactured by nonstandardized methods. They therefore may contain a variety of impurities and other substances difficult to characterize. The development of accurate risk data in characterizing the adverse drug reaction-prone individual is presently receiving increased attention [Cohen, 1965; Witts 1965; Wilson 1966]. Classical epidemiological concepts of host, agent, and environment have been utilized in studies of adverse drug reactions (ADR), and this experience should be helpful in dealing with some of the problems surrounding acute and chronic health effects of drug abuse. Some host factors of importance in ADR studies include age, sex, race, genetic predisposition, atopic history, and concurrent illnesses. Agent or drug factors include chemical structure, pharmacologic class, antigenicity, route of administration, dosage, duration of use, and physical as well as pharmacologic incompatibilities. Environmental factors include diet, occupational and household exposures, sunlight, temperature, and humidity as some items of importance.

2.1. Usual Methods for Reporting Adverse Drug Reactions

Zbinden [1963] has reviewed 215 articles evaluating approximately 100 different drugs in 21,200 patients. In these studies, 7.3 percent of the patients had an observable ADR. Over 50 percent involved the skin as the organ system of primary involvement. In another review of ADR case reports, 169 articles were analyzed again involving approximately 100 different drugs. The total number of ADR noted was 450, of which the most commonly involved organ systems were hematopoietic, liver, and skin.

A major problem is this type of ADR study is that of defining the drug reaction itself. Reports which have concerned themselves with ADR incidence in hospitalized patients have reported incidences ranging from 0.35 to 18 percent (Table 6). This range primarily reflects variability in the definition as to what constitutes an ADR.

The risk of carcinogenicity, mutagenicity, and teratogenicity from the use of prescription drugs is thought to be prevented of diminished considerably by drug evaluation

Table 6. Incidence of Adverse Drug Reactions

Source	Population at Risk	No. of Individuals with ADR	% ADR
Friend [1962]: Peter Bent Brigham Hospital, 1958	6,629	31	0.48
MacDonald and MacKay [1964]: Mary Fletcher Hospital, 1962	9,557	98	1.0
Schimmel [1964]: Grace-New Haven Hospital, 1964	1,014	119	12.0
Cluff et al. [1965]: Johns Hopkins Hospital, 1964	714	97	13.6
Smith [1969]: Johns Hopkins Hospital, 1965	900	97	10.8
Hurwitz and Wade [1969]: Belfast City Hospital, 1965–66	1,160	118	10.2
Oglivie and Ruedy [1967]: Montreal General Hospital, 1965–66	731	132	18.0
Borda et al. [1968]: Lemuel Shattuck Hospital, 1966	830	—	35.0

required by law. In fact, rare reactions and those which take many years or generations to become manifest are very difficult to prevent by any reasonable program, and many ADR are not dramatic or unique enough to be reported with any consistency [Meyler 1960]. This dilemma has been amply demonstrated in the case of chloramphenicol [Smick et al. 1964; Wallerstein 1969). This drug was administered to over 8 million patients prior to the general recognition of its hematopoietic effects. As a result of this experience the American Mediacl Association initiated a Registry on Blood Dyscrasias which eventually evolved into its Registry on Adverse Reactions (Friend 1962; Wintrobe, 1965; De Nosaquo 1966).

Lasagna [1964] has succinctly stated the problems inherent in interpreting data collected in this manner in referring to adverse effects of oral contraceptives. "If one does not know the incidence of drug-related mortality from thrombo-embolism, and one does not know the incidence of thrombo-embolic disease in a comparable population not taking Enovid, one cannot possibly determine accurately the presence of increased risk, even by applying the most sophisticated statistical techniques." Unfortunately, studies of drug abuse epidemiology have even greater handicaps.

2.2 Proposed Studies of ADR and Their Possible Application to Drug Abuse Epidemiology

A drug reaction monitoring system has recently been instituted by the Kaiser-Permanente Medical Group in the San Francisco Bay Area [Collen 1967]. This study is expected "to provide data on 250,000 individuals each year who utilize approximately 35,000 hospital admissions and one million office visits." Current plans include use of Kaiser-Plan outpatient pharmacies for outpatient denominator data. This goal will be accomplished by direct feed-in from these

pharmacies into a central computer. Inpatient denominator data will be obtained directly from nursing stations by visual-display input terminals. Diagnosis including ADR, working diagnosis, and abnormal laboratory results will provide numerator data. These data will also be read into the central computer by input terminals located in the outpatient department and on hospital wards.

Finney [1964, 1965] has discussed the need for adequate channels of information and the types of data required to make statistical inferences regarding ADR. Because of the low incidence of ADR associated with many drugs, he places special emphasis on the necessity for developing an international monitoring system. If appropriate host, agent, and environmental data are collected, analysis of several different sets could be accomplished using automatic data-processing systems.

Experience with drugs of abuse should be characterized, as with ADR studies, into first that of persons receiving specific drugs to develop drug risk data (drug sets); second, monitoring of all persons with a specific disease or health condition, e.g., pregnancy, diabetes, glucose 6-phosphate dehydrogenase deficiency, etc., could be undertaken to determine if different risks occur in certain populations (population sets); third, events or diagnoses such as leukemia, mongolism, anencephaly, and buccal cancer could be monitored to determine whether specific drugs have contributed to the event (events sets). Although the utilization of drug sets is particularly appropriate to hospital-based epidemiologic studies of ADR such as those discussed here, all three mechanisms are applicable to the use of clinical rosters and population rosters.

3. Methods and Recommended Guidelines

When case reports or the results of animal studies suggest that drug abuse leads to specific pathology, then such effects must be looked for in susceptible groups to test the indicated hypothesis. This method is generally referred to as *specific hypothesis testing*.

In this approach it is essential that appropriate population rosters be available for sample selection; in addition to this, control populations which have differing drug use patterns, but which are otherwise comparable, are of considerable importance. For drug abuse studies, such rosters can be based upon surveyed populations, upon those identified at clinics or other health facilities, or upon law enforcement rosters. This sequence is also the sequence of desirability, since large biasing factors may determine whether drug abuse experience leads to entry to a health facility or to law enforcement rosters. Specific hypothesis testing requires appropriate-sized populations and the use of adequate statistical procedures in light of the anticipated frequency of the morbid event [WHO Scientific Group 1968].

An example of the above approach is provided in a study by Leck et al. [1969]. These investigators examined birth certificates of women who had been exposed to A2 influenza epidemics during the early months of their pregnancy. Table 7 compares numbers of malformations in infants with high-risk and low-risk births in 1962–1965 for 17 standard metropolitan statistical areas. The high-risk group comprised cases in which according to the birth dates recorded, the period of high mortality from influenza in the city concerned might have coincided with early pregnancy. The last column of Table 7, Standardized Incidence Ratio, refers to the correction applied for season of the year when children were born, since there are seasonal and secular variations unrelated to influenza in the frequency of malformed births. The hypothesis of an effect of influenza upon certain types of malformations appears to be substantiated. It is obvious that specific hypothesis testing with respect to drug ex-

posures might raise questions of defining a high-risk group that would be much harder to answer than is the case for this example.

Another epidemiologic method which is applicable to defining effects of drug abuse is the *surveillance* approach. The surveillance approach assumes an adequate recording of general vital data, as well as types of morbidity and mortality data which could reflect alterations of mutagenic, carcinogenic, or teratogenic rates. It also assumes knowledge about temporospatial variations in drug abuse experience and requires appropriate controls for evaluation of relevant variables, such as smoking, radiation, and other environmental exposures. This epidemiologic method can thus serve a variety of needs but has generally been neglected.

Table 8 is an example of data which can be utilized for surveillance studies [Dental Health Center 1966]. An obvious problem with data of this sort is that there may be differing levels of precision and validity to the diagnoses. The three diagnoses shown in Table 8, however, are relatively unlikely to be subject to diagnostic error. It is interesting to note that in those with anencephaly, spina bifida, and hydrocephaly there are wide fluctuations in the male-female ratio during this period. Presumably any biases of diagnosis and reporting would not differ between sexes in different years. Data such as this raise the question as to whether any environmental or drug exposures might influence such rates. The study of problems of this sort already has an extensive literature; for example, Naggan and MacMahon [1967] have reported ethnic differences in the prevalence of anencephaly and spina bifida. They also report a higher rate with populations of lower socioeconomic status. Such an effect of socioeconomic status, again, could possibly be a reflection of environmental exposures, or drug or food use patterns.

There is presently no surveillance of the sex

Table 7. Numbers of Selected Malformations reported among Live Births in 17 Standard Metropolitan Statistical Areas, 1962–65 According to Risk of Exposure to Influenza during Early Pregnancy

Type of Malformation	a High-Risk Births	b Low-Risk Births	Crude incidence ratio $\left(\dfrac{a}{200,000} \div \dfrac{b}{1,884,100}\right)$	Standardized Incidence Ratio
Anomalies of Nervous System				
Anencephalus	52	466	1.05	1.32
Spina bifida, encephalocele	126	1,097	1.08	1.13
Hydrocephalus	57	579	.93	.93
Microcephalus	2	105	.18	.24
Anomalies of Digestive System				
Cleft palate	55	556	.93	.93
Cleft lip	62	464	1.26	1.47[1]
Cleft palate with cleft lip	74	779	.89	1.10
Esophageal defects	11	135	.77	1.12
Anorectal defects	39	378	.97	.80
Hypospadias	123	1,218	.95	.93
Anomalies of Musculoskeletal System				
Clubfoot	232	2,247	.97	.89
Reduction deformities				
Upper lims only	51	320	1.50[2]	1.91[2]
Lower lims only	13	129	.95	1.23
Upper and lower limbs	6	45	1.26	1.32
Limbs unspecified	2	22	.86	.75
Congenital dislocation of hip	14	150	.88	.77
Diaphragmatic hernia	10	114	.83	1.01
Down's Disease	92	810	1.07	1.16
Exomphalos	26	272	.90	1.16

[1]$0.05 > \frac{P}{2} > 0.01$; [2]$0.01 > \frac{P}{2} > 0.001$. Source: Leck, 1969.

Table 8. Live-Born White Infants with Congenital Malformations in California—1961–65

Year	Live Births	Cases All Forms of Congenital Malformations	Rate per 1,000	Anencephaly			Spina Bifida			Hydrocephaly		
				Male	Female	Ratio Male/Female	Male	Female	Ratio Male/Female	Male	Female	Ratio Male/Female
1961	381,198	4306	11.30	28	43	0.65	82	78	1.05	58	42	1.38
1962	378,347	4187	11.07	36	37	0.97	82	95	0.86	43	43	1.00
1963	380,505	4243	11.15	23	37	0.62	71	90	0.79	51	38	1.34
1964	374,587	3994	10.66	43	44	0.98	72	83	0.87	51	35	1.46
1965	355,074	3851	10.85	29	49	0.59	64	89	0.72	39	42	0.93

Source: Dental Health Center, 1966.

Table 9. Overall Pregnancy Loss-Disability (12 weeks or More Gestation) by Selected Medical Conditions Diagnosed Shortly Before or During Pregnancy (Single Deliveries)

Condition[1]	Interval between First Diagnosis and LMP			
	0–3 Months Prior		0–11 Weeks Post	
	No. of women	L-D rate per 100[2]	No. of women	L-D rate per 100[2]
I. L-D rate 25% or more above overall rate of 17.97 per 100 in either of two intervals				
Rubella	*	*	14	35.71
Gastroenteritis, colitic	68	13.24	65	23.08
Urinary tract infections	59	22.03	48	27.08c
Accidents, poisoning, violence	189	22.75c	140	22.86
Benign neoplasm, excl. gyn.	47	25.53	30	20.00
Any allergic disease	279	17.20	88	22.73
Mental, psychoneurotic/personality disorders, nervousness	234	19.23	171	23.98b
Chronic rheumatic heart disease	*	*	41	24.39
Gynecological Disorders (noninfectious)				
Malposition of uterus	26	30.77c	78	23.08
Uterine fibromyoma	33	33.33b	94	26.60b
Other gynecological conditions	83	25.30a	102	20.59
Disorder of menstruation	184	26.09c	—	—
Antepartum bleeding, staining or spotting	—	—	732	39.21a
Rising Rh titer	—	—	12	41.67c
Edema of ankles and feet	—	—	22	27.27
II. L-D rate less than 25% above overall rate of 17.97 per 100 (includes L-D rates below overall rate)				
Infections or Inflammations				
Upper respiratory infections, sinusitis, pharyngitis	812	20.32	701	16.12
Bronchitis	67	11.94	56	21.43
Influenza, viral disease of respiratory and G.I. tract	165	20 00	146	19.86
Infection of reproductive organs and genitalia	284	19.37	270	17.41

Conditions[1]	Interval between First Diagnosis and LMP			
	0–3 Months Prior		0–11 Weeks Prior	
	No. of women	L-D rate per 100[2]	No. of women	L-D rate per 100[2]
Other Selected Conditions				
Hay fever	194	17.53	54	18.52
Disease of thyroid	46	15.22	45	11.11
Obesity	287	17.07	182	20.88
Anemia	52	15.38	46	21.74
Haemorrhoids	36	22.22	28	21.43
Arthritis, rheumatism, synovitis, bursitis, and tenosynovitis	166	19.88	86	13.95
Varicose veins of lower extremities	24	20.83	83	15.66
Immunizations and Injections				
Gamma globulin injections	—	—	129	21.71
Polio immunization	402	14.68	456	13.82
Influenza immunization	*	*	59	16.95
Allergy injection	176	17.05	*	*

[1] Conditions under medical treatment in HIP during specified periods related to LMP.
[2] Fetal deaths (12 weeks or more gestation), neonatal deaths, low birth-weight infants, plus children with "S" anomalies per 100 pregnancies of 12 weeks or more gestation.
*Less than five loss-disability events in category.
Note: Conditions of special interest are included in table even where the frequencies are low, provided five or more loss-disability events occurred in one of the time intervals. Asterisks (*) indicate a cell with fewer than five L-D events. Probability that a difference between the L-D rate for a selected condition and the overall L-D rate, as large or larger than observed, is due to chance factors is indicated by
[a] for $P \leq .01$;[b] for $.01 < P.05$;[c] for $.05 < P \leq .10$.

Source: S. Shapiro and M. Abramowicz, "Pregnancy Outcome Correlates Identified through Medical Record-Based Information," *American Journal of Public Health* 59 : 9 (1969), pp. 1644–1645.

ratio or its change in human populations. It is conceivable that considerable changes in this ratio could occur which would pass unnoticed. For example, in order to determine if a change in the male-female ratio from 0.51 to 0.47 was significant, we would require a study population of at least 1,250 of each sex. If the shift was smaller (0.51 to 0.50), a population of 20,000 of each sex would be required to determine whether it was significant at the 5 percent level.

A study relevant to the general problem of fetal-loss surveillance has recently been reported by Shapiro and Abramowicz [1969]. They have examined physician's reports and medical charts in the Health Insurance Plan of Greater New York to determine the relationship between maternal conditions and pregnancy outcome. Congenital malformations and pregnancy loss have been combined to indicate overall rates of pregnancy loss-disability (Table 9). They have included all pregnancies of 12 or more weeks gestation by selected medical conditions in mothers diagnosed shortly before or during pregnancy. The overall rate of pregnancy loss-disability was found to be 17.97 per 100. The highest excess rate occurred in the presence of increasing Rh titers, but significant elevations occurred in the post-last menstrual period (LMP) interval with urinary tract infections, mental disorders, uterine fibromyoma, and symptoms of antepartum bleeding. Significant conditions occuring in the pre-LMP interval were accidents, poisoning, or violence and gynecological disorders. The second part of Table 9 shows a number of other conditions with lower loss-disability rates. It is of considerable interest to question whether the excess rates with urinary tract infections and mental disorders might have been related to drugs used for the management of these conditions or otherwise associated with their presence.

We believe that the reports cited provide useful guidelines for the types of studies which should be undertaken for surveillance of nonpsychiatric effects of drug abuse on offspring. Clearly there is room for great improvement in the reporting of congenital abnormalities and pregnancy losses. The intensive effort to do this in selected communities would be justified for a number of purposes of which the long-term effects of drug use would be only one.

4. Discussion

A number of recommendations thus emerge from the material presented. It is possible to obtain clinical data from hospitals or clinics concerning the occurrence of drug reactions, but it is unlikely that most acute reactions in the population at risk will be seen in established medical facilities. Support for improved data handling from local community clinics which have the confidence of drug-using populations may improve this current situation.

In some instances it may be valuable to provide mortality data such as that available from local medical examiners on a real time basis rather than several years later. Systematic surveillance of changes in mortality by sex, age, and cause of death may then provide some useful clues with regard to acute adverse effects of drugs.

No useful mechanism for increasing the ease of reporting adverse reactions due to legally prescribed as well as illicit drugs is available. Current attempts to obtain this information in hospital-based studies may provide some information, but the extent to which these data are applicable to individuals in the drug-using community is at present unresolved.

Surveillance of newborns for changes in sex ratio, fetal deaths, and congenital abnormalities has usually been carried out only for short periods of time and upon relatively small population sets. Registries which also obtain data on drug taking by parents may eliminate the likelihood that large numbers of adverse effects may occur in newborns before the recognition that such events are taking place.

5. Summary

This review is primarily concerned with the long-term health effects of various drugs used without medical sanction. We have attempted to provide an appraisal of the potential role of epidemiologic research in future programs related to the problem of drug abuse. Epidemiologic studies are for the most part inadequate at present. Basic information is required to characterize the groups of people who use drugs as well as the types of drugs and the quantities and methods of administration.

A review of the literature pertaining to drug use in normal adult populations, high school students, college students, and other special groups indicates that there is a wide range of drug-taking behavior.

Epidemiologic methods which may be appropriate to the drug abuse problem have been developed in areas such as occupational and environmental cancer, congenital abnormalities, effects of radiation, and tobacco-smoking exposures. A brief presentation of some epidemiological approaches to adverse drug reactions and its relevancy to drug abuse is also discussed.

A review of current research proposals indicates that insufficient effort is being directed toward longitudinal studies necessary to determine the long-sterm consequences of drug abuse. Without implementation of appropriate studies we may well assume that the same lack of information which existed with regard to the effects of alcohol, tobacco, community air pollution, and many other substances is likely to develop. Several epidemiologic approaches are recommended including a specific hypothesis testing approach and a surveillance approach.

References

Blackford, L. S. (1969). *California's Health* 27 : 3.

Blum, R. H. (1969). *Students and Drugs.* San Francisco : Jossey-Bass Inc.

Borda, I. T., D. Slone, and H. Jick (1968). *J.A.M.A.* 205 : 645.

Brown, R., R. Craemer, and I. Babow (1968). Patterns of Sedative and Tranquilizer Use Among Male Alcoholics at Napa State Hospital. State of California Division of Research, Department of Public Health. Mimeo.

Brown, R. V. (1968). Conejo Narcotics Study : Preliminary Report. Mimeo.

Cederlof, R., L. Friberg, E. Jonsson, and K. Lennart (1965). *Arch. Environ. Health* 10 : 346.

Cluff, L. E., G. Thornton, L. Seidl, and J. Smith (1965). *Trans. Ass. Amer. Physicians* 78 : 255.

Cohen, Lord of Birkenhead. (1965). *J. Roy. Inst. Public Health* 28 : 97.

Cohen, S. I., and M. Deane (1969). Berkeley : California State Department of Public Health. Unpublished data.

Collen, M. F. (1967). Personal communication.

De Nosaquo, N. (1966). *Ann. Intern. Med.* 64 : 1325.

Demos, G. D., and J. W. Shainline (1967). Drug Use on the College Campus : Pilot Survey : Committee for the Study of Drugs at California State College at Long Beach. Mimeo.

Dental Health Center, San Francisco (1966). National Cleft Lip and Palate Intelligence Service 1 : 3.

Devonshire, C. M. (1969). Cited in R. H. Blum, *Students and Drugs.* San Francisco : Jossey-Bass Inc.

Dickenson, F. (1967). *Reader's Digest,* November, 114.

Eells, K. (1967). A Survey of Student Practices and Attitudes with Respect to Marijuana and LSD. California Institute of Technology. Unpublished.

Finney, D. J. (1964). *J. Chron. Dis.* 17 : 565.

Finney, D. J. (1965). *J. Chron. Dis.* 18 : 77.

Fort, J. (1968). *Berkeley Gazette,* December 13.

Friend, D. G., and R. G. Hoskins (1960). *Med. Clin. N. Amer.* 44 : 1381.

Friend, D. G. (1962). *J.A.M.A.* 181 : 111.

Gallup poll. (1969). *San Francisco Chronicle,* May 26.

Goldberg, L. (1968). *Bull. Narcotics* 20 : 1.

Goldberg, L. (1968). *Bull. Narcotics* 20 : 9.

Hekimian, L. J., and S. Gershon (1968). *J.A.M.A.* 205 : 75.

Hollister, L. E. (1965). *Postgrad. Med.* 37 : 94.

Hurwitz, N., and O. L. Wade (1969). *Brit. Med. J.* 1 : 531.

Imperi, L. L., H. D. Kleber, and J. S. Davie (1968). *J.A.M.A.* 204 : 87.

Jackson, D. (1969). *A Preliminary Report on the Attitudes and Behavior of Toronto Students in Relation to Drugs.* Addiction Research Foundation, 344 Bloor St. West, Toronto.

Lambert, D., and J. Price (1967). Pub. Castro Valley Unified School District. Mimeo.

Lasagna, L. (1964). *Perspect. Biol. Med.* 7 : 457.

Leck, I., S. Hay, J. J. Witte, and J. C. Greene (1969). *Public Health Rep.* 84 : 971.

MacDonald, M. G., and B. R. MacKay (1964). *J.A.M.A.* 190 : 115.

Manheimer, D. I., G. D. Mellinger, and M. B. Balter (1968). *California Medicine* 109 : 445.

Menachem, F. K., P. M. Densen, and D. C. Krug (1968). *Int. J. Addictions* 3 : 139.

Meyler, L. (ed.). (1960). *Side Effects of Drugs.* Amsterdam : Excerpta Medica Foundation.

Miller, J. L. (1969). Cited in R. H. Blum. *Students and Drugs.* San Francisco : Jossey-Bass, Inc.

Naggan, L., and B. MacMahon (1967). *New Eng. J. Med.* 277 : 1119.

Oglivie, R. I., and J. Ruedy (1967). *Canad. Med. Ass. J.* 97 : 1445.

Pearlman, S. (1967). *Amer. J. Orthopsych.* 37 : 297.

Polonsky, D., G. F. Davis, and C. F. Roberts (1967). *A Follow-Up Study of the Juvenile Drug Offender.* Sacramento : Institute for the Study of Crime and Delinquency.

Rhodes, G. (1968). *San Francisco Examiner and Chronical,* June 2.

Robins, L. N., H. S. Darvish, and G. E. Murphy (1969). The Long-Term Outcome for Adolescent Drug Users : A Follow-Up Study of 76 Users and 146 Non-Users. In J. Zubin and A. Freedman, eds., *Psychopathology of Adolescence,* Grune and Stratton. To be published.

————, and G. E. Murphy (1967). *Amer. J. Public Health* 57 : 1580.

Roney, J. G., and M. L. Nall (1967). *California Medicine* 107 : 452.

Sadusk, J. F. (1966). *J.A.M.A.* 196 : 119.

Schimmel, E. M. (1964). *Ann. Intern. Med.* 60 : 100.

Seidl, L. G., C. F. Thornton, and L. E. Cluff (1965). *Amer. J. Public Health* 55 : 1170.

Shapiro, S., and M. Abramowicz (1969). *Amer. J. Public Health* 59 : 1629.

Shapiro, S., and S. H. Baron (1961). *Public Health Rep.* 76 : 481.

Sir Francis Drake High School *Jolly Roger.* (1968). San Anselmo, Calif. Vol. 18 (April).

Smick, K. M., P. K. Condit, R. L. Proctor, and V. Suther (1964). *J. Chron. Dis.* 17 : 899.

Smith, D. E. (1969a). *California Medicine* 110 : 472.

———— (1969b). *California Medicine* 110 : 151.

Smith, J. W., L. G. Seidl., and L. E. Cluff (1966). *Ann. Intern. Med.* 65 : 629.

Suchman, E. A. (1968). *J. Health Soc. Behav.* 9 : 146.

Thomas, M. L. (1967). Report of Narcotics Survey-Secondary Schools, Fresno City Unified School District, Dept. of Guidance and Testing. October. Mimeo.

United States National Committee on Vital and Health Statistics (1968). National Center for Health Statistics, Series 4, No. 7, Washington, D.C. : Public Health Service.

WHO Scientific Group Report (1968). *WHO Tech. Rep.* No. 401.

Wallerstein, R. O. (1969). *J.A.M.A.* 208 : 2045.

Wilson, G. M. (1966). *Brit. Med. J.* 5495 : 1065.

Wintrobe, M. M. (1965). *Ann. Intern. Med.* 62 : 170.

Witts, L. J. (1965). *Brit. Med. J.* 5470 : 1081.

Yanese, T. (1962). In *The Use of Vital and Health Statistics for Genetic and Radiation Studies.* New York : United Nations, pp. 119–133.

Zbinden, G. (1963). In S. Garattini and D. Shore eds. *Advances in Pharmacology,* vol. 2, New York : Academic Press.

3 Nonbehavioral Pharmacology

M. H. Joffe and W. Martin

For the purposes of this discussion, we classify the nonnarcotic drugs into several categories and subcategories based on a peculiar combination of chemical and pharmacological properties. Narcotic drugs occupy a separate section of this paper. Neither classification by itself serves to cover the differences, nor is there a really clear-cut structure-activity theory that deals with more than one type of compound. Shulgin [1969] has provided the SAR theory in the phenethylamine group, and Szara [1967] has done considerable work in the area of tryptamines, while the classic papers of Rothlin [1957] cover the indole compounds related to LSD.

The major problem faced by the pharmacologist as we see it in this area is that his biological tools are either not adequate as presently constructed, or nonexistent for a proper evaluation.

We are still, no matter how sensitive the detector is, dependent on the animal to provide information on the effects. If these effects are at a molecular level that present tools are not sufficiently sensitive to detect, they will be missed. If the effects are perhaps buffered by cellular constituents, they are again difficult to detect. If they involve enzyme systems we are ignorant of, they again may be undetectable. This latter situation is probably the most important consideration of all, for to date there is no real link between action identifiable at the physiological level and action at the psychiatric level. True, at toxic levels there are observable physiological disturbances, but at doses which are behaviorally active for LSD or THC, there are no pathognomonic relationships.

LSD does have ergot-like sympathomimetic effects, but these are so overwhelmed by psychiatric influences on the same portion of the autonomic system that they are easily masked.

One area of activity in which a reasonably holistic theory has been constructed is that of the sympathomimetic stimulants—cocaine, amphetamine, methamphetamine, the stimulant hallucinogens in the phenethylamine class (MDA, DOM, TMA, etc.) as outlined by Snyder [1967]. However, we may point out that as comprehensive as this theory is, it is being vigorously challenged, not on the basis of the involvement of norepinephrine in central nervous processes, but on its real role —is it stimulant, as the Brodie-Axelrod hypothesis would have us consider, or depressant, as the animal data would suggest? In all instances of intracerebral administration of exogenous norepinephrine to animals, a depressant action is noted, rather than a stimulant one. In two recent papers, Mandell [1968] has shown the action of the tricyclic antidepressant imipramine to be antagonistic to norepinephrine in the chick, and postulates that perhaps the antidepressant action of imipramine is manifested via the interference with the behaviorally depressant norepinephrine's access to postsynaptic membranes. But here again we are faced with the fact that these are baby chicks we are experimenting with, not clinically depressed humans. How far can the parallel go between animal and man?

In spite of all this pro and con discussion on the actual role of norepinephrine in the central nervous system, the involvement of the biogenic amines is pretty firmly established. Stein and Wise [1970] have shown that the addition of amphetamine to the animal excites both physiological and psychological processes. Increase in heart rate, respiration, dilatation of the pupils, the classical signs of a sympathomimetic compound, one which produces the effects of discharge of the adrenal medulla, are all to be found after the administration of these stimulant compounds. Strangely enough, however, there develops a rather good tolerance to the physiological effects of the amphetamines, and just to complicate things a little, the psychiatric

excitation produced by amphetamines reverses to a depression just shortly before the occurrence known as the toxic psychosis sets in [Griffiths et al. 1970]. Does this now represent the depressant effect of excess norepinephrine, epinephrine, a metabolite, exhaustion of the amine oxidase mechanism, or something entirely different?

The hallucinogens of the tryptamine or indolealkylamine series N,N-DMT, N,N-DET, psilocin, psilocybin, etc., are not only synthetics; they are also found in many plants, particularly among South American Indians [Holmstedt and Lingrea 1967]. The cohoba snuff is a product containing DMT, and the 5-methoxy-N-methyltryptamine has also been found in certain snuff as well as in several species of a grass, *Phalaris tuberosa* by Marczynski [1959] and *P. arundinacea* by Wilkinson [1958], that is associated with a disease in sheep, manifesting both neurological and behavioral changes. In this group of compounds, structure-activity relationships have also been proposed, the dimethyl derivatives having greater potency than the monomethyl, possibly because they are more resistant to monoamine oxidase action. However, the dimethyl tryptamine bufotenine is still a matter of controversy, its blood pressure-raising properties being so pronounced that its psychotropic powers were not manifested to Isbell et al. [1968] because of the potential danger due to the physiological effects. But bufotenine with a CH_3O substituted for its OH becomes 5-methoxy DMT and a very potent psychotropic.

There are many modifications of this basic tryptamine nucleus, and contrary to expected fact, the shorter side-chain $CH_2—COOH$ which is found in Gramine, instead of in the longer $—CH_2—CH_2—N\text{\Large<}^{CH_3}_{CH_3}$ of DMT, produces a compound showing antagonism to some of the effects of LSD, a higher toxicity, and the ability to cause convulsions than the dimethylated derivatives, and its 5 methoxy derivative was less potent than Gramine itself [Airaksinen and McIsaac, 1968].

The potent tryptamines produce copious salivation, increased activity, confusion, and near convulsive activity among the South American Indians. The interest in the group mainly revolves around the metabolic fate, for while the end product is 5-hydroxyindole-acetic acid (5 HIAA) and glucuronides, disturbances of the pathway of tryptamine metabolism may produce compounds closely related or causal to the natural disease of schizophrenia. The adrenolutin theory is well known as a consequence of such studies [Osmond and Smythies 1952].

In general the tryptamines are sympathomimetic, raising blood pressure, dilating pupils, and causing nausea and thick, stringy salivation. Increased and incoherent speech are also found, which puts primitive man in communication with the beyond, and modern man beyond communication. Seitz [1967] has described the phenomenon; the product itself was analyzed by Holmstedt [1965]. An allied group of hallucinogens is the LSD type, whose chemical nucleus incorporates the indole structure and is closely allied to the tryptamines. There are many diverse actions of this group— the best known, other than the psychiatric, being the inhibition of serotonin, hyperreflexia, piloerection, and the raising of body temperature—in general the signs of an ergot-like sympathomimetic.

Probably the most unusual finding with this group of compounds is the remarkable drop in effectiveness in one or more properties if the molecule is tampered with in any fashion. Most remarkable of all is the total lack of any activity, biochemical, psychiatric, or behavioral, when the l-compound is used rather than the d-compound [Pfeiffer 1959]. The separation of activities among the various modifications of this latter group is really remarkable. The d- iso-LSD has the same lack of activity as the l- form and is the product identifiable in urine; the compound MLD-41 (d-1-methyl-LSD) has only 40 percent of the psychotropic properties of the d-LSD 25 but it has almost 4 times the serotonin-antagonizing property (on rat uterus) and about 5 percent of the pyretogenic effect. The Brom LSD cpd, Bol 148, has 5 percent of the pyretogenic activity, equal or slightly greater serotonin-inhibiting powers, and no psychological effect in humans. The MBL 61 or methylbrom LSD has no pyretogenic effects, but it inhibits serotonin about 5 times better than either BOL or LSD 25. The d-monethylamide and the d-dimethylamide share all the properties of the diethylamide, but in lesser potency, as might be expected.

The most provokingly strange finding is that the effects of optical isomerism is so very pronounced, both psychiatrically and physiologically. If one wishes to examine almost any effect of d-LSD 25 to the exclusion of other effects, it is quite probable that other members of the series could be found which have an exacerbation of one effect and a diminution of other effects. A recent paper demonstrates that AMT (d-1-α-methyltyrosine), a compound known to interfere with norepinephrine metabolism and to reverse the effects of amphetamine, can also reverse the sympathetic manifestations of LSD in rabbits. The excitation of motor activity, pupil dilation, and salivation are abolished, but the hyperthermia remains. The involvement of LSD in catecholamine metabolism is thus demonstrated, as one suspects from its gross actions, but another mechanism must be responsible for the hyperthermia. Recent studies have also shown the presence of discrete serotoninergic neurones within the central pathways of the brain [Aghajanian et al. 1968]. Whether such discrete groups of cells within one or another area of the brain can be the mechanism by which seemingly diverse functions are carried out is as yet unknown—or even whether a different dose level of drug is a necessary factor when the mechanism itself is the same is not known.

Another group of compounds that is found by Abood and Biel [1962] to be hallucinogenic, and that is used by the drug culture in a pleasureable fashion, is the strong anticholinergics. We use this phraseology purposely, for many groups of psychiatrically normal individuals have expressed not only an unwillingness to repeat the exposure but a dissatisfaction with the previous episode. In this chemical group are compounds like Ditran and other glycollic acid esters whose action is classically anticholinergic—dry mouth, pupillary dilation with paralysis of accommodation (cycloplegia), increased heart rate, red dry hot skin due to inhibition of sweating, inhibition of gastric motility and secretion, and bronchodilation. The psychiatric aspects in the case of the glycollates appear at minimal doses, but they are very closely followed by the physical manifestations, in striking contrast to the next group of compounds that we would like to discuss.

The pharmacology of marijuana and its constituent cannabinol derivatives at the present time is a diffuse mass of what might be called organized chaos. There are almost innumerable reports on the subject, and but one fact shines through the darkness. No one has yet had a sufficiently large sample to perform animal experiments that are definitive, replicatable, and within the realm of reality in the sense that a finding can be made at a dose level relatable to that of the human showing psychological effects; and except for one or two experiments done with a sample of synthetic Δ^9 by Isbell et al. [1967] at Lexington, there have been no instances where pure, identifiable material has been used on humans. Since Isbell's conclusions were that respiration, reflexes, and blood pressure did not change, and that only after

statistical analysis of before, during, and after heart rates could a change be seen, there is little pharmacological information available. A definitive toxicity study on animals is now in progress.

At the present time it is not possible to identify the level of THC in body fluids. To make a long story short on this matter, it is not a question of being able to get sufficient instrument sensitivity but of knowing to what the THC is converted before it enters the blood stream, because the compound per se is not to be found. When one administers a mixture of compounds, such as occurs in either the plant or extracts of the plant, it is impossible to determine which of the cannabinols came from the administered mixture or was metabolically converted. The provision of adequate amount of chemically pure synthetic material will serve to make it possible to determine some true facts about the effects of THC. The biggest job in this field is the separation of fact from fancy.

Before concluding remarks on the stimulants and hallucinogens, we would like to comment on a group of drugs about which considerably more information exists. The narcotics and barbiturates differ from most therapeutic agents in that they have several additional dimensions. In addition to organ toxicity, certain drugs of abuse induce compulsive drug-seeking behavior. Further, abuse of drugs is characterized by social toxicity. In defining the abuse potentiality of drugs, which is closely related to the concept of a malevolence or a hazard index as suggested by Drs. Lederberg and Shulgin, Martin [1965; in press] has viewed it as having the following three related dimensions.

1. Compulsive Drug-Seeking Behavior
Narcotic drugs of abuse give rise to compulsive drug-seeking behavior through several mechanisms. Most drugs of abuse produce subjective changes that are thought to re-

present some positive gain to the individual. The work of Hill et al. [1963] in assessing subjective effects of drugs suggests that a variety of drugs of abuse, including narcotic analgesics, barbiturates, LSD-like psychotogens, and amphetamines, produce an enhancement of self-image and a feeling of well-being in appropriate doses and settings.

Several types of agents when administered chronically induce tolerance and physical dependence. When patients who are tolerant to and dependent on morphine and barbiturate-like drugs are withdrawn, they experience signs and symptoms of abstinence which are associated with feelings of discomfort and pain. These are needs which are reduced by the drugs of abuse. These needs, like the need to avoid pain or hunger, permit the establishment of conditioned behavior. Wikler and Pescor [1967] have suggested that conditioned abstinence and conditioned drug-seeking behavior may be responsible for relapse of dependent subjects following treatment.

Recently, and perhaps more directly related to the purpose of this monograph, it has been observed that chronic administration of morphine induces physiological changes that persist for many months after morphine has been withdrawn [Martin and Jasinski 1969], and these changes are associated with increased excretion of epinephrine [Eisenman et al. 1969] and hypersensitivity of the psychogalvanic skin response to hypercapnia [Jones et al. 1969]. These observations may be related to those of Himmelsbach [1941], who found that the abstinent addict exhibited hyperresponsivity to the cold pressor test.

2. Organ Toxicity

A variety of overt and covert types of toxicity are induced by drugs of abuse. The respiratory depressant effects of narcotic analgesics are well known. Narcotic addicts have a very high death rate, probably in excess of 2 percent per annum, which would be over 10 times that of appropriate general populations of the same age, sex, and race. Patients who have a high level of dependence on alcohol or on sedative-hypnotics such as barbiturates may have a withdrawal mortality of 10 to 20 percent if not adequately treated. Cirrhosis of the liver, polyneuritis, and Wernicke-Korsakoff syndromes are well-known consequences of alcoholism. LSD-like hallucinogens, amphetamine-like agents, and marihuana are capable of inducing a toxic psychosis.

The use of unsterile techniques in administering drugs by most addicts is responsible for the transmission of infectious diseases, including hepatitis, subacute bacterial endocarditis, and tetanus.

3. Social Toxicity

The abuse of drugs is commonly associated with increased criminal activity, decreased productivity, and a serious disruption of interpersonal relationships. The most overt and serious toxic effects of common drugs of abuse are summarized in Table 1.

One further statement we would like to make regarding the nonpsychiatric pharmacology of the nonnarcotic compounds we have been discussing is that they represent a whole new order of investigation. The minimal effective dose response is manifested via behavioral change, not in the area of physiological changes that the pharmacologist is accustomed to measuring. Furthermore, the physiologically toxic dose is either far above the psychiatrically toxic dose, or perhaps it will be found only after chronic administration; the identification and characterization of acute physiological effects is also in areas not previously entered into. One example is surely the genetic effects which the classical pharmacologist would not have looked at, but which are apparent at drug doses comparable to the psychiatric effects. The argument developing concerning genetic effects is, we

Table 1. Toxic Effects of Common Drugs.

Drugs	Acute Toxicity	Chronic Toxicity
Narcotic analgesics	Respiratory depression, pulmonary edema, convulsions, phlebitis, tissue inflammation	Physical dependence with both early and protracted abstinence
Sedative-hypnotics (barbiturates, minor tranquilizers)	Ataxia, impaired judgment, emotional lability, coma	Physical dependence with convulsions, delirium, and hyperpyrexia as abstinence signs
LSD-like hallucinogens	Toxic psychoses and persisting psychotic reactions	
Amphetamine-like agents	Psychotic episodes	Psychotic episodes

believe, based on whether significant numbers of individuals of a group show statistical evidence of numbers of chromosome changes. This in no way denies that certain subjects demonstrate profound chromosomal and reproductive changes [Jacobson 1969]. It is necessary to look at other areas such as enzymes at the molecular level, the detailed biochemical and anatomical architecture of the brain itself, and areas yet unknown before we can identify the physiological correlates of psychiatric action. That they exist we have no doubt; we have never believed that central nervous system function is dependent on other than physiological events. It is our job to identify and describe the events so that understanding and therefore control of them is the end result. Since the gene is the controller of where, what, and how much activity is to go on, it certainly should be a fertile area to investigate to help make the correlation between physiological events and psychiatric manifestations.

References

Abood, L. G., and J. H. Biel (1962). *Int. Rev. Neurobiol.* p. 217.

Aghajanian, G. K. et al. (1968). *Science* 164:402.

Airaksinen, M. M., and W. M. McIssac (1968) *Amer. Med. Exp. Fenn.* 46:367.

Eisenman, A. J., J. W. Sloan, W. R. Martin, D. R. Jasinski, and J. W. Brooks (1969). *J. Psychiat. Res.* 7:19.

Griffiths, J. D., J. H. Cavanaugh, and J. A. Oates (1970). In D. Efron, ed., *Psychotomimetic Drugs,* Workshop Series No. 4, NIMH, p. 287.

Hill, H. E., C. A. Haertzen, A. B. Wolbach, and E. J. Miner (1963). *Psychopharmacologia* 4:167.

Himmelsbach, C. K. (1941). *J. Pharmacol. Exp. Ther.* 73:91.

Holmstedt, B. (1965). *Arch. Int. Pharmacodyn.* 156:285.

———, and Jan Erik Lingrea (1967). In D. Efron, B. Holmstedt, and N. S. Kline, eds., *Ethnophamacologic Search for Psychoactive Drugs,* PHS Publication No. 1645, GPO, Washington, D.C., pp. 339–373.

Isbell, H., C. W. Gorodetsky, D. Jasinski, U. Claussen, F. V. Spulak, and F. Korte (1967). *Psychopharmacologia* 11 : 184.

——— (1968). Personal communications.

Jacobson, C. (1969). Unpublished contractor reports to BNDD.

Jones, B. E., W. R. Martin, and D. R. Jasinski (1969). *Psychopharmacologia* 14 : 394.

Mandell, A. (1968). *Science* 162 : 1442.

Marczynski, T. (1959). *Bull. Acad. Pol. Sci.* 7 : 151.

Martin, W. R. (1965). In J. R. DiPalma, ed., *Drill's Pharmacology in Medicine*. New York: McGraw-Hill, vol. 3, pp. 274–285.

——— (in press). In L. Brill and E. Harms, eds., *Yearbook of Drug Abuse,* New York: Behavioral Publishers.

———, and D. R. Jasinski (1969). *J. Psychiat. Res.* 7 : 9.

Osmond, H., and J. R. Smythies (1952). *J. Ment. Sci.* 98 : 309.

Pfeiffer, C. (1959). Unpublished results.

Rothlin, E. (1957). *J. Pharm. Pharmacol.* 9 : 569.

Seitz, G. J. (1967). In D. Efron, B. Holmstedt, and N. S. Kline, eds., *Ethnophamacologic Search for Psychoactive Drugs, PHS Publication No. 1645,* Washington, D.C.: GPO. pp. 315–338.

Shulgin, A. (1969). *Nature* 221 : 537.

Snyder, S. (1967). *Amer. J. Orthopsych.* 37 : 864.

Stein, L., and C. David Wise (1970). In D. Efron, ed., *Psychotomimetic Drugs,* Workshop Series No. 4, NIMH, p. 123.

Szara, S. (1967). *Amer. J. Psychiat.* 123 : 1513.

Wikler, A., and F. T. Pescor (1967). *Psychopharmacologia* 10 : 255.

Wilkinson, S. (1958). *J. Chem. Soc.* (London), p. 2079.

4 Drug Interactions—Principles and Problems in Relation to Drugs of Abuse

G. J. Mannering

The modern trend in medicine is to administer more and more drugs simultaneously. This practice, sometimes referred to as polypharmacy, has its counterpart in the increasing frequency with which more than one drug is used simultaneously or interchangeably to control or otherwise modify their pleasure-producing effects. While the surreptitious use of drugs for purposes other than the treatment of disease is automatically labeled "drug abuse," polypharmacy is frequently a form of drug abuse in itself. Indeed, polypharmacy is often employed by the therapist and by the illicit user of drugs for the same reasons. Periodic shortages of favored drugs on the illicit market has also led to experimentation with new drugs and consequent polypharmacy. The drug abuser may be obtaining drugs from both legitimate and illegitimate sources. He is not likely to inform his physician of his illegal use of drugs, and this factor may complicate the physician's ability to assess the efficacy or toxicity of the prescribed drugs. The drug abuser is not infrequently under psychiatric surveillance. This almost always means he is receiving one or more psychotropic drugs, some of which are notorious for their interactions with other drugs.

Adverse reactions resulting from drug interactions increase in proportion to the number of drugs given and the duration of administration. It is estimated that the average inpatient receives six drugs daily [Smith et al. 1966]. Knowledge of adverse effects of drugs due to drug interactions has been slow to accumulate for a number of reasons, including failure of physicians to recognize that such interactions are possible, a general lack of objective criteria as to what comprises a reaction, a natural reluctance of the physician to recognize that he may have prescribed the wrong treatment, and the lack of controlled studies of drug interactions employing quantitative measurements. Evaluation of the problem is even more difficult when we consider the effects of multiple drug use on the drug abuser. We have no accurate picture of the number or kinds of drugs he uses, the purity of the drugs, the doses employed, or the effects experienced. We can only assume that polypharmacy creates the same kinds of problems for the drug abuser as for the patient.

Before a compound can perform as a drug it must possess various properties. If taken orally it must be capable of passing through the membranes lining the gastrointestinal tract into the blood in which it is transported to tissues where it is desired that it produce its effects. During transport it may be bound to serum proteins, in which combination it is inert, and an equilibrium is established between drug bound to serum protein, free circulating drug, and drug bound to tissues or otherwise taken up by tissues. The drug may then produce its effect on the surface of the cells of the tissue, or more commonly it will enter the cell and react with receptors causing changes in the cell physiology such that a desirable or undesirable pharmacologic effect is elicited. It may also react with cell constituents but not produce pharmacologic changes, at least not in that tissue; or it may react with a metabolic site and be biotransformed to a product of lesser or greater pharmacologic activity, generally the former. In most cases the receptor site associated with drug action is not the metabolic site. Drug action and drug degradation occur concomitantly, usually in different tissues. Most drugs are weak acids or bases and thus exist to some degree in un-ionized form at body pH. This nonpolarity of drugs permits their penetration of the many membranes they must transgress in order to reach their sites of action, but it also retards their excretion. The lipoidal nature of the kidney tubule ensures that drugs contained in the glomerular filtrate will return to the blood stream. It has

been calculated that many drugs would have half lives of months, or even years, if it were required that they be excreted unchanged by the kidney [Brodie, Cosmides, et al. 1965]. Almost all biotransformations of drugs result in compounds that are more polar, and thus more excretable, than their parents. In view of the many biological hurdles a compound must clear before it can serve as a drug, it is small wonder that of the many compounds tested, so few find their way to the pharmacist's shelf.

The picture becomes more complicated exponentially as more and more drugs are used simultaneously, because each may compete with the other at all or any of the many sites of drug reactions encountered as the drugs course through the body from their point of absorption to their point of excretion. Thus, drugs may interact before or during absorption, they may compete for binding sites on serum proteins, for binding sites on or in cells, or for receptor and metabolic sites; and each drug may influence the excretion of the other.

A drug may alter the action of another drug in several ways: by producing one or more effects similar or opposite to those of the drug in question; by direct chemical or physical interaction of drugs; by displacement of drugs bound to plasma or other proteins; by altered renal clearance of drugs; through conditioning by previous drug effects; by interaction of drugs with receptor sites; and by inhibition or stimulation of the metabolic site. A few examples of the various kinds of drug interaction will be given, but because of the great current interest in interactions involving the metabolic site and the view that interactions occurring at this site will prove to be more common than those occurring at other sites, this category of interactions will receive special attention here. Several reviews of various aspects of drug interaction have appeared in the literature [Barber 1965;

Brodie 1965 ; Burns and Conney 1965 ;
Dollery 1965 ; Lasagna 1965 ; Macgregor
1965 ; Milne 1965 ; Shepherd 1965 ; Sjöqvist
1965 ; Zubrod 1965 ; McIver 1965, 1967 ;
Conney 1967 ; Gillette 1967 ; Mannering
1968a, 1968b ; Morrelli and Melmon, 1968].

1. Interaction Through the Elicitation of Similar or Opposite Effects

The additive or antagonistic effect of one drug
on the action of another through the elicita-
tion of a similar or opposite effect is probably
the most widely known of the drug interactions. The combined administration of two
drugs having similar effects to enhance the
desired overall effect is a common practice.
Depressant drugs such as barbiturates and
alcohol are used in combination for desired
combined effects, sometimes with fatal consequences. The heroin user may substitute
barbiturates or alcohol when heroin is not
available. Both physicians and drug abusers
use drugs having opposing pharmacologic
effects to antidote toxic effects due to overdosage. Thus the physician uses a barbiturate
as a depressant to counteract excessive
stimulant effects of amphetamine and the
drug abuser employs the same drug to
"down" the effects of the same stimulant
"head." A classical example of the alternate
use of drugs having opposite effects is that
of the habituated cocaine user who employs
heroin so frequently as an antidote to over-
doses of cocaine that he becomes addicted to
heroin.

2. Direct Chemical or Physical Interaction

Cholestyramine alleviates the pruritus of
biliary cirrhosis by binding bile salts in the
gastrointestinal tract, thus preventing their
reabsorption. It also binds a variety of drugs
and prevents their absorption [Gallo et al.
1965]. Tetracyclines are chelating agents,
and the gastrointestinal absorption of these
antibiotics is retarded when given simultan-

eously with antacids containing multivalent
cations [Dearborn et al. 1957]. Many drugs
are incompatible chemically or physically
and cannot be used together in solutions to
be employed intravenously. Sometimes interactions may be useful, as for example in the
treatment of lead poisoning and selected cases
of hypercalcemia with the chelating agent
ethylenediaminetetraacetate, or in the restora-
tion of coagulation when protamine is used
to bind heparin.

3. Interaction by Displacement of Drugs Bound to Plasma and Other Proteins

The distribution of a drug between blood and
other tissues can be altered by drug interaction.
Many drugs are reversibly bound to plasma
proteins. Certain drugs would seem to be
bound to the same binding sites because they
can displace one another. In the bound state,
drugs are pharmacologically inert. Displacement of the drug from its binding protein
permits it to act; it also makes the drug
available for metabolism and excretion. The
net effect of displacement is that of increasing
the dose of the drug, and this can result in
toxic reactions. Sulfonylureas, which are
bound avidly to protein [Wishinsky et al
1962], are displaced by sulfonamides.
Tolbutamide released in this manner may
cause hypoglycemia. Certain long-acting
sulfonamides are displaced from serum
albumin by phenylbutazone [Anton 1960].
The sulfonamides released in this manner
diffuse into the tissues and phenylbutazone
thus enhances the antibacterial action of the
sulfonamides even though their plasma levels
are decreased. Phenylbutazone can also displace warfarin and cause bleeding [Aggeler
et al. 1967]. Methotrexate, useful in leukemias, and sometimes used for severe psoriasis,
may be displaced by highly acidic, protein-
bound drugs such as salicylates and sulfonamides, causing pancytopenia [Dixon et al.
1965]. Quinacrine is highly bound to protein.

If pamaquine is given simultaneously or shortly after quinacrine during the course of treatment of malaria, binding sites which normally inactivate the pamaquine are not available, and pamaquine toxicity may be seen [Zubrod et al. 1948].

Gillette [1968] cautions against over-emphasis of the role of drug displacement: "Displacement of drugs from binding sites, therefore, will be pharmacologically important only when a drug is eliminated at an abnormally slow rate and only when more than 90 percent of the drug in plasma is bound, or it distributes with the extracellular water, or it is displaced from other tissues in addition to plasma proteins, or when the level of unbound drug is near threshold levels before administration of the displacing substance. In most instances, displacement merely tends to confuse investigators, who attempt to relate pharmacologic effects with plasma levels of the drug." Many acidic drugs (e.g., phenylbutazone, sulfonamides, coumarin anticoagulants) are highly bound to plasma proteins; they appear to possess the other necessary properties outlined by Gillette, causing them to create problems when they are displaced from their binding sites by other drugs.

Certain drugs may act through their ability to combine with certain proteins rather than intrinsic activity. Corticosteroids are transported in plasma by a special globulin, transcortin. Brodie [1965] has produced evidence suggesting that antirheumatic drugs may cause their effects by combining with transcortin, thereby releasing cortisol.

4. Interactions through Altered Renal Clearance

Changes in urinary pH, such as may be caused by disease or therapy with ammonium chloride, sodium bicarbonate, thiazides, or acetazolamide, may influence the excretion of drugs that are weak acids and bases, which includes most drugs. Ionized drugs are poorly reabsorbed from the glomerular filtrate by the tubules, whereas the nonpolar forms of drugs are rapidly reabsorbed. Thus drugs that are weak acids are reabsorbed poorly from alkaline glomerular filtrates and rapidly when the filtrates are acid; the reverse is true for drugs that are bases. Probenizid delays the excretion of penicillin by direct action on the tubule.

5. Interactions as a Result of Conditioning by Previous Drug Effects

The example best known to drug abusers of a drug interaction by conditioning as a result of previous drug effects is the tolerance that develops to opiate narcotics through chronic use. Similar, although less marked, tolerance is also seen with barbiturates and alcohol. Cross tolerance is seen between individual members of the natural and synthetic opiates, between different barbiturates, and between barbiturates and alcohol. The reasons for the development of tolerance to the opium alkaloids and to alcohol remain unkown, but barbiturates produce tolerance, at least in part, by stimulating their own rates of metabolism.

Thiazide diuretics cause potassium loss and thereby may predispose patients to digitalis toxicity. Reserpine depletes myocardial stores of potassium and this may cause undue bradycardia when digitalis is given [Roberts et al. 1963]. Catecholamine-depleting agents, like guanethidine and reserpine, may render patients refractory to pressor agents that depend upon catecholamine release for their activity [Morrelli and Melmon 1968]. Reserpine may prevent uptake of administered catecholes by storage sites and thus render patients hypersensitive to infused norepinephrine [Dollery 1965].

Barbiturates and digitalis become less effective during hormonal replacement in patients with hypothyroidism [Lowenthal and Fisher

1957]. At the same time there is a more rapid turnover of blood-clotting factors and a decrease in the dose requirements of anticoagulant drugs [Doherty and Perkins 1966]. Antibiotics may diminish the vitamin K-synthesizing capacity of the intestinal flora and thereby reduce the prothrombinopenic dose of anticoagulant. Spironolactone antagonizes the effects of potassium salts and may result in hyperkalemia if potassium salts are given [Morrelli and Melmon 1968].

6. Interaction at Receptor Sites

Drug effects are determined largely by the binding of drugs to cellular receptors. These receptors may be employed by the cell to combine with natural substrates. A drug may react with a receptor and simulate the action of the natural substrate, or it may form an inert combination with the receptor and thus interfere with the interaction of the receptor with its natural substrate. The best understood model of this kind of receptor-drug relationship is that of the receptor for acetylcholine. Many acetylcholine derivatives are known to combine with this receptor to produce many of the effects of acetylcholine, while other compounds like atropine have a high affinity for the acetylcholine receptor but possess no pharmacologic action of their own. Knowledge of the mechanism of action of such drugs at the receptor level is the basis for the intelligent use of drugs and the understanding of adverse effects. The understanding of interactions at specific receptor sites also enables the proper design of antidotal drugs.

Nalorphine (Nalline), the N-allyl derivative of morphine, which appears to react with the same receptors for morphine and related narcotic analgesics, is a dramatic antidote for overdosage of the opiates. The administration of a small dose of nalorphine causes minor withdrawal symptoms (e.g., pupil dilation) in subjects who are using opiate narcotics; this phenomenon has proved valuable in the monitoring of convicted drug abusers who have been paroled.

7. Interaction at the Metabolic Site

The termination of drug action is as important as the action itself, for only in special cases is it desired that the action be permanent. Drug action is most frequently terminated as a result of drug biotransformation. Thus anything that accelerates or decelerates the rate of drug biotransformation will decrease or prolong drug action. Because drug metabolism may be going on rapidly while the remainder of one dose or the whole of a subsequent dose are being absorbed and distributed, its rate may determine the concentration of the drug reached at the site of action. Thus, the intensity as well as the duration of drug action may be affected by the rate of drug biotransformation. During the last fifteen years, three major concepts have emerged which greatly increase our understanding of the role that drug metabolism plays in the therapeutic application of drugs: (1) a common enzyme system responsible for the biotransformation of many drugs exists in the endoplasmic reticulum (microsomal fraction) of the liver; (2) many drugs stimulate this common enzyme system to metabolize drugs more rapidly; and (3) many drugs inhibit this common drug-metabolizing system. The role that the interaction of drugs may play in the acceleration or deceleration of the rates of drug metabolism takes on greater significance as the practice of polypharmacy grows and as increasing numbers of drugs are given for long periods of time, frequently for the remaining life span of the patient.

7.1. The Metabolic Site

The first description of the metabolism of a foreign compound by hepatic microsomes was given by Mueller and Miller [1949, 1953]. They showed that the microsomal fraction of a liver homogenate catalyzed the reductive splitting of the azo linkage and the oxidative N-demethylation of aminoazo dyes. The reactions required TPN, DPN, and molecular oxygen. Shortly afterward, Brodie and associates [1955] showed that the enzymes responsible for the metabolism of many drugs were localized in hepatic microsomes. Recombination of the various cellular fractions was needed for activity. The observations that the reaction was stimulated by glucose-6-phosphate (G-6-P) and that the soluble fraction was a good source of G-6-P dehydrogenase led to the finding that TPN is required in its reduced form. Further studies revealed that the soluble fraction can be replaced by a TPNH-generating system consisting of TPN and G-6-P dehydrogenase, or by TPNH itself. Magnesium ion is required for full activity. The requirements of both a reducing agent and molecular oxygen locate these enzymes in Mason's [1957, 1965] classification of oxygenases as external mixed-function oxidases; that is, the enzymes catalyze the consumption of one molecule of oxygen per molecule of substrate with one atom of oxygen appearing in the product and the other undergoing two-equivalent reduction. Direct support of this view was given by Posner and coworkers [1961] who employed $^{18}O_2$ and $H_2^{18}O$ to show that the oxygen utilized in the hydroxylation of acetanilide is derived from molecular oxygen rather than from water.

A wide variety of oxidative reactions are known to occur in microsomes: deamination, O-, N-, and S-dealkylation, hydroxylation of alkyl and aryl hydrocarbons, epoxidation, formation of alkylol derivatives, N-hydroxylation, N- and S-oxidation, and dehalogenation. Azo- and nitro-reductase activities are also found in hepatic microsomes. The great versatility of the microsomal drug-metabolizing system seems less remarkable when the reactions are visualized simply as different kinds of hydroxylation reactions [Brodie,

Gillette et al. 1958; Gillette 1963, 1966), frequently followed by rearrangement.

In the mechanism proposed by Brodie and coworkers [Brodie, Gillette et al. 1958; Gillette 1966] TPNH reduces a component in the microsomes which reacts with molecular oxygen to form an "active oxygen" intermediate. The active oxygen is then transferred to the drug.

1. $TPNH + A + H^+ \longrightarrow AH_2 + TPN^+$
2. $AH_2 + O_2 \longrightarrow$ active oxygen
3. Active oxygen + drug $\longrightarrow$
   oxidized drug + $A + H_2O$

$TPNH + O_2 + drug =$
   $TPNH^+ + H_2O + $ oxidized drug

Key enzymes in the overall reaction are NADPH-cytochrome c reductase, the flavin enzyme involved in the oxidation of TPNH, cytochrome P-450, and cytochrome P-450 reductase, which functions in the reduction of oxidized cytochrome P-450. Figure 1 shows typical examples of oxidative reactions performed by the TPNH-dependent hepatic microsomal system: oxidations of an analgesic agent, a carcinogen, and a steroid hormone. The sequence of biochemical events involving TPNH and cytochrome P-450 as visualized by Omura and coworkers [1965] is shown in Figure 2.

7.2. Stimulation of the Metabolic Site
3-Methylcholanthrene is one of the many polycyclic hydrocarbons used to produce experimental skin tumors. The aminoazo dyes resembling butter yellow (p-dimethylaminoazobenzene) are potent inducers of liver cancer. For reasons not stated, Richardson and Cunningham [1951] administered 3-methyl-4-dimethylaminoazobenzene and 3-methylcholanthrene together and found a great reduction in the incidence and severity of primary liver-cell carcinoma caused by the dye. The solution to the problem posed by this apparently serendipitous finding was soon

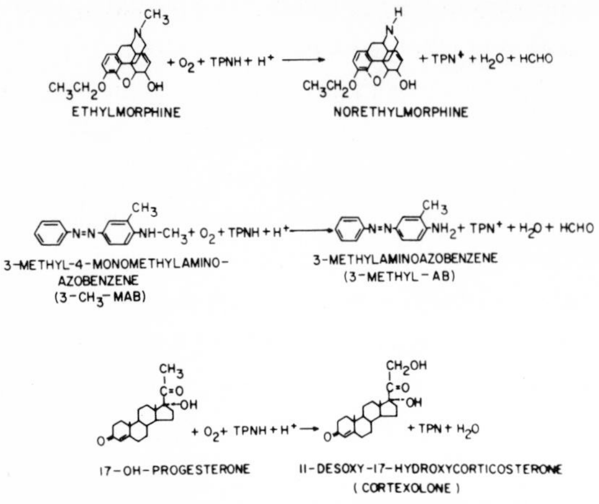

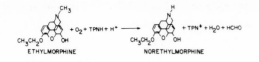

Figure 1. Examples of oxidative reactions performed by the TPNH-dependent hepatic microsomal system; oxidation of an analgesic agent, a carcinogen, and a steroid hormone.

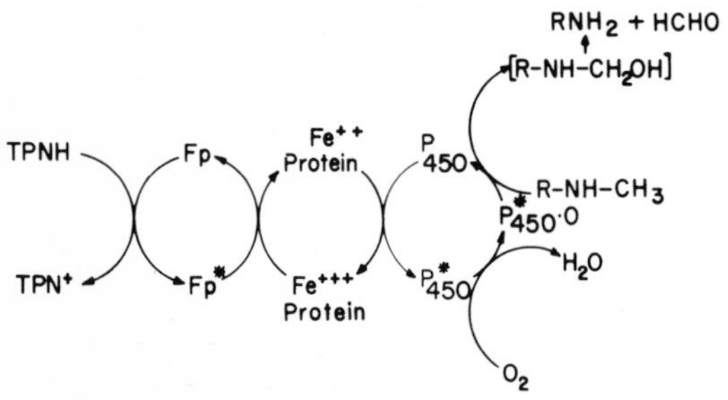

Figure 2. Proposed electron transfer system employed in the metabolism of drugs.

forthcoming from the laboratory of James and Elizabeth Miller, who showed that polycyclic hydrocarbons increase the activity of the hepatic endoplasmic reticulum to biotransform aminoazo dyes to noncarcinogenic metabolites. Polycyclic aromatic hydrocarbons, such as 3-methylcholanthrene, 3,4-benzpyrene, and 1,2,5,6-dibenzanthracene, induce greatly increased activities of the hepatic microsomal enzymes that N-demethylate and reduce the azo linkage of aminoazo dyes [Conney et al. 1956] and hydroxylate 3,4-benzpyrene, 2-acetylaminofluorene, and several drugs [Conney et al. 1957, 1959; Cramer et al. 1960].

The stimulatory effect of barbiturates and other drugs on drug metabolism was discovered by Remmer [Remmer 1958, 1959a, 1959b; Remmer and Alsleben 1958] while searching for mechanisms responsible for barbiturate tolerance and also by Conney, Burns, and associates [Conney and Burns 1959; Conney, Davison, et al. 1960; Conney, Bray, et al. 1961a, Conney, Michaelson, et al. 1961b] during investigations on the effects of barbiturates and several unrelated drugs on ascorbic acid biosynthesis and drug metabolism.

More than two hundred drugs and other compounds are known to stimulate drug metabolism [Mannering 1968a]. Induction relates to no particular pharmacologic classification of drugs; hypnotics, sedatives, central nervous system stimulators, anticonvulsants, tranquilizers, hypoglycemic agents, antiinflammatory agents, muscle relaxants, analgesics, antihistaminics, anesthetic agents, and steroid hormones all have been shown to induce drug metabolism. Halogenated insecticides are particularly potent inducing agents.

Induction has been demonstrated in all mammalian species studied. In general, agents that induce the increased metabolism of a drug in one species will also do so in another.

There is also good correlation between inductive effects measured in vivo and in vitro. However, it would be unwise to place complete confidence in these generalizations because notable exceptions do exist. The degree to which an inducing agent will act, or in some cases, whether it will act at all, may depend upon such factors as sex, strain, and age of the species under investigation, and even on the interval of time between the administration of the agent and the measurement of the response. Many good inducing agents actually inhibit drug metabolism during the first six hours after administration [Brazda and Baucum 1961; Serrone and Fujimoto 1961, 1962; Kato, Chiesara, et al. 1962b; Remmer 1962a, 1962b; Rümke 1963].

Evidence based on the use of known inhibitors of protein synthesis suggests that the inductive process involves the synthesis of increased amounts of drug-metabolizing enzymes. The inductive effects of phenobarbital and 3-methylcholanthrene are prevented by ethionine [Conney, Miller, et al. 1956, 1957; Conney, Davison, et al. 1960; Fujimoto and Plaa 1961; Kato 1961,] puromycin [Conney and Gilman 1963; Gelboin and Blackburn 1964; Orrenius and Ernster 1964] and actinomycin D [Gelboin and Blackburn, 1964; Orrenius and Ernster 1964; Conney 1965; Orrenius et al. 1965], substances known to block protein synthesis by different mechanisms. Inducing agents stimulate drug metabolism by increasing levels of cytochrome P-450 [Orrenius and Ernster 1964; Ernster and Orrenius 1965; Remmer and Merker 1965; Kato 1966; Schmid et al. 1966; Sladek and Mannering 1966, 1969a, 1969b] and TPNH-cytochrome c reductase [Orrenius and Ernster 1964; Ernster and Orrenius 1965; Kato 1966; Sladek and Mannering 1969a, 1969b] in the hepatic endoplasmic reticulum. In many cases, the increase in cytochrome P-450 after phenobarbital administration, and the subsequent decline to the normal level after the effect of the barbiturate had run its course, paralleled the gradual increase and subsequent decline in the rate of drug metabolism that occurred.

Induction most frequently reduces the effectiveness or toxicity of a drug, but in a few cases the drug is made more active as a result of biotransformation, and induction increases its effectiveness. Acetanilide, acetophenetidin, chloral hydrate, chlorguanide, and prontosil are transformed in man from inactive or relatively inactive drugs to metabolites of therapeutic value [Williams 1963]. Mephobarbital, primidone, aspirin, and phenylbutazone are active drugs per se, but they are converted to metabolites that are also active [Williams 1963]. Octamethyl pyrophosphoramide (Schradan), and Guthion are relatively nontoxic as such, but they are metabolized to potent cholinesterase inhibitors. Inducing agents increase the toxicity of these insecticides [Kato 1961]. Tremorine produces tremors only because it is metabolized to oxotremorine [Cho et al. 1961; Welch and Kocsis 1961; George et al. 1962]. These studies are of special interest because they illustrate how induction experiments can reveal the active species in certain cases.

The list of drugs known to induce drug metabolism in man is short but growing. Evidence for induction has not always been obtained by measurement of the rate of drug metabolism, but frequently by following the effectiveness of a given dose of the drug with and without the inducing agent, as for example, the effect of an anticoagulant on the coagulability of blood with or without the administration of an inducing agent such as phenobarbital. However, in most cases these indirect evaluations of inducing agents in man support what has already been learned about the same inducing agents in lower animals using more rigorous criteria. The inductive effects of drugs on the rate of metabolism of the coumarin anticoagulants have received a great deal of study, probably because the response to the coumarins can be readily assessed and because of the vital necessity of maintaining blood levels of these drugs within relatively narrow limits. The following drugs have been shown to induce increased rates of metabolism of coumarins in man: barbiturates, including phenobarbital, secobarbital, amobarbital, butabarbital, and heptabarbital [Corn and Rockett 1965; Cucinell, Conney, et al. 1965; Goss and Dickhous 1965; Robinson and MacDonald 1966; Antlitz et al. 1968; Hunninghake and Azarnoff 1968; MacDonald and Robinson 1968]; chloral hydrate [Cucinell, Odessky, et al. 1966]; griseofulvin [Catalano and Cullen 1966]; glutethimide [Hunninghake and Azarnoff 1968]; and meprobamate [Hunninghake and Azarnoff 1968]. In clinical studies, phenobarbital has been shown to stimulate the metabolism of diphenylhydantoin [Cucinell, Conney, et al. 1965], griseofulvin [Busfield et al. 1963], digitoxin [Jelliffe and Blankenhorn 1966] and the glucuronidation of salicylamide [Crigler and Gold 1966]. Phenylbutazone increases the metabolism of aminopyrine in man [Chen et al. 1962] and meprobamate [Douglas et al. 1963] and glutethimide [Remmer 1962a] enhance their own rates of metabolism in man.

Chlorinated insecticides are known to be potent inducers of drug metabolism [Conney, Welch, et al. 1967]. Studies by Hart and Fouts [Hart and Fouts 1963, 1965; Hart, Shultice, et al. 1969] showed that treatment of rodents with a variety of halogenated hydrocarbons increased the rate of metabolism of drugs such as hexobarbital, aminopyrine, and chlorpromazine. The compounds studied were chlordane, DDT, DDD, perthane, kelthane, and methoxychlor. Long-lasting effects were obtained with a diet containing only 5 ppm of DDT, a level which can be found in human foods. Recently Kolmodin et al.

[1969] showed that 26 men who were occupationally exposed to insecticides, mainly Lindane and DDT, had significantly shorter plasma half-lives of antipyrine than 36 control subjects. These studies point out the need for further investigation of the possible contribution that pesticides and other environmental contaminants may make to the great variability of drug effects seen in individual subjects.

The smaller number of compounds known to induce drug metabolism in man does not mean that man is less subject to induction than other species, but simply that relatively few compounds have as yet been tested clinically. All the drugs shown to be inducing agents in man have also been shown to induce drug metabolism in lower animals. Until shown not to be the case, it would be well to assume that any drug that produces an inductive effect in lower animals will also do so in man. If this is a correct assumption, a great number of drugs in common use act as inducing agents in man.

The loss of a previously established inductive effect can result in overdosage. The effectiveness of anticoagulants depends largely on the rate at which they are metabolized, and this action may vary as much as fourteenfold among individuals [Brodie, Cosmides, et al. 1965]. It is thus necessary to establish the dose of an anticoagulant on an individual basis. Frequently, while the dose is being adjusted to fit the patient, phenobarbital is also administered. The rate of detoxication of the anticoagulant increases during phenobarbital treatment, and the dose is adjusted not only to the initial rate of drug metabolism of the individual but to inductive changes as well. This presents no problem as long as both drugs are given, but after a time phenobarbital is usually withdrawn and the use of the anticoagulant is continued. The induction acquired as a result of the chronic administration of phenobarbital is lost after a few days, and the patient is now overdosed with the anticoagulant, possibly with fatal consequences.

7.3. Tests for Induction of Drug Metabolism

The inductive properties of an agent can be demonstrated in various ways: by determining the effect of the agent on the duration of action of a drug; the effect of the agent on the rate of metabolism of a drug in vivo; the effect of the agent on the urinary excretion of certain normal metabolites (e.g., L-ascorbic acid, D-glucaric acid, 6β-hydroxycortisol); the effect of the administered agent on the drug-metabolizing enzymes of the liver measured in vitro; the effect on the binding of drugs to microsomal hemoprotein; the effect of the agent on the amount and kind of cytochrome P-450 in the hepatic microsomes; and by electron microscopic examination of the hepatic endoplasmic reticulum of animals treated with the agent. Not all of these tests are required to establish the inductive status of an agent, but it would be wise not to rely on a single test. Both in vivo and in vitro tests should be employed, for it does not necessarily follow that an agent that shows an inductive effect in vitro will show a similar effect in vivo, even though this is usually the case. It should also be remembered than an agent may induce the increased metabolism of one drug, but not that of another.

Numerous in vitro and in vivo studies have provided many variations of procedures with respect to the age, species, and strain of the animals employed, dosages of the inducing agent and the drug being studied, time interval between the injection of the agent and the performance of the test, incubation mixtures, duration of incubation, and other factors. Each laboratory has its favorite test or battery of tests; a list of tests that have been used or which conceivably might be used is given in Table 1.

7.3.1. Tests that Depend on the Effect of an Inducing Agent on the Duration of Action of a Drug

Hexobarbital sleeping time and zoxazolamine paralysis time are the tests most frequently employed. The action of hexobarbital is terminated through its biotransformation to ketohexobarbital, and zoxazolamine is hydroxylated to 6-hydroxy-zoxazolamine, a product that has little or no muscle relaxant activity. After the administration of a given inducing agent for several days, rats are injected intraperitoneally with test doses of hexobarbital or zoxazolamine. The time required for an animal to elicit its righting reflex spontaneously is recorded as the sleeping time or the paralysis time.

The hexobarbital sleeping time test can be performed with a minimum of equipment, time, and talent. However, it has the disadvantage of not being applicable to the detection of all inducing agents; 3-methylcholanthrene, 3,4-benzpyrene, and probably other polycyclic hydrocarbons do not stimulate the rate of hexobarbital metabolism [Conney, Davison, et al. 1960; Arcos et al. 1961]. The test is also not applicable when the agent itself alters sleeping time.

The zoxazolamine paralysis test differs from the hexobarbital sleeping time test in that 3-methylcholanthrene and 3,4-benzpyrene, as well as many drugs, stimulate the rate of zoxazolamine metabolism. Because it is possible that certain agents may induce an increased rate of hexobarbital metabolism, but not that of zoxazolamine metabolism, it is recommended that both the hexobarbital test and the zoxazolamine test be employed when a new agent is under investigation.

7.3.2. Tests that Depend on the Effect of an Inducing Agent on the Rate of Metabolism of a Drug In Vivo

Metabolism of hexobarbital. The overall conditions for the demonstration of induction using the determination of hexobarbital in

Table 1. Tests for Measuring Induction of Drug Metabolism.

Test	Measurement	Species	References
1. Duration of hexorbital action	Righting reflex	Rat	Conney, Davison, et al. 1960; Anders and Mannering, 1966
2. Duration of zoxazolamine action	Righting reflex	Rat	Conney, Davison, et al. 1960
3. Metabolism of hexobarbital in vivo	Disappearance of hexobarbital from blood	Rat, dog	Conney and Burns 1963; Anders 1966; Anders and Mannering 1966b; Remmer and Siegart 1964
4. Metabolism of antipyrine in vivo	Disappearance of antipyrine from blood	Rat, dog, man	Brodie and Axelrod 1950; Cucinell, Conney, et al. 1965
5. Metabolism of aminopyrine in vivo	a. Disappearance of aminopyrine from blood	Man	Chen et al. 1962
	b. Urinary excretion of 4-aminoantipyrine	Rat, dog, man	Remmer, 1962b; Remmer, 1964; Remmer and Siegart 1964; Siegart et al. 1964
6. Metabolism of phenylbutazone in vivo	Disappearance of phentylbutazone from blood	Dog	Burns et al. 1963; Cucinell, Koster, 1963
7. Urinary excretion of ascorbic acid	Ascorbic acid in urine	Rat	Conney and Burns, 1959; Burns, Conney, et al. 1960; Conney, Bray, et al. 1961a
8. Urinary excretion of D-glucaric acid	D-glucaric acid in urine	Rat, guinea pig, man	Marsh and Reid 1963; Aarts, 1965
9. Urinary excretion of 6β-hydroxycortisol	6β-hydroxycortisol in urine	Man	Bledsoe et al. 1964; Werk et al. 1964; Burstein and Klaiber 1965; Conney 1967; Kuntzman et al. 1966
10. Metabolism of drugs in vitro			
a. N-demethylation of ethylmorphine	Formaledhyde formation by hepatic microsomes	Rat	Takemori and Mannering 1958; Mannering 1968a; Sladek and Mannering 1966
b. N-demethylation of 3-methyl-4-aminoazobenzene	Formaldehyde formation by hepatic microsomes	Rat	Takemori and Mannering 1958; Mannering, 1968a; Sladek and Mannering 1966
11. Binding of drugs to microsomal hemoprotein			
a. Aniline binding	Difference spectra	Rat	Imai and Sato 1966a; Remmer, Schenkman, et al. 1966
b. Hexobarbital binding	Difference spectra	Rat	Imai and Sato 1966a; Remmer, Schenkman, et al. 1966
12. Measurement of microsomal P-450 levels			
a. Carbon monoxide as a ligand	Difference spectra	Rat	Omura and Sato 1962; Sladek and Mannering 1966
b. Ethyl isocyanide as a ligand	Difference spectra	Rat	Imai and Sato 1966b; Sladek and Mannering 1966

vivo are the same as those employed in the hexobarbital sleeping time test. At one or more time intervals after the administration of hexobarbital, the rats are anesthetized with ether, 1.5 ml of blood is taken from each rat by aortic puncture, and hexobarbital analyses are performed.

Gas chromatography. This method was employed recently by Anders [1966] for the determination of hexobarbital and other barbiturates in blood. The procedure has several advantages. Because only a very small sample (0.1 ml) of tail blood is used, duplicate samples can be taken sequentially from the same animal, thus reducing the number of animals required in the test. The extraction procedure is very simple, and the problem of the considerable blank reading that exists with other tests is eliminated.

Metabolism of antipyrine. The determination of the rate of antipyrine metabolism in vivo has been used in rats, dogs, and man as a test for induction. Antipyrine has the advantages of distributing evenly throughout body water and of being only slightly bound to plasma proteins. Protein binding and distribution to fat complicate the use of many drugs, including many barbiturates. In addition, antipyrine produces minimal pharmacologic effects and is therefore more acceptable for use in man than many other drugs that could be used to study induction.

Metabolism of aminopyrine. Chen and co-workers [1962] studied the inductive effect of phenylbutazone on aminopyrine metabolism in man. Subjects were given an intravenous dose of 800 mg of aminopyrine; six hours later, plasma levels of aminopyrine were measured. The same subjects were treated daily with phenylbutazone for periods ranging from four to 21 days, and the aminopyrine test was repeated.

The urinary excretion of 4-aminoantipyrine. This substance, the major metabolite of aminopyrine and dipyrone, has been used by

Remmer and associates to evaluate inductive effects in rats, dogs, and man [Remmer 1962b; Conney and Burns 1963; Remmer and Siegert 1964; Siegert et al. 1964].

Metabolism of phenylbutazone in vivo. The phenylbutazone test is very useful in measuring induction in the dog. The small dose of phenylbutazone used in the test has the advantage of producing no noticeable pharmacologic effects.

7.3.3. Tests That Depend on the Effect of an Inducing Agent on the Urinary Excretion of a Normal Metabolite

Excretion of ascorbic acid. Drugs that induce microsomal enzymes also increase the urinary excretion of ascorbic acid in those species capable of synthesizing the vitamin [Conney and Burns 1959; Burns, Conney, et al. 1960; Conney, Bray, et al. 1961a]. The biochemical features common to these two seemingly unrelated inductive phenomena are not known. Increased ascorbic acid synthesis results from the stimulation of the metabolism of glucose and galactose via the glucuronic acid pathway. Ascorbic acid synthesis is stimulated not only by many drugs commonly employed therapeutically, but by the polycyclic hydrocarbons as well. The effect is marked; rats that normally excreted less than 1 mg of ascorbic acid per day excreted 20 mg per day after 3-methylcholanthrene (100 mg i.p. for 5 days) was injected, and 23 mg per day after barbital (100 mg orally for 5 days) was fed (Burns et al 1960).

Excretion of D-glucaric acid. The inability to synthesize ascorbic acid excludes the possibility of using ascorbic acid excretion as a measure of the induction of an enhanced glucuronic acid pathway in guinea pigs and in man and other primates. However, the excretion of D-glucaric acid, which, like ascorbic acid, is also formed through the glucuronic acid pathway, was found to be elevated in rats [Marsh and Reid 1963] and guinea pigs [Aarts 1965] after the administration of phenobarbital or aminopyrine. Aarts [1965] observed the daily excretion of D-glucaric acid to increase about fourfold in a subject who had been given 300 mg of phenobarbital daily for seven days. He suggested that the determination of the urinary excretion of D-glucaric acid may be useful as an indicator of induction in man.

Excretion of 6β-hydroxycortisol. Drugs that stimulate drug metabolism also stimulate the rate of hydroxylation of steroids by the hepatic endoplasmic reticulum [Conney and Klutch 1963; Bledsoe et al. 1964; Werk et al. 1964; Burstein and Klaiber 1965; Conney, Jacobson, et al. 1965a; Conney, Schneidman, et al. 1965b; Kuntzman et al. 1966]. Phenobarbital, diphenylhydantoin, and phenylbutazone increase the urinary excretion of 6β-hydroxycortisol in man without causing a corresponding increase in the total 17-hydroxycorticoids in urine [Bledsoe et al. 1964; Werk et al. 1964; Burstein and Klaiber, 1965; Kuntzman et al. 1966; Conney 1967]. Conney [1967] has suggested that the ratio of 6β-hydroxycortisol to total 17-hydroxycorticoids in urine may be a useful index of liver microsomal hydroxylase activity in man.

7.3.4. Tests that Depend on the Effect of an Inducing Agent on the Rate of Metabolism of a Drug In Vitro

A large number of compounds might be used as substrates in in vitro studies designed to reveal induction. However, for a variety of reasons, certain of these compounds are preferred over others. In our laboratory the N-demethylations of ethylmorphine and 3-methyl-4-methylaminoazobenzene (3-methyl-MAB) are the reactions employed most frequently in induction studies. Product formation (HCHO) is measured in both reactions. The measurement of formaldehyde has the advantages of accuracy, sensitivity, specificity, and simplicity. Ethylmorphine was chosen largely because only a single

reaction is measured, N-demethylation. O-deethylation also occurs, but the acetaldehyde thus formed does not interfere with the determination of formaldehyde, and the enzyme system responsible for O-demethylation does not appear to be the same as that which catalyzes N-demethylation [Axelrod 1956; Elison and Elliott 1964]. Ethylmorphine is preferred to morphine because it is demethylated much more rapidly [Takemori and Mannering 1958]. 3-Methyl-MAB was selected to represent those substrates that are induced both by phenobarbital and many other drugs and by the polycyclic hydrocarbons. It has the advantage over certain other aminoazo dyes of having a single N-methyl group, of not being hydroxylated measurably, and of being resistant to the microsomal azoreductase that cleaves the azo linkage [Mueller and Miller 1953]. The disadvantages of 3-methyl-MAB are its water insolubility and its commercial unavailability.

7.3.5. Tests That Depend on the Effect of an Inducing Agent on the Amount and Kind of Cytochrome P-450 Contained in Hepatic Microsomes

Good correlation is found between the levels of microsomal cytochrome P-450 and the activity of certain drug-metabolizing enzymes. On the strength of this correlation, it is possible to determine the inductive properties of an agent simply by determining the amount of cytochrome P-450 in the microsomes.

There are exceptions to the rule that a rise in the level of cytochrome P-450 will reflect a rise in the activity of the microsomal drug-metabolizing enzymes. For example, 3-methylcholanthrene increases microsomal P-450 levels and 3-methyl-MAB N-demethylase activity, but not ethylmorphine N-demethylase activity [Sladek and Mannering 1966, 1969a, 1969b]. This was explained as being due to a qualitative change in the cytochrome P-450 that results when 3-

methylcholanthrene is administered [Sladek and Mannering 1966, 1969a, 1969b]. This change is recognizable spectrally when ethyl isocyanide rather than carbon monoxide is employed as a ligand for reduced cytochrome P-450; instead of a single peak at 450 mμ, peaks at 430 mμ and 455 mμ are observed. The heights of the 430 mμ and 455 mμ peaks depend upon the pH of the solution, with very little of the 455 mμ peak existing at pH 6, and very little of the 430 mμ peak being seen at pH 8. Microsomes from untreated and phenobarbital-treated rats exhibit 430 mμ and 455 mμ peaks of equal heights at pH 7.6, whereas microsomes from 3-methylchol-anthrene treated rats show equal heights of the two peaks when the pH is 6.9.

7.3.6. Electron Microscopic Studies

Many drugs that induce increased drug metabolism also cause a morphological change in the hepatic parenchymal cell. This is observed under the electron microscope as a marked proliferation of the smooth-surfaced endoplasmic reticulum [Remmer and Merker 1963, 1965; Fouts and Rogers 1965; Ortega 1966]. The polycyclic hydro-carbons produce a much smaller effect [Fouts and Rogers 1965]. Although the technique requires expensive equipment and special training, in laboratories where the electron microscope is used routinely it may be useful in the detection of inductive effects produced by drugs.

7.4. Inhibition at the Metabolic Site

The relative lack of substrate specificity of the microsomal drug-metabolizing system is considered to be due to the function of a single oxidase system involving cytochrome P-450, or to that of a limited number of oxidase systems involving one or more cyto-chromes [Mannering 1968a]. If structurally unrelated drugs are metabolized by a single enzyme system, or if a single rate-limiting compoment is common to the system or systems involved in the metabolism of these drugs, then each drug should inhibit competitively the metabolism of the other. In studies conducted in our laboratory, this proved to be the case [Rubin et al. 1964a]. Hexobarbital, chlorpromazine, zoxazolamine, phenylbutazone, and acetanilide all were competitive inhibitors of the N-demethylation of ethylmorphine; and ethylmorphine, hexobarbital, and chlorpromazine were mutually inhibitory, also competitively. The inhibitor and Michaelis constants of these reactions supported the view that drugs in combination can act as alternative substrates for the microsomal drug-metabolizing en-zymes. Butler and coworkers [1965] con-cluded from similar studies that trimethadione and metharbital each inhibit the N-demethyla-tion of the other by competing for the same microsomal enzyme or enzymes. Amino-pyrine competitively inhibits the O-demethyla-tion of p-nitroanisole [Booth and Gillette 1966]. Inhibition is not always competitive; for example, inhibition of the microsomal parahydroxylation of diphenylhydantoin by isoniazid and p-aminosalicylic acid was non-competitive [Kutt, Verebely, et al. 1968]. Kato, Chiesara, and associates [1962a, 1964] found that the microsomal metabolism of pentobarbital, hexobarbital, meprobamate, carisoprodol, and strychnine was inhibited by 36 drugs.

These studies suggest that the inhibition of drug metabolism by the interaction of drugs as substrates at the metabolic site may play a general role in drug therapy and in drug abuse. The so-called potentiating effects of certain drugs may well be due to their ability to compete as substrates with other drugs. Until recently, little attention has been paid in either man or lower animals to the possible role that interactions of drugs at the metabolic site may have in prolonging drug action, but the few studies that have been performed suggest that this type of drug interaction may be quite common. Studies in man were largely prompted by clinicians who noted dramatic reactions to certain drugs when they were given in combination, and who refused to dismiss such incidents as allergic or idiosyncratic responses.

The metabolism of pentobarbital and meprobamate were inhibited by chlorcyclizine, glutethimide, phenaglycodol, imipramine, and phenylisopropylhydrazine during the first 30 minutes following their administration to rats [Kato, Chiesara, et al. 1964]. Ethylmorphine and codeine inhibit the metabolism of hexobarbital by rats in vivo [Rubin et al. 1964b]. Imipramine and desmethylimipramine inhibit the oxidation of tremorine to oxotremorine in the rat [Sjöqvist and Gillette 1965; Hammer and Sjöqvist 1966; Sjöqvist, Hammer, et al. 1968]. Desmethylimipramine inhibits oxotremorine metabolism in the rat, but not in the mouse [Sjöqvist, Hammer, et al. 1968].

The coumarin group of anticoagulants have been implicated in a number of interactions involving inhibition of drug biotransformation. Elevated plasma levels and toxic symptoms were noted in patients who had received either diphenylhydantoin [Hansen et al. 1966] or tolbutamide [Kristensen and Hansen 1967] in addition to bishydroxycourmarin. Bishydroxycoumarin was also shown to double the half life of chlorpropamide in man [Kristensen and Hansen 1968]. On the other hand, phenyramidol inhibits the metabolism of bishydroxycoumarin and thereby increases the effectiveness and toxicity of the anticoagulant [Carter 1965; Solomon and Schrogie 1966]. Other interactions in man known to be mediated by inhibition include the inhibition of the metabolism of diphenylhydantoin by disulfiram [Kiørboe 1966; Olesen 1966, 1967] and isoniazid [Murray 1962; Kutt, Winters, et al. 1966] and that of tolbutamide by sulphaphenazole and phenylbutazone [Christensen et al. 1963].

The hydrazine monoamine oxidase (MAO)

inhibitors have been more widely implicated in inhibitory drug interactions than any other group of drugs. They are thought to produce their mood-elevating effects and other stimulatory actions, at least in part, by elevating levels of naturally occurring amines such as norephedrine and serotonin in the central nervous system. The mechanisms involved are complex and not entirely understood. For example, the MAO inhibitors have a greater effect in prolonging the actions of indirectly acting amines such as amphetamine or tyramine than upon the directly acting catecholamines such as epinephrine and norepinephrine, which owe their destruction more to catechol-O-methyl transferase than to MAO. Interactions from hydrazides resulting in fatalities have led to warnings that great caution should be exercised when MAO inhibitors are used with other drugs and with certain foods. It is not unusual for an abuser of drugs to have had psychiatric problems anteceding his problem with drugs, in which case he may be receiving a MAO inhibitor as part of his treatment. This could prove fatal if he were to self-administer one of the commonly used sympathomimetic drugs such as amphetamine or one of its congeners. Sjöqvist [1965] has listed numerous clinical examples of interactions between MAO inhibitors and other drugs. Amphetamine [Zeck 1961], metamphetamine [Dally 1962; A. Mason 1962; Stark 1962; McDonald 1963] and ephedrine [Low-Beer and Tidmarsh 1963] have caused fatal interactions with MAO inhibitors. Lloyd and Walker [1965] describe a patient who had been treated with MAO inhibitors (phenelzine and trifluoperizine) for about five weeks and then given two 10-milligram tablets of dexamphetamine by a "friend." Their consumption led to an elevated blood pressure which resulted in cerebral hemorrhage and death. Tonks and Lloyd [1965] warn against the use of nonprescription drugs when MAO inhibitors are used. A patient receiving phenelzine went into status epilepticus after consuming phenylpropanolamine, an ephedrine-like drug, and isopropamide, an anticholinergic drug, contained in a common cold remedy. Imipramine, amitriptylline, and other dibenzazepine derivatives, which are widely used for the treatment of depression, are considered particularly risky when taken with MAO inhibitors. The signs and symptoms experienced with such combinations are like those seen in severe atropine poisoning, including convulsions, coma, hyperpyrexia, and marked spasm. Appetite suppressants are frequently amphetamine-like drugs, and their intake with MAO inhibitors should be avoided.

In addition to those effects of the MAO inhibitors which are more or less predictable from their better understood modes of action, these drugs produce effects not directly attributable to their effect on the metabolism of amines. That MAO inhibitors inhibit enzymes other than MAO was first suggested by Brodie and coworkers [Cooper et al. 1954; Fouts and Brodie 1956; Laroche and Brodie 1960], who showed that hydrazides (iproniazid, nialamide, and β-phenylisopropylhydrazine) prolonged hexobarbital hypnosis in rats by interfering with the metabolism of hexobarbital. The effect on hexobarbital was short-acting; that on MAO, long-acting. It is now known that MAO inhibition by hydrazides is irreversible and enzyme activity is restored only by synthesis of new enzyme. In studies employing hepatic microsomes, iproniazid was shown to inhibit the metabolism of hexobarbital, amphetamine, and acetanilide [Fouts and Brodie 1956; Rogers and Fouts 1964]. Iproniazid inhibits the N-demethylation of ethylmorphine competitively [Anders and Mannering 1966a].

Numerous cases of the incompatibility of meperidine (Demerol) and MAO inhibitors have been reported [Mitchell 1955; Papp and Benaim 1958; Palmer 1960; Shee 1960; Pells-Cocks and Passmore-Rowe 1962; Tayler 1962; Vigran 1964]. The toxic manifestations, which frequently appear within minutes of the administration of meperidine, consist of excitation, both hypotension and hypertension, impaired respiration, hyperpyrexia, shock, rigidity, coma, and death. The temptation is to explain the reaction as being due to the inhibition of the enzymes responsible for meperidine biotransformation. That this may be the case, at least in part, is suggested by recent studies of Eade and Renton [1970], in which the MAO inhibitors, phenelzine and tranylcypromine, retarded the degradation of meperidine in intact animals. However, the rapid onset of the potentiated effects of meperidine and the abnormal pharmacological characteristics of some of these effects can hardly be explained on the basis of a decelerated metabolic degradation of meperidine [Sjöqvist 1965]. The claim is made that the incompatible response of combined meperidine and MAO inhibitor therapy is seen in only a small percentage of patients [Churchill-Davidson 1965]. In any event, meperidine addicts or opiate addicts who substitute meperidine for morphine or heroin risk severe reactions if they are also receiving MAO inhibitors.

Undoubtedly the most bizarre of incompatibilities is that of the MAO inhibitors and certain foods. Early in the 1960s numerous reports were published of serious side effects associated with the intake of MAO inhibitors, including sudden, severe headaches, photophobia, neck stiffness, hypertension, and collapse. These severe symptoms were seen only sporadically among users of MAO inhibitors, and no reason for their occurrence could be found until Blackwell [1963] become interested in the observation that a pharmacist's wife who was under treatment with MAO inhibitors experienced typical side effects shortly after eating cheese. He investigated the diet of other patients receiving MAO inhibitors and found that eight of ten patients experienced headache after eating cheese. Asatoor and coworkers [1963] suggested from chemical investigation into various cheeses that tyramine was the dietary factor involved. They postulated that under normal conditions tyramine was broken down by MAO contained in the gut, but after enzyme inhibition with a MAO inhibitor, tyramine was absorbed and exerted its known pressor effect. Subsequent studies leave little doubt that tyramine is the culprit. Certain wines and beer also contain sufficient tryptamine to produce the effect. DOPA, contained in broad beans, produces a similar interaction with MAO inhibitors [Hodge et al. 1964]. Tyramine has been generally supposed to be detoxified by MAO contained in the mitochondria of the intestinal wall, the liver, and other tissues. However, Rand and Trinker [1968] have provided rather convincing evidence that MAO inhibitors potentiate the effects of tyramine and other indirectly acting sympathomimetic amines, not by interfering with the metabolism of endogenous noradrenaline, but by retarding the binding or breakdown of these amines by the hepatic microsomal enzyme system.

Inhibitors of microsomal enzymes have been used as insecticidal synergists. Certain methylenedioxyphenyl compounds, particularly piperonyl butoxide, are widely used to increase the toxicity of pesticides by inhibiting their inactivation [Metcalf 1967]. Methylenedioxybenzenes have been shown to inhibit the metabolism of insecticides such as parathion [Nakatsugawa and Dahm 1965, 1967], carbamides [Hodgson and Casida 1961], naphthalene [Philleo et al. 1965], and chlorinated hydrocarbons [Nakatsugawa, Ishidar et al. 1965b; Wong and Terriere, 1965; Lewis et al. 1967]. Insecticidal synergists may be pharmacologically important to man because they are known to inhibit

drug metabolism in mammals. A large number of these compounds have been examined both in vivo and in vitro for their inhibitory effects [Fine and Molloy, 1964; Epstein et al. 1967a, 1967b, 1970; Anders 1968; Fujii et al. 1968, 1970; Jaffe et al. 1968, 1969].

Any discussion of inhibitors of drug metabolism would be incomplete without some mention of SKF 525-A (2-diethyl-aminoethyl 2,2-diphenylvalerate-HCl). A congener of adiphenine, it was originally synthesized as a possible parasympatholytic agent. It proved not to be important for this purpose, but showed the interesting property of prolonging the hypnotic action of hexo-barbital while lacking any sedative activity of its own [Cook et al. 1954]. The answer to the way in which SKF 525-A produced its effects was soon forthcoming from Brodie's laboratory, where it was shown to inhibit the metabolism of a wide variety of drugs both in vivo and in vitro [Axelrod, Reichenthal, et al. 1954; Cooper et al. 1954; Fouts and Brodie 1955, 1956; Brodie 1956; Gaudette and Brodie 1959]. The inhibitor is not used therapeutically, but it has been of great value as a tool for investigating drug metabolism. SKF 525-A was only the first of many compounds of minimal pharmacologic activity now known to inhibit drug metabolism [Mannering 1968a]. After studying the inhibition kinetics of 11 of these compounds, Anders and Mannering [1966a] concluded that they were inhibiting microsomal drug metabolism, at least in part, by serving as alternative substrates. SKF 525-A differs from other drugs that have been studied in that it combines irreversibly with microsomes [Rogers and Fouts 1964; Anders, Alvares, et al. 1966a]; this may endow the compound with special inhibitory properties quite different from that which is explainable on the basis of its being a substrate.

The chronic administration of morphine to

rats causes a reduction in the capacity of hepatic microsomes to N-demethylate narcotic analgesics [Axelrod 1956b]. The suggestion was made that this tolerance to metabolism could be likened to the tolerance to the drug effect that develops when morphine is given repeatedly, and that the metabolic site for morphine therefore resembled the receptor site for morphine. This concept has been abandoned largely as a result of the observation that chronic morphine administration causes a reduction in the metabolism of many drugs not related to the narcotic analgesics either in structure or pharmacologic action. Recently it has been shown that morphine reduces drug metabolism only in the adult male rat; no response to morphine was seen in mature females or in immature rats of either sex [Chaplin et al. 1968]. Females and immature males behaved like mature males with respect to the morphine effect when testosterone was administered; ergosterol eliminated the effect in mature males [Chaplin et al. 1970]. Whether or not this sex difference in the response to morphine occurs in other species is not known.

7.5. Tests for Inhibition of Drug Metabolism

Tests 1, 2, 3, 4, 5, 6, and 10 (Table 1) can be used to determine whether or not a given drug is a general inhibitor of drug metabolism. Tests 1 and 2 cannot be used if the drug in question itself has an effect on hexobarbital sleeping time or zoxazolamine paralysis time. Drugs are not usually tested to determine whether they are general inhibitors of drug metabolism, but rather, because clinical findings suggest that drugs may be interacting. This leads to experimental designs that will test the interaction of the two drugs in question. Because an elevated blood level of a drug may be due to displacement of the drug from protein-binding sites as well as from a reduced rate of metabolism, it is necessary to determine drug levels at several time intervals to establish the rate of disap-

pearance of drug from the blood. The results of such a study are given in Figure 3.

In vitro studies employing hepatic microsomes can provide information regarding the inhibitory interactions of drugs, but the results are frequently not applicable to the experience in vivo. Thus, triparanol and chlorpromazine did not affect the metabolism of pentobarbital or meprobamate, and phenobarbital did not inhibit meprobamate metabolism [Kato, Chiesara, et al. 1964]. The in vivo metabolism of hexobarbital by rats was not inhibited by morphine, norcodeine, dextromethorphan, levomethorphan, meprobamate, or acetanlilde [Rubin, Tephly, et al. 1964a]. Because of the many factors that may affect accumulation of drugs at the metabolic site in the whole animal, these results were not unexpected. In order for a drug to inhibit the metabolism of another drug at the metabolic site, a number of conditions must be met. The effectiveness of a substrate inhibitor will relate to its Michaelis constant (K_m); inhibitory capacity is increased as the ratio of the K_m of the inhibiting drug to the K_m of the inhibited drug is decreased. The maximal velocity (V) of the inhibiting drug should not greatly exceed that of the drug being inhibited, or its presence at the metabolic site will not be maintained long enough to produce a sustained effect. Other factors being equal, the inhibitory capacity of the drug is increased as V approaches zero. Knowledge of the overall metabolic disposition of the drugs will also provide some predictability as to whether one drug will inhibit the metabolism of another. The biotransformation studied in vitro may not represent the major metabolic route in vivo, and drugs metabolized by separate routes cannot interfere with each other's metabolism as alternative substrates unless rate-limiting cofactors or other endogenous intermediates are shared by both metabolic pathways. Potency of the drugs in

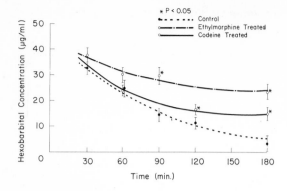

Figure 3. Inhibition of metabolism of hexobarbital in vivo by ethylmorphine (52 µmoles per kg). or codeine (52 µmoles per kg). Hexobarbital was administered at a dose level of 320 µmoles per kg. The values given represent the means ($\pm$ S.E.) obtained from at least 4 rats. (Reprinted by permission from A. Rubin, T. R. Tephly, and G. R. Mannering (1964). *Biochemical Pharmacology* 13:1053–1057.)

question is also of great importance in this regard. Very potent drugs are not likely to interfere with much less potent drugs simply because their concentrations at the metabolic site are likely to be very different, although this factor would be offset if the K_m of the more potent drug were much less than that of the drug of lesser potency. Most of this information is seldom available, and the quickest and most reliable way to determine if one drug will prolong the metabolism of another is to do the in vivo experiment.

Data from in vitro inhibition studies are too frequently reported in units that do not permit comparisons. It should be remembered that the I_{50} (the amount of compound required to produce 50 percent inhibition) are arbitrary values that depend upon the concentration of substrate employed. Inhibitor constants (K_i) are much more meaningful data for purposes of comparison.

8. Unexplained and Multiple Interactions

The attempt was made in this chapter to categorize examples of drug interactions where mechanisms have been established with reasonable documentation. This might create the impression that individual drug interactions can be explained by only one of the possible ways that drugs may interact. It is rather more probable that a given drug may interact in several ways. Thus, for example, a drug might interact at both the receptor and metabolic sites and at the same time displace a drug bound to protein. The example has been given of MAO inhibitors which appear to inhibit both MAO and the microsomal enzymes responsible for drug metabolism and which also seem to affect receptors not associated with these enzymatic sites. A large number of drugs are known to be incompatible with each other, but their modes of interaction have not been studied sufficiently to permit an understanding of the mechanisms involved. An example of this that may be pertinent to the problem of drug abuse is the interaction of hexobarbital and amphetamine with tetrahydrocannabinols, the active ingredients of marihuana. In mice, tetrahydrocannabinols increased the hypnotic effect of hexobarbital and the activity induced by amphetamine [Garriott et al. 1967]. The mechanisms of these interactions are not known, but the fact that the activities of two opposite acting drugs were enhanced by tetrahydrocannabinols suggests that the biotransformations of hexobarbital and amphetamine had been inhibited. Attempts are being made to catalog the numerous drug interactions of both established and unknown etiology [McIver 1965, 1967; Hansten, 1969a, 1969b]. The many drugs available and the persistent increase in the average number of drugs taken per patient have not only set the scene for many new drug inter-actions, but communication with those re-sponsible for drug therapy has not kept pace with the problem. Dunphy [1969] has suggested a system for recording information on drug interactions on index cards for rapid monitoring of drug usage.

9. Summary

Polypharmacy in therapeutics has its counter-part in the increasing frequency with which more than one drug is used simultaneously or interchangeably by drug abusers to control or otherwise modify their pleasure-producing effects. Adverse reactions resulting from drug interactions increase in proportion to the number of drugs used and the duration of administration. Evaluation of the problem is difficult under ideally controlled clinical conditions; in the case of the drug abuser, we have no accurate picture of the number or kinds of drugs used, the purity of drugs, dosage of drugs, or the effects experienced. We can assume only that in general the problems faced by the physician are those experienced by the drug abuser in his practice of polypharmacy.

A drug may alter the action of another drug in several ways: by producing one or more effects similar or opposite to those of the drug in question; by direct chemical or physical interaction of drugs; by displace-ment of drugs bound to plasma or other proteins; by altered renal clearance of drugs; through conditioning by previous drug effects; by interaction of drugs with receptor sites; and by inhibition or stimulation of the metabolic site. Examples of all of these inter-actions are given, but because it can be pre-dicted from evidence already gathered that interactions occurring at the metabolic site will be many times more numerous than those seen in other categories, this part of the discussion was dealt with in considerable depth.

References

Aarts, E. M. (1965). *Biochem. Pharmacol.* 14:359.

Aggeler, P. M., R. A. O'Reilly, L. Leong, and P. E. Kowitz (1967). *New Engl. J. Med.* 276:496.

Anders, M. W. (1966). *Anal. Chem.* 38:1945.

———— (1968). *Biochem. Pharmacol.* 17:2367.

————, A. P. Alvares, and G. J. Mannering (1966a). *Mol. Pharmacol.* 2:328.

————, and G. J. Mannering (1966b). *Mol. Pharmacol.* 2:319.

————, and G. J. Mannering (1966c). *Mol. Pharmacol.* 2:341.

Antlitz, A. M., M. Tolentino, and M. F. Kosai (1968). *Current Ther. Res.* 10:70.

Anton, A. H. (1960). *J. Pharmacol. Exp. Ther.* 129:282.

Arcos, J. C., A. H. Conney, and N. P. Buu-Hoi (1961). *J. Biol. Chem.* 236:1291.

Asatoor, A. M., A. J. Levi, and M. D. Milne (1963). *Lancet* 2:733.

Axelrod, J. (1956a). *Biochem. J.* 63:634.

———— (1956b). *Science* 124:263.

————, J. Reichenthal, and B. B. Brodie (1954). *J. Pharmacol. Exp. Ther.* 112:49.

Barber, M. (1965). *Proc. Roy. Soc. Med.* 58:990.

Blackwell, B. (1963). *Lancet* 2:414.

Bledsoe, T., D. P. Island, R. L. Ney, and G. W. Liddle (1964). *J. Clin. Endocrinol. Metab.* 24:1303.

Booth, J., and J. R. Gillette (1966). Unpublished observations cited by J. R. Gillette, *Advan. Pharmacol.* 4:219.

Brazda, F. G., and R. Baucum (1961). *J. Pharmacol. Exp. Ther.* 132:295.

Brodie, B. B. (1956). *J. Pharm. Pharmacol.* 8:1.

——— (1965). *Proc. Roy. Soc. Med.* 58:946.

———, and J. Axelrod (1950). *J. Pharmacol. Exp. Ther.* 98:97.

———, J. Axelrod, J. R. Cooper, L. Gaudette, B. N. LaDu, C. Mitoma, and S. Udenfriend (1955). *Science* 121:603.

———, G. J. Cosmides, and D. P. Rall (1965). *Science* 148:1547.

Brodie, B. B., J. R. Gillette, and B. N. LaDu (1958). *Ann. Rev. Biochem.* 27:427.

Burns, J. J., and A. H. Conney (1965). *Proc. Roy. Soc. Med.* 58:955.

———, A. H. Conney, P. G. Dayton, C. Evans, G. R. Martin, and D. Taller (1960). *J. Pharmacol. Exp. Ther.* 129:132.

———, A. H. Conney, and R. Koster (1963). *Ann. N.Y. Acad. Sci.* 104:881.

Burstein, S., and E. L. Klaiber (1965). *J. Clin. Endocrinol. Metab.* 25:293.

Busfield, D., K. J. Child, R. M. Atkinson, and E. G. Tomich (1963). *Lancet* 2:1042.

Butler, T. C., W. J. Waddell, and D. T. Poole (1965). *Biochem. Pharmacol.* 14:937.

Carter, S. A. (1965). *New Eng. J. Med.* 273:423.

Catalano, P. M., and S. I. Cullen (1966). *Clin. Res.* 14:266.

Chaplin, M. D., N. E. Sladek, and G. J. Mannering (1968). *Fed. Proc.* 27:349.

——— (1970). Unpublished observations.

Chen, W., P. A. Vrindten, P. G. Dayton, and J. J. Burns (1962). *Life Sci.* 1:35.

Cho, A. K., W. L. Haslett, and D. J. Jenden (1961). *Biochem. Biophys. Res. Commun.* 5:276.

Christensen, L. K., J. M. Hansen, and M. Kristensen (1963). *Lancet* 2:1298.

Churchill-Davidson, H. C. (1965). *Brit. Med. J.* 1:520.

Conney, A. H. (1965). In B. B. Brodie and J. R. Gillette, eds., *Proceedings of the Second International Pharmacological Meeting, Prague.* London: Pergamon Press, vol. 4, p. 277.

——— (1967). *Pharmacol. Rev.* 19:317.

———, G. A. Bray, C. Evans, and J. J. Burns (1961a). *Ann. N.Y. Acad. Sci.* 92:115.

———, and J. J. Burns (1959a). *Nature* 184:363.

———, and J. J. Burns (1963a). *Advan. Enzyme Regulation* 1:189.

———, C. Davison, R. Gastel, and J. J. Burns (1960). *J. Pharmacol. Exp. Ther.* 130:1.

———, J. R. Gillette, J. K. Inscoe, E. G. Trams, and H. S. Posner (1959b). *Science* 130:1478,

———, and A. G. Gilman (1963b). *J. Biol. Chem.* 238:3682.

———, M. Jacobson, K. Schneidman, and R. Kuntzman (1965a). *Life Sci.* 4:1091.

———, and A. Klutch (1963c). *J. Biol. Chem.* 238:1611.

———, I. A. Michaelson, and J. J. Burns (1961b). *J. Pharmacol. Exp. Ther.* 132:202.

———, E. C. Miller, and J. A. Miller (1956). *Cancer Res.* 16:450.

———, E. C. Miller, and J. A. Miller (1957). *J. Biol. Chem.* 228:753.

———, K. Schneidman, M. Jacobson, and R. Kuntzman (1965b). *Ann. N.Y. Acad. Sci.* 123:98.

———, R. M. Welch, R. Kuntzman, and J. J. Burns (1967). *Clin. Pharmacol. Ther.* 8:2.

Cook, L., J. J. Toner, and E. J. Fellows (1954). *J. Pharmacol. Exp. Ther.* 111:131.

Cooper, J. R., J. Axelrod, and B. B. Brodie (1954). *J. Pharmacol. Exp. Ther.* 112:55.

Corn, M., and J. F. Rockett (1965). *Med. Ann. D.C.* 34:578.

Cramer, J. W., J. A. Miller, and E. C. Miller (1960). *J. Biol. Chem.* 235:250.

Crigler, J. F., and N. I. Gold (1966). *J. Clin. Invest.* 45:998.

Cucinell, S. A., A. H. Conney, M. Sansur, and J. J. Burns (1965). *Clin. Pharmacol. Ther.* 6:420.

———, R. Koster, A. H. Conney, and J. J. Burns (1963). *J. Pharmacol. Exp. Ther.* 141:157.

———, L. Odessky, M. Weiss, and P. G. Dayton (1966). *J.A.M.A.* 197:366.

Dally, P. J. (1962). *Lancet* 1:1235.

Dearborn, E. H., J. T. Litchfield, Jr., H. J. Eisner, J. J. Corbett, and C. W. Dunnett (1957). *Antibiot. Med. Clin. Therapy* 4:627.

Dixon, R. L., E. S. Henderson, and D. P. Rall (1965). *Fed. Proc.* 24:454.

Doherty, J. E., and W. H. Perkins (1966). *Ann. Intern. Med.* 64:489.

Dollery, C. T. (1965). *Proc. Roy. Soc. Med.* 58:983.

Douglas, J. F., B. J. Ludwig, and N. Smith (1963). *Proc. Soc. Exp. Biol. Med.* 112:436.

Dunphy, T. W. (1969). *Am. J. Hosp. Pharm.* 26:367.

Eade, N. R., and K. W. Renton (1970). *J. Pharmacol. Exp. Ther.* 173:31.

Elison, C., and H. W. Elliott (1964). *J. Pharmacol. Exp. Ther.* 144:265.

Epstein, S. S., J. Andrea, P. Clapp, and D. Mackintosh (1967b). *Toxicol. Appl. Pharmacol.* 11:442.

———, R. G. Csillag, H. Guerin, and M. A. Friedman (1970). *Biochem. Pharmacol.* 19:2605.

———, S. Joshi, J. Andrea, P. Clapp, H. Falk, and N. Mantel (1967a). *Nature* 214:526.

Ernster, L., and S. Orrenius (1965). *Fed. Proc.* 24:1190.

Fine, B. C., and J. O. Molloy (1964). *Nature,* 204:789.

Fouts, J. R., and B. B. Brodie (1955). *J. Pharmacol. Exp. Ther.* 115:68.

———, and B. B. Brodie (1956). *J. Pharmacol. Exp. Ther.* 116:480.

———, and L. A. Rogers (1965). *J. Pharmacol. Exp. Ther.* 147:112.

Fujii, K., H. Jaffe, Y. Bishop, E. Arnold, D. Mackintosh, and S. S. Epstein (1970). *Toxicol. Appl. Pharmacol.* 16:482.

———, H. Jaffe, and S. S. Epstein (1968). *Toxicol. Appl. Pharmacol.* 13:431.

Fujimoto, J. M., and G. L. Plaa (1961). *J. Pharmacol. Exp. Ther.* 131:282.

Gallo, D. G., K. R. Bailey, and A. L. Sheffner (1965). *Proc. Soc. Exp. Biol. Med.* 120:60.

Garriott, J. C., L. J. King, R. B. Forney, and F. W. Hughes (1967). *Life Sci.* 6:2119.

Gaudette, L. E., and B. B. Brodie (1959). *Biochem. Pharmacol.* 2:89.

Gelboin, H. V., and N. R. Blackburn (1964). *Cancer Res.* 24:356.

George, R., W. L. Haslett, and D. J. Jenden (1962). *Life Sci.* 1:361.

Gillette, J. R. (1963). *Progr. Drug. Res.* 6:11.

——— (1966). *Advan. Pharmacol.* 4:219.

——— (1967). In P. E. Siegler and J. H. Moyer III, eds., *Animal and Clinical Pharmacological Techniques in Drug Evaluation.* Chicago: Year Book Medical Publishers, p. 48

——— (1968). In D. H. Tedeschi and R. E. Tedeschi, eds., *Importance of Fundamental Principles in Drug Evaluation.* New York: Raven Press, p. 69.

Goss, J. E., and D. W. Dickhaus (1965). *New Eng. J. Med.* 273:1094.

Hammer, W., and F. Sjöqvist (1966). In 1st Symposium Antidepressant Drugs, Milan, *Excerpta Med. Int. Congr.,* series 122, p. 279.

Hansen, J. M., M. Kristensen, L. Skovsted, and L. K. Christensen (1966). *Lancet* 2:265.

Hansten, P. D. (1969a). *Hosp. Formular. Manage.* 4:20.

——— (1969b). *Hosp. Formular. Manage.* 4:28.

Hart, L. G., and J. R. Fouts (1963). *Proc. Soc. Exp. Biol. Med.* 114:388.

———, and J. R. Fouts (1965). *Arch. Exp. Pathol. Pharmakol.* 249:486.

——— R. W. Shultice, and J. R. Fouts (1963). *Toxicol. Appl. Pharmacol.* 5:371.

Hodge, J. V., E. R. Nye, and G. W. Emerson (1964). *Lancet* 1:1108.

Hodgson, E., and J. E. Casida (1961). *Biochem. Pharmacol.* 8:179.

Hunninghake, D. B., and D. L. Azarnoff (1968). *Arch. Intern. Med.* 121:349.

Imai, Y., and R. Sato (1966a). *Biochem. Biophys. Res. Commun.* 22:620.

——— (1966b). *Biochem. Biophys. Res. Commun.* 23:5.

Jaffe, H., K. Fujii, H. Guerin, M. Sengupta, and S. S. Epstein (1969). *Biochem. Pharmacol.* 18:1045.

———, K. Fujii, M. Sengupta, H. Guerin, and S. S. Epstein (1968). *Life Sci.* 7:1051.

Jelliffe, R. W., and D. H. Blankenhorn (1966). *Clin. Res.* 14:160.

Kato, R. (1961). *Arzneimittel-Forsch.* 11:797.

——— (1966). *J. Biochem.* 59:574.

———, E. Chiesara, and P. Vassanelli (1962a). *Experientia* 18:269.

——— (1962b). *Med. Exp.* 6:254.

——— (1964). *Biochem. Pharmacol.* 13:69.

Kiørboe, E. (1966). *Epilepsia* 7:246.

Kolmodin, B., D. L. Azarnoff, and F. Sjöqvist (1969). *Clin. Pharmacol. Ther.* 10:638.

Kristensen, M. D., and J. M. Hansen (1967). *Diabetes* 16:211.

—— (1968). *Acta Med. Scand.* 183:83.

Kuntzman, R., M. Jacobson, and A. H. Conney (1966). *Pharmacologist* 8:195.

Kutt, H., K. Verebely, and F. McDowell (1968). *Neurology* 18:706.

——, W. Winters, and F. McDowell (1966). *Neurology* 16:594.

Laroche, M., and B. B. Brodie (1960). *J. Pharmacol. Exp. Ther.* 130:134.

Lasagna, L. (1965). *Proc. Roy. Soc. Med.* 58:978.

Lewis, S. E., C. F. Wilkinson, and J. W. Ray (1967). *Biochem. Pharmacol.* 16:1195.

Lloyd, J. T. A., and D. R. H. Walker, (1965). *Brit. Med. J.* 2:168.

Low-Beer, G. A., and D. Tidmarsh (1963). *Brit. Med. J.* 2:683.

Lowenthal, I., and L. M. Fisher (1957). *Experientia* 13:253.

MacDonald, M. G., and D. S. Robinson (1968). *J.A.M.A.* 204:97.

MacDonald, R. (1963). *Lancet* 1:269.

Macgregor, A. G. (1965). *Proc. Roy. Soc. Med.* 58:943.

McIver, A. K. (1965). *Pharm. J.* 195:609.

—— (1967). *Pharm. J.* 199:205.

Mannering, G. J. (1968a). In A. Burger, ed., *Selected Pharmacological Testing Methods,* New York: Marcel Dekker, p. 51.

—— (1968b). In D. H. Tedeschi and R. E. Tedeschi, eds., *Importance of Fundamental Principles in Drug Evaluation,* New York: Raven Press, p. 105.

Marsh, C. A., and L. M. Reid (1963). *Biochim. Biophys. Acta* 78:726.

Mason, A. (1962). *Lancet* 1:1073.

Mason, H. S. (1957). *Science* 125:1185.

—— (1965). *Ann. Rev. Biochem.* 34:595.

Metcalf, R. L. (1967). *Ann. Rev. Entomol.* 12:229.

Milne, M. D. (1965). *Proc. Roy Soc. Med.* 58:961.

Mitchell, R. S. (1955). *Ann. Intern. Med.* 42:417.

Morrelli, H. F., and K. L. Melmon (1968). *California Medicine* 109:380.

Mueller, G. C., and J. A. Miller (1949). *J. Biol. Chem.* 180:1125.

—— (1953). *J. Biol. Chem.* 202:579.

Murray, F. J. (1962). *Am. Rev. Respirat. Dis.* 86:729.

Nakatsugawa, T., and P. A. Dahm (1965a). *J. Econ. Entomol.* 58:500.

——, and P. A. Dahm (1967). *Biochem. Pharmacol.* 16:25.

——, M. Ishida, and P. A. Dahm (1965b). *Biochem. Pharmacol.* 14:1853.

Olesen, O. (1966). *Acta Pharmacol. Toxicol.* 24:317.

—— (1967). *Arch. Neurol.* 16:642.

Omura, T., and R. Sato (1962). *J. Biol. Chem.* 237:1375.

——, R. Sato, D. Y. Cooper, O. Rosenthal, and R. W. Estabrook (1965). *Fed. Proc.* 24:1181.

Orrenius, S., J. L. E. Ericsson, and L. Ernster (1965). *J. Cell Biol.* 25:627.

——, and L. Ernster (1964). *Biochem. Biophys. Res. Commun.* 16:60.

Ortega, P. (1966). *Lab. Invest.* 15:657.

Palmer, H. (1960). *Brit. Med. J.* 2:944.

Papp, C., and S. Benaim (1958). *Brit. Med. J.* 2:1070.

Pells-Cocks, D., and A. Passmore-Rowe (1962). *Brit. Med. J.* 2:1545.

Philleo, W. W., R. D. Schonbrod, and L. C. Terriere *J. Agr. Food Chem.* 13:113.

Posner, H. S., C. Mitoma, S. Rothberg, and S. Udenfriend (1961). *Arch. Biochem.* 94:280.

Rand, M. J., and F. R. Trinker (1968). *Brit. J. Pharmacol.* 33:287.

Remmer, H. (1958). *Naturwissenschaften* 45:189.

—— (1959a). *Arch. Exp. Pathol. Pharmakol.* 235:279.

—— (1959b). *Arch. Exp. Pathol. Pharmakol.* 237:296.

—— (1962a). In B. B. Brodie and E. G. Erdos, eds., *Proceedings of the First International Pharmacological Meeting, Stockholm,* London: Pergamon Press, vol. 6, p. 235.

—— (1962b). In J. I. Mongar and A. V. S. DeReuck, eds., *Ciba Foundation Symposium on Enzymes and Drug Action,* Boston: Little, Brown, p. 276.

—— (1964). In *Proceedings of the European Society for the Study of Drug Toxicity*, Excerpta Medica International Congress Series no. 81, London: Excerpta Medica Foundation, p. 57.

——, and B. Alsleben (1958). *Klin. Wochschr.* 36:332.

——, and H. J. Merker (1963). *Klin. Wochschr.* 41:276.

——, and H. J. Merker (1965). *Ann. N.Y. Acad. Sci.* 123:79.

——, J. Schenkman, R. W. Estabrook, H. Sasame, J. Gillette, S. Narasimhulu, D. Y. Cooper, and O. Rosenthal (1966). *Mol. Pharmacol.* 2:187.

——, and M. Siegert (1964). *Arch. Exp. Pathol. Pharmakol.* 247:522.

Richardson, H. L., and L. Cunningham (1951). *Cancer Res.* 11:274.

Roberts, J., R. Ito, J. Reilly, and V. J. Cairoli (1963). *Circulation Res.* 13:149.

Robinson, D. S., and M. G. MacDonald (1966). *J. Pharmacol. Exp. Ther.* 153:250.

Rogers, L. A., and J. R. Fouts (1964). *J. Pharmacol. Exp. Ther.* 146:286.

Rubin, A., T. R. Tephly, and G. J. Mannering (1964a) *Biochem. Pharmacol.* 13:1007.

—— (1964b). *Biochem. Pharmacol.* 13:1053.

Rümke, C. L. (1963). *Arch. Exp. Pathol. Pharmakol.* 244:519.

Schmid, R., H. S. Marver, and L. Hammaker (1966). *Biochem. Biophys. Res. Commun.* 24:319.

Serrone, D. M., and J. M. Fujimoto (1961). *J. Pharmacol. Exp. Ther.* 133:12.

—— (1962). *Biochem. Pharmacol.* 11:609.

Shee, J. C. (1960). *Brit. Med. J.* 2:507.

Shepherd, M. (1965). *Proc. Roy. Soc. Med.* 58:964.

Siegert, M., B. Alsleben, W. Liebenschutz, and H. Remmer (1964). *Arch. Exp. Pathol. Pharmakol.* 247:509.

Sjöqvist, F. (1965). *Proc. Roy. Soc. Med.* 58:967.

——, and J. R. Gillette (1965). *Life Sci.* 4:1031.

——, W. Hammer, H. Schumacher, and J. R. Gillette (1968). *Biochem. Pharmacol.* 17:915.

Sladek, N. E., and G. J. Mannering (1966). *Biochem. Biophys. Res. Commun.* 24:668.

——, (1969a). *Mol. Pharmacol.* 5:174.

——, (1969b). *Mol. Pharmacol.* 5:186.

Smith, J. W., L. G. Seidl, and L. E. Cluff (1966). *Ann. Intern. Med.* 65:629.

Solomon, H. M., and J. J. Schrogie (1966). *J. Pharmacol. Exp. Ther.* 154:660.

Stark, D. C. D. (1962). *Lancet* 1:1405.

Takemori, A. E., and G. J. Mannering (1958). *J. Pharmacol. Exp. Ther.* 123:171.

Tayler, D. C. (1962). *Lancet* 2:401.

Tonks, C. M., and A. T. Lloyd (1965). *Brit. Med. J.* 1:589.

Vigran, I. M. (1964). *J.A.M.A.* 187:953.

Welch, R. M., and J. Kocsis (1961). *Proc. Soc. Exp. Biol. Med.* 107:731.

Werk, E. E., Jr., J. MacGee, and L. J. Sholiton (1964). *J. Clin. Invest.* 43:1824.

Williams, R. T. (1963). *Clin. Pharmacol. Ther.* 4:234.

Wishinsky, H., E. J. Glasser, and S. Perkal (1962). *Diabetes* 11:18.

Wong, D. T., and L. C. Terriere (1965). *Biochem. Pharmacol.* 14:375.

Zesk, P. (1961). *Med. J. Australia* 2:607.

Zubrod, C. G. (1965). *Proc. Roy. Soc. Med.* 58:988.

—— T. J. Kennedy. and J. A. Shannon (1948) *J. Clin. Invest.* 27:114.

II. Chronic Biological Hazards

5 Carcinogenic Hazards

J. A. Miller

1. The General Nature and Causes of Neoplasms

Tumors or neoplasms are abnormal masses of host-derived tissue which grow in a manner uncoordinated with normal tissues and organs. Neoplasms occur in a very wide variety of tissues in many species, and they generally persist and grow more or less continuously even after removal of any known causative agents. Neoplasms which invade adjacent tissue and spread or metastasize to other parts of the organism are known as *malignant neoplasms* or *cancers*. These malignant tumors frequently exhibit rapid growth, atypical structures, many mitotic figures, and invasive destruction of the host. Benign neoplasms lack these features, especially the ability to metastasize, and are usually encapsulated. However, benign neoplasms may kill the host through pressure or gross mass. Progression from benign neoplasms to malignant neoplasms or cancers is a frequent but not invariable occurrence.

Many neoplasms occur without known causes, and the majority of these "spontaneous" neoplasms occur in the last third of the life span in man and in other animals. The incidences of these neoplasms vary with the species and strain, and it may be markedly lowered or raised by selective breeding. Most selective breeding studies have employed the laboratory mouse and rat.

Many agents will cause neoplasms to develop in a variety of species more rapidly and in greater incidence than would occur spontaneously. It is not known if these varied carcinogenic agents induce neoplasms de novo, if they hasten the processes leading to the "spontaneous" tumours, or if either mechanism may apply in specific cases.

Three principal classes of carcinogenic agents exist. A large number of viruses containing DNA or RNA are known that can induce cancer in experimental animals. Viral carcinogens for man probably exist, particularly in the induction of the leukemias, but none has been demonstrated unequivocally. The carcinogenic viruses cannot yet be distinguished from other viruses by their physical, chemical, or genetic characteristics. Many nonviral chemicals, some of which are of biological or natural origin but most of which are of synthetic origin, are known which will induce cancer in experimental animals after the application of sufficient dosage and after an adequate latent period. These chemicals are generally small organic molecules with molecular weights below 500. A third class of carcinogenic agents consists of ultraviolet light and a variety of ionizing radiations.

Man has the dubious distinction of being the first species in which carcinogenesis by chemicals and by radiation was demonstrated. The first clear finding, by Pott in 1775, was derived from observations on the unusually high occurrence of scrotal skin cancer in chimney sweeps who had gross and prolonged contact with coal soot. A number of other compounds, organic and inorganic, have been found to be carcinogenic in man, usually in industrial situations; frequently these tumors followed exposure to large amounts of these agents for many years. Most skin cancer in man results from overexposure to solar ultraviolet light. Modern studies on the geographical pathology of cancer [Oettle 1964; Higginson 1969] suggest that a large fraction of nonskin cancer in the human also results from carcinogenic agents in the environment—possibly chemicals, viruses, or radiations.

Neoplasms obviously result from defects in growth control among cells and tissues in the organism. These defects do not invariably give rise to gross neoplasms, and the cellular alteration may remain latent. The interplay of many factors (e.g., hormonal or immunological) may be required to permit the appearance of gross tumors following dosage with carcinogens. The cellular and molecular mech-anisms by which carcinogenic viruses, chemicals, and radiations induce neoplasms are not known. Most of the hypotheses proposed for these mechanisms are based on the proposition that these agents, directly or indirectly, induce heritable and apparently irreversible alterations in the content, or expression, or both, of genetic information needed for the control of growth in a cooperative community of cells. Natural selection among the altered cells and their progeny for those with proliferative advantages favors the progression and growth of these cells into gross neoplasms that are under little or no host control.

2. Cancer in Man—Therapeutic and Prophylactic Prospects

Cancer is second only to the combined cardiovascular and circulatory diseases as a cause of death in the developed countries, where medical and nutritional advances have permitted long life spans. Surgery and radiotherapy remain the primary forms of treatment of cancer, although considerable progress has been made in the chemotherapy of certain types of cancer. Early diagnosis of many forms of cancer is still uncertain or unavailable. It has been estimated that *full* utilization of present diagnostic and therapeutic procedures could lead to cures in about 50 percent of all human cancer. Actually only about one-half of this rate is achieved under the best present conditions.

The prevention of cancer in man has been possible in a few situations where certain chemical and radiation hazards have been recognized and removed. Most of these instances have been industrial or medical situations, and they have not involved large population groups. The modern epidemic of bronchogenic carcinoma in man apparently has a principal cause in the excessive inhalation of cigarette smoke, but the elimination of this habit will at best be slow. Hopefully, through multidisciplinary research, we can look forward to progress on the identification and diminution or removal of the major carcinogenic viral, chemical, and radiation hazards to which man is subject.

3. The Role of Methods for the Detection and Evaluation of the Carcinogenic Hazards of Chemicals for Man

Man, like all other living organisms, is composed of chemicals and is nourished by chemicals in a world consisting of chemicals and radiations, some of them harmful to living cells. In previous times these harmful agents were generally not a product of man's own activities. Modern man lives in a truly chemical age in which he possesses, and frequently employs on a large scale, great abilities to alter his chemical environment and his own body. Some of the chemicals man employs in these ways pose certain hazards to man and other living forms. Furthermore, there is now a renewed awareness of toxicants, including carcinogens, that may occur naturally in food and in drugs. Principally through the use of acute and chronic tests of these synthetic and natural chemicals in experimental animals and sometimes in man, it has been possible to ascertain many toxicological hazards and control the use of these toxic chemicals. Our increasing awareness of the carcinogenic properties of certain synthetic and natural chemicals makes it necessary that we ensure in a practical manner that the chemicals we encounter or use in our modern environment do not pose significant carcinogenic hazards for man. This is a very complex problem, and we do not know its full dimensions or solution. The following paragraphs present various aspects of this problem, particularly our present knowledge of chemical carcinogenesis and the procedures now available for the detection and evaluation of the carcinogenic hazards for man of chemicals such as drugs of abuse.

4. Chemical Carcinogens—Structural Variety, Classes, and Biochemical Reactivity

4.1. Synthetic Organic Compounds

The carcinogenic activities of certain tars and oils for the skin of man and of certain aromatic amines for the human urinary bladder were early hints of the structural variety later found among the chemical carcinogens. The first laboratory demonstration of the carcinogenicity of chemicals was accomplished in Japan with the induction by coal tar of skin neoplasms in rabbits (1915) and mice (1918). This led to the discovery by British workers in 1930 of the carcinogenic polycyclic aromatic hydrocarbons. Similarly, Japanese workers in the 1930's discovered the carcinogenic aromatic aminoazo dyes, which are active primarily in the liver of the rat and mouse. During this time the activity of the human urinary bladder carcinogen 2-naphthylamine was confirmed in the dog. An important addition to the class of carcinogenic aromatic amines was made in 1941 with the finding that the proposed insecticide 2-acetylaminofluorene was carcinogenic in a variety of tissues in the rat.

In the quarter century that followed these initial findings, numerous non aromatic substances of very diverse structure were found to produce neoplasms in a variety of species and tissues. Some of the wide variety of structure seen among the synthetic chemical carcinogens is shown in Figures 1 and 2. Many of the compounds shown are representative of large groups of similar carcinogenic agents.

4.2. Natural Products

At present about a dozen fungal and green plant metabolites are known to be carcinogenic [Miller and Miller 1965] ; the structures of some of these compounds are shown in Figure 3. The aflatoxins, the toxic pyrrolizidine alkaloids, and cycasin are among the most potent chemical carcinogens known.

4.3. Inorganic Compounds

A variety of inorganic carcinogens is known :

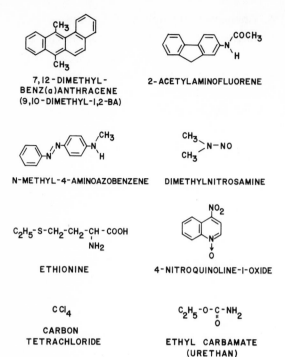

7,12-DIMETHYL-BENZ(a)ANTHRACENE (9,10-DIMETHYL-1,2-BA)

2-ACETYLAMINOFLUORENE

N-METHYL-4-AMINOAZOBENZENE

DIMETHYLNITROSAMINE

$C_2H_5-S-CH_2-CH_2-CH-COOH$
|
NH_2

ETHIONINE

4-NITROQUINOLINE-1-OXIDE

CCl_4

CARBON TETRACHLORIDE

$C_2H_5-O-C-NH_2$
‖
O

ETHYL CARBAMATE (URETHAN)

Figure 1. Some synthetic chemical carcinogens.

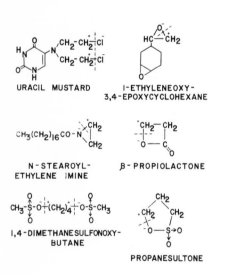

URACIL MUSTARD

1-ETHYLENEOXY-3,4-EPOXYCYCLOHEXANE

$CH_3(CH_2)_{16}CO-N$

N-STEAROYL-ETHYLENE IMINE

β-PROPIOLACTONE

$CH_3-S-O-(CH_2)_4-O-S-CH_3$

1,4-DIMETHANESULFONOXY-BUTANE

PROPANESULTONE

Figure 2. Some synthetic carcinogenic alkylating agents.

asbestos material (Mg, Fe, Na silicates); As derivatives (?); BeO; Cd powder; Co powder; CaCrO$_3$; Ni powder; Ni$_2$S$_3$; Pb(OAc)$_2$; and Se derivatives (?). Agents such as asbestos and chromate were first suspected as carcinogens from studies in humans. Arsenic compounds are under suspicion as carcinogens in man, but trials in experimental animals have been negative.

4.4. Chemicals Recognized as Carcinogens in Man

The list of known compounds in this category (Table 1) is small but varied and includes aromatic hydrocarbons, aromatic amines, an alkylating agent, and several inorganic compounds.

4.5. Smooth-Surface Carcinogenesis ("Film," "Solid-State," or "Polymer" Carcinogenesis)

In rats and some other species carcinogenesis occurs in connective tissue cells near intact implants of almost every substance tried (cellophane, nylon, Teflon, ivory, silver, platinum, etc.), provided that the implant has a sufficient surface area. In general, the formation of sarcomas as a consequence of exposure to these implants occurs late (after 1 year in the rat), but the incidence of tumors may eventually approach 50 percent. The possible role of smooth-surface carcinogenesis must be considered when tumors develop in the subcutaneous tissue of rodents at the site of often repeated injections of chemicals, especially in vehicles (e.g., oils) which remain at the site of injection for long times [Grasso and Golberg 1966].

4.6. Biochemical Reactivity of Chemical Carcinogens and Their Metabolites

For carcinogenesis to occur with chemical carcinogens it is axiomatic that these agents or their metabolites must react in some manner, directly or indirectly, covalently or noncovalently, with critical molecules in cells. Many chemical carcinogens are known to

form covalent nucleic acid-bound and pro-
tein-bound derivatives in target cells [Miller
and Miller 1966]. Only the reactive carcinogenic alkylating agents and possibly some
of the carcinogenic metal ions appear to be
carcinogenic per se. Chemically these compounds and ions are electrophilic reactants.
The other carcinogenic chemicals appear to
require conversion inside cells to final reactive carcinogenic forms which also are electrophilic reactants. This has been documented
to various degrees for both aliphatic and aromatic carcinogens [Miller and Miller 1969].
The metabolic activation reactions for dimethylnitrosamine [Magee and Barnes
1967] and the aromatic amines [Miller and
Miller 1969] are known in considerable detail. Information is also accumulating on the
nucleophilic sites in proteins and nucleic
acids that are attacked by the carcinogenic
electrophilic reactants [Magee and Barnes
1967; Miller and Miller, 1969]. The importance of these aspects of the biochemical
reactivity of chemical carcinogens is that they
bring order into the variety of structures with
carcinogenic activity. They may further provide a basis for the future recognition of
carcinogenic chemicals from their structures
and metabolic products. However, at present
one cannot predict the carcinogenicity of a
given structure with much assurance.

4.7. Carcinogenic Mechanisms of Action

As noted above, the cellular and molecular
mechanisms of action are not known for any
class of carcinogen—viral, chemical, or physical. However, the characterization of the reactive forms of chemical carcinogens as electrophilic reactants suggests several reasonable
molecular mechanisms of action. Several of
these mechanisms, direct and indirect, genetic
and epigenetic, are shown in Figure 4. It is of
interest that the active forms of chemical
carcinogens, where tested, have been found
to be mutagenic [Magee and Barnes 1967;
Miller and Miller 1969].

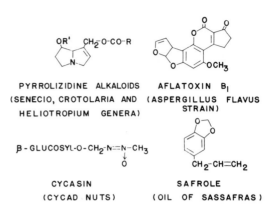

Figure 3. Some naturally occurring carcinogens.

Table 1. Chemicals Recognized as Carcinogens in Man.

Soots, tars, oils	Skin, lungs
Cigarette smoke	Lungs
2-Naphthylamine	Urinary bladder
4-Aminobiphenyl	Urinary bladder
Benzidine	Urinary bladder
N,N-bis(2-chloroethyl)-2-naphthylamine	Urinary bladder
Bis(2-chloroethyl)sulfide	Lungs
Nickel compounds	Lungs, nasal sinuses
Chromium compounds	Lungs
Asbestos	Lungs, pleura

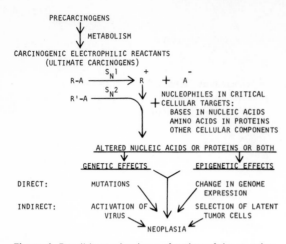

PRECARCINOGENS

$\downarrow$ METABOLISM

CARCINOGENIC ELECTROPHILIC REACTANTS
(ULTIMATE CARCINOGENS)

$$R\text{-}A \xrightarrow{S_N1} R^+ + A^-$$

$$R'\text{-}A \xrightarrow{S_N2}$$

NUCLEOPHILES IN CRITICAL
CELLULAR TARGETS:
   BASES IN NUCLEIC ACIDS
   AMINO ACIDS IN PROTEINS
   OTHER CELLULAR COMPONENTS

ALTERED NUCLEIC ACIDS OR PROTEINS OR BOTH

GENETIC EFFECTS   EPIGENETIC EFFECTS

DIRECT: MUTATIONS   CHANGE IN GENOME
                                EXPRESSION

INDIRECT: ACTIVATION OF   SELECTION OF LATENT
             VIRUS   TUMOR CELLS

NEOPLASIA

Figure 4. Possible mechanisms of action of the reactive electrophilic forms derived from chemical carcinogens.

5. Biological Aspects of Carcinogenesis by Chemicals

5.1. Similarity of Spontaneous Tumors and Those Induced by Chemicals, Radiations, and Viruses

Within a given histologic type, tumors which develop spontaneously or as a consequence of known exposure to a carcinogenic chemical, virus, or radiation are generally not distinguishable from each other in growth pattern, morphology, or chemical or biochemical properties [Clayson 1962; Hueper and Conway 1964; Klein 1969]. As a corollary the nature of the inciting agent cannot usually be determined from examination of the tumor. Virus-induced tumors usually carry some manifestation of the causative virus, e.g., specific antigens, viral nucleic acid, messenger RNAs, etc. The detection of these viral characters may, in a few laboratory cases, be relatively easy; in most other cases the detection of the cause, even a viral carcinogen, may be difficult or impossible. The lack of viral characters is unconvincing evidence for the lack of involvement of a virus in the causation of a tumor. Likewise, detection of viral characters is not a priori evidence of a causative agent since passenger viruses are a common finding in tumors. Chemical carcinogens are only rarely detectable in the induced tumors.

Tumor-specific antigens are detectable in many chemically induced and spontaneous neoplasms. Antigenic variability of these tumors seems to be the rule, and even different tumors induced in the same animal with the same chemical will exhibit different tumor-specific antigens. Virus-induced tumors exhibit specific cross-reacting antigens when induced by the same virus; these antigens are coded for by information in the virus. However, virus-induced tumors are now being found to contain a background of individual tumor-specific antigens similar to those found in chemically induced tumors.

5.2. Irreversibility of the Malignant Conversion

At the gross tissue level the malignant conversion is essentially irreversible. Thus, few cases of regression of malignant human tumors, in the absence of therapy, have been documented. Whether or not the malignant conversion is also irreversible at the cellular level is not clear. Neoplastic cells which reverted to nonneoplastic cells before they developed into clones would not be easily detected. Likewise, the reversion of a few malignant cells within a large clone would have little detectable effect on the progressive growth of a malignant mass.

5.3. Specificities of Chemical Carcinogens with Respect to Tissues, Species, Age, Sex, and Other Factors

Historically certain carcinogens, especially the alkylating agents and the polycyclic aromatic hydrocarbons, have been recognized as agents which induce tumors primarily at sites of application. Other chemical carcinogens, such as the aromatic amines, have been noteworthy for their low activities at sites of application and their predilection for inducing tumors in specific internal organs. Likewise, large differences have been recorded frequently in the susceptibilities to specific carcinogens of tissues of different species, in male vs. female animals, and in young vs. adult animals.

A major factor in determining the susceptibility of a tissue to a carcinogen is the level of the ultimate reactive carcinogen which reaches a tissue or which is formed in it. When an ultimate carcinogen is administered, as in the case of the alkylating agents, the cells near the site of application can be expected to receive the highest doses. With other chemical carcinogens the levels of the ultimate carcinogens formed in the various tissues will depend on the transport of the ad-ministered chemical and its proximate carcinogenic forms and on the relative activities of the tissues for metabolism to the ultimate carcinogen as compared to metabolism to noncarcinogenic products.

Other factors probably also modify the susceptibility of tissues. Thus, promotion of cell growth (as in fetal or newborn animals or in rapidly proliferating tissues) may provide cells with more sites or more accessible sites for the critical reactions between macromolecules and ultimate carcinogens which lead to neoplasia. Endocrine stimulation could function in a similar manner or could accelerate the appearance of tumors through facilitating the growth of neoplastic cells.

5.4. Routes of Application

Carcinogens which are administered as the ultimate carcinogenic form or which can be metabolized to such a form at the injection site are usually more efficiently administered by subcutaneous injection. Either single injections or repeated injections can be employed. However, when low to moderate incidences of tumors with long latent periods are induced after very large numbers of injections, the possible contributions of "smooth surface carcinogenesis," as contrasted to carcinogenesis by the specific chemical employed, must be considered. Chemicals which are carcinogenic at sites of subcutaneous injection also often induce tumors of the skin following topical application to mice, especially if the administration of the carcinogen is followed by repeated applications of a promoting substance (e.g., croton oil or its active ingredients, the phorbol esters). The carcinogenicity of the aromatic amines has been most readily demonstrated by administration of the compounds in the diet for many months; the total amounts of compound required are often large, probably because of the inefficient conversion of the amines to the ultimate carcinogenic metabolites and limited delivery to the critical targets. Intraperitoneal and intravenous injections have also been employed, as well as the direct injection or implantation of compounds within specific tissues.

5.5. Dose Response

In general the incidence of tumors increases and the latent period decreases as the dose of a carcinogenic chemical is increased. With small doses the latent period may be too long to permit development of gross tumors within the life-span of the animal; high doses may kill the animal before tumors become apparent.

5.6. Combined Effects of Two or More Carcinogens

Doses of the same or different carcinogens administered either simultaneously or sequentially may produce additive, synergistic, or inhibitory effects. Inhibitory effects can result from altered metabolic patterns which reduce the effective levels of one or both carcinogens; inhibition of amine carcinogenesis by administration of polycyclic hydrocarbons is an example. Competition for reactive sites may be a factor in other situations.

The best documented synergistic responses are found in mouse skin tumorigenesis. Thus, some initiating agents (e.g., urethan) and some promoting agents (e.g., croton oil) induce very few tumors when administered alone, but administration of the initiator and then the promoter results in high tumor yields.

5.7. Rapid Tests for Carcinogenic Activity

At present only studies on the production of tumors in vivo are recognized as valid tests of carcinogenic activity. Since these tests require many months or years, more rapid assays to predict the possible carcinogenic hazards of chemicals have been sought. To date no test with good predictive value for chemicals of different types has been achieved, although in some cases correlations have been achieved within limited classes of compounds.

Chemical transformation of cells cultured in vitro has been studied in this context, since in some systems these transformed clones grow as tumors in vivo. Other proposed short-term tests have been assays for destruction of sebaceous glands of mouse skin and various mutagenicity and toxicity tests with plants, Drosophila, microorganisms and mammals. Two major questions exist with regard to all of these tests: (1) Are the key intermediate(s) in the assay under consideration the same reactive form(s) operative in the carcinogenic action of the chemical? and (2) Are the capabilities of the test cells and the various tissues of man to make and respond to the reactive metabolite(s) similar?

6. Test Procedures in the Detection of Carcinogenic Activity of Drugs

6.1. General Recommendations

Guidelines on the general principles for the detection of carcinogenicity and the evaluation of carcinogenic hazards have been outlined by several expert committees and others in the past decade [Food Protection Committee 1959; FAO/WHO Expert Committee 1961; Clayson 1962; Hueper and Conway 1964; Arcos et al. 1968; Weisburger and Weisburger 1968; WHO Scientific Committee 1969]. It has been generally agreed that the minimum requirements for a bioassay of carcinogenicity are as follows: biometrically adequate numbers of animals of at least two species and both sexes, with adequate controls, subjected for their lifetimes to a suitable dose range of the test compound including doses considerably higher than those proposed for or experienced by the human. In the following paragraphs specific aspects of such tests are considered as they would relate to the properties and uses of drugs of abuse.

In principle, tests on experimental animals which are to be used in the assessment of the carcinogenic hazard of a chemical for man should, as far as possible, simulate the conditions which might obtain during human exposure. This principle would determine that the compounds should be administered by the same routes (oral, subcutaneous, etc.) and in the same or similar vehicles, as those employed by the human subject. Likewise, in addition to tests on both male and female animals from weaning through adult life, consideration should also be given to special conditions of immaturity, pregnancy, diet, other drugs or exposures, etc. Further, if drugs are administered to pregnant animals, the young as well as the primary treated animals should be retained for lifetime examination. Neonatal animals may have special advantages in tests on drugs of abuse since they have exhibited high sensitivity to the action of several chemical carcinogens [Toth 1968; Della Porta and Terracini 1969]. Thus, in some cases where high pharmacologic activity may preclude prolonged testing of a drug of abuse, it is possible that administration to neonatal animals may permit more adequate tests than short-term administration to adult animals.

The possible effects of the use of more than one drug by some individuals is of particular importance in the present problem, since some drugs of abuse, for instance certain of the barbiturates, induce higher levels of various drug-metabolizing enzymes in the rodent liver and other tissues than occur normally. These altered enzyme activities may serve to either enhance or diminish the carcinogenic and other toxic properties of the same drug administered subsequently or of other drugs administered simultaneously or subsequently.

Dosage levels exceeding by a factor of from 10 to 1,000 times the probable human exposure level are generally employed in animal tests for carcinogenicity, and these doses are generally administered for the major share of the life span. The highest level would usually be one which will produce a minimal to moderate amount of short-term toxicity, but one which will permit most of the animals to survive for at least one year. At least one or two lower doses, which do not cause a large reduction in life span, are also recommended. Data on animals exposed to several dose levels help in the development of information on the relationship between tumor incidence and dose, if tumors occur. The high dose levels are *essential* to help to compensate for two major deficiencies in the feasible experimental designs. The first of these is the practical impossibility of using large enough groups of animals to detect, with statistical significance, increases in tumor incidences of less than a few percent over those of the negative controls. The second problem is the possibly extreme difference in the level of active forms of the carcinogen in the tissues of man and the experimental animal as a consequence of species differences in the transport and metabolism of the compound. The latter problem can also be approached by the use of several experimental species, and at least two, in the hope that at least one of them may approach man with respect to the extent of formation of ultimate carcinogenic forms from the compound administered. Metabolic studies of the test compounds in man and experimental animals and an attempt to match the metabolic patterns of man and the test animals should receive more consideration.

In view of the above considerations, it is clear that the experimental groups should be as large as possible, but practical considerations rarely permit the use of groups larger than, if as large as, 100 animals. It is critical that all animals be maintained for the major share of their life span. Furthermore, all animals should be subjected at death or upon termination of the experiment to careful gross and microscopic examination. Of equal importance is the maintenance at the same time of large groups of both negative and positive control animals. The animals should be randomized from the same source as the experimental groups, and they should receive identical treatment to that of the experimental groups except for the compound under test. This includes the administration of the same diet and application of the same amounts of the vehicles used for administration of the test compound. In the case of positive controls this vehicle would contain a compound known to be carcinogenic by the route administered. All of the control animals must receive comparable autopsies to those of the experimental groups.

6.2. Oral Administration

The oral route appears to be a major mode of entry of certain drugs of abuse into man. These materials should therefore be tested by oral application, and gastric intubation would appear to be the method of choice. This procedure permits accurate dosage and, by virtue of the pulse-dosing, probably approximates the human model of drug administration better than administration in the diet or drinking water. However, the latter procedures are convenient and may permit the testing of higher levels of drug. Diets containing test compounds should be made up frequently and stored in a manner to prevent rancidity or destruction of the test compound; drinking water containing test compounds should be changed daily. In all cases records should be kept at intervals of the consumption of drug, so that approximate total intakes of the test compound can be calculated.

The rat, mouse, and hamster have been most widely used in studies on the carcinogenicity of orally administered compounds; for this reason and because of their relatively short life spans they are probably the animals of choice for these and the following tests.

6.3. Inhalation

Drugs which are administered by inhalation or sniffing should ideally be tested for car-

cinogenic activity by these procedures. In practice, however, this ideal has been difficult to attain, since experimental animals cannot be forced to inhale in a manner comparable to that used by man in inhaling smoke from drug-containing cigarettes. Similarly, procedures of sniffing or snorting, akin to those used for the inhalation of amyl nitrite or certain solvent-containing products such as glues, have not been attained with small experimental animals.

The experimental models for administration of respiratory toxicants include exposure to gases or aerosols in closed chambers or intratracheal administration. The latter technique has generally been applied to such materials as dusts and hydrocarbons, and it would appear to be a reasonable model for any drug which might gain entry to the lungs in a finely suspended solid form. Adaptations of this model might permit the intratracheal administration of drugs to the lungs in gaseous form. Exposure to gases or aerosols in closed chambers may also be useful in the latter problem, but to attain similar exposures to those obtained on inhalation, much larger concentrations of the toxicant in the air would be necessary.

The products of incomplete combustion of many organic substances appear to contain carcinogenic hydrocarbons such as benzo(a)-pyrene. On this basis marijuana smoke would be expected to contain these combustion products. Thus it will be desirable to ascertain the carcinogenic potency of tars from the combustion of drugs of abuse that are smoked. Topical applications of the tars to the skin of mice may suffice for this purpose.

6.4. Intravenous Injection

Certain drugs of abuse are injected by their users into the peripheral circulation. The most satisfactory animal counterpart appears to be the injection of the drug into the tail vein of the rat or mouse. Such injections should be made in the same solvent(s) used for administration to human users and should be made repeatedly to simulate the exposure of a chronic user. The ear veins of the rabbit are also satisfactory for repeated intravenous injections, but there is little literature on the carcinogenicity of chemicals other than the polycyclic hydrocarbons and a few amines for this species.

6.5. Subcutaneous and Intramuscular Injection

Those drugs of abuse administered to humans in this manner should be tested by subcutaneous or intramuscular injection into animals. Subcutaneous injection, often including some intramuscular injection, has been widely used as an assay for carcinogenic activity, especially with rats, mice, and hamsters, and an extensive literature is available on the use of this assay system. While the tumors often develop at the site of injection, subcutaneous injections of carcinogens can also result in tumor induction in a wide spectrum of tissues. Both the tumors which develop at the injection site and those which arise at distant sites are important indicators of carcinogenic activity, but tumor induction only or largely at distant sites can be taken as preliminary evidence of the need for metabolic activation to a proximate carcinogenic form.

While rapid induction of a significant incidence of tumors at the site of injection of one or a few small doses of a compound appears to be unequivocal evidence for its carcinogenic activity, the development of low to moderate incidences of sarcomas with long latent periods as a consequence of many injections at the same site is more difficult to interpret. Thus, often-repeated injections into a subcutaneous site of aqueous or oily preparations may give rise to low to moderate incidences of sarcomas with long latent periods. Large numbers of comparably treated controls become especially important in these studies.

6.6. Other Routes

Other routes of administration of compounds to experimental animals have been used for specific purposes in carcinogenicity studies and may have some value in tests on the carcinogenicity of some drugs of abuse. Two of these methods are the intraperitoneal injection of aqueous or oily preparations, and the implantation of pellets of carcinogens or of threads impregnated with carcinogens into selected tissues. Topical application, especially to the skin of mice and rabbits, has received considerable study in the experimental laboratory, especially as a model for the two-stage (initiation and promotion) model of carcinogenesis.

6.7. Pathological Examinations

Regardless of the species, compound, or route of administration, pathological examination of all animals is of paramount importance. For this purpose it is essential that moribund animals or those with large tumors be killed, and that dead animals be removed for necropsy as soon as possible. All animals should receive complete necropsies, which include careful gross examination of the skin and its underlying structures, the mammary tissue, the organs of the abdominal, thoracic, and oral cavities, and the brain and its associated structures. All tumors or possible tumors, together with any suspected gross metastases, should be fixed and examined by a competent pathologist experienced with the species under study. The benign or malignant nature of each neoplasm should be determined, if possible. Control animals must receive comparable examinations in order that the significance of the tumors observed in the experimental groups can be ascertained.

6.8. Evaluation of the Experimental Data

Where moderate to high incidences of a given type of tumor are observed in treated experimental animals as compared to low incidences of the same type of tumor in the negative controls, the conclusion that the compound causes tumors to develop can be made with reasonable certainty, provided that the experimental design was adequate.

The more difficult problem is the question of whether or not low incidences of tumors at one or more sites are significantly different from the incidences of tumors at these sites in the control groups. As the margin between the incidences in the control and experimental groups is narrowed, the statistical significance of the observation with a given number of animals per group becomes less certain; or, conversely, larger experimental groups are needed to establish the significance of the result. Even if no tumors develop among the experimental animals or if the number of tumors in the control and experimental groups are equal, it cannot be stated that the compound is not carcinogenic. Rather, one can only conclude that the upper limit of the possible carcinogenic activity for the compound under question is that incidence which would have been statistically different from the control incidence under the conditions of the experiment. These statistical problems have received careful consideration by Mantel and Bryan [1961].

7. Evaluation of Carcinogenic Hazards of Drugs of Abuse for Man

On both moral and practical grounds the possible carcinogenic effects of chemicals to which humans might be exposed must be determined in experimental animals, generally in short-lived species. The extension of the results of these determinations to man appears reasonable on two grounds. First, it appears that despite a great variety of studies no significant aspect of the natural occurrence, induction, and properties of cancer in man appears to differ fundamentally from similar aspects of neoplasia in experimental animals with either short or long life spans. Second, some assurance of the general applicability of the tests can be derived from the fact that

the chemicals known to be carcinogenic in man also induce neoplasia in experimental animals; the only exception known is that certain arsenical compounds may have activity in man, but they have not exhibited carcinogenicity in the experimental animals studied. However, many clear differences in the activities of chemical carcinogens in various species exist, and the unpredictable occurrence of species differences is the principal limitation in the extrapolation of the results on experimental animals to man.

In order to minimize the species or metabolic differences that might exist between man and experimental animals in their responses to a given chemical compound, the tests for carcinogenicity must be conducted with dosages at the highest practical levels and in more than one test species. In the future, as knowledge of the mechanisms of chemical carcinogenesis increases, it may be possible by comparative metabolic experiments with tissue preparations from humans and experimental animals to select the proper species for the life-time test of a given chemical. However, at present the uncertainty in the extrapolation of experimental tests in chemical carcinogenesis to man makes it necessary to evaluate both positive and negative results in these tests with considerable caution.

Positive results on the carcinogenicity of a substance in one or more experimental species raise suspicion of a similar activity in man, and great prudence is indicated in the exposure of humans to such compounds. Despite the probable existence of noncarcinogenic dosage levels in the experimental species in which a compound is carcinogenic, there is no practical basis for the quantitative extrapolation of such data to man.

Of greater importance, from a practical standpoint, is the uncertainty in the safety of a substance not found to be carcinogenic in experimental species. The degree of this uncertainty must be judged for each compound on the basis of the stringency of the tests which indicate no carcinogenic hazard and the extent to which humans will be exposed to the compound in question.

Thus tests for carcinogenicity form a necessary part of the examination for safety of any substance to which humans are exposed. These tests become more urgent when large numbers of humans of all ages will be exposed for appreciable portions of their life spans; and they require the expert appraisal of each substance on its own merits on the basis of sound experimental data and a knowledge of its use.

8. Extant Data on the Carcinogenicity of Drugs of Abuse

No relevant studies on the carcinogenicity of the important drugs of abuse were revealed in a close search of the literature. There may be unpublished observations, but it seems un-likely that any useful information on the carcinogenicity of these drugs now exists. Some information is available on a few minor drugs of abuse. Thus, toxic solvents such as chloroform and carbon tetrachloride are hepatocarcinogenic in the mouse, and in-dustrial benzene inhalation is suspected of causing leukemia in the human [Clayson 1962; Hueper and Conway 1964].

9. Recommendations

Information on the carcinogenic risks which may be imposed on the human user of drugs of abuse and on her progeny should be avail-able. For this purpose priorities should be established as to the order of importance of these drugs with respect to determination of carcinogenicity, and those compounds for which the information is deemed most urgent should be tested as soon as possible. A major factor in the determination of the priorities should be the prevalency of use of the compound. Further, positive results in biological tests such as those for muta-

genicity or teratogenicity should also be given weight, since at least some compounds show activity in more than one of these tests.

Since the experiments on the administration of the drugs to humans are already under way, retrospective and prospective epidemiological studies on the incidences of neoplasms in persons who have subjected and will subject themselves to these compounds should be instigated. Statistically adequate studies of this nature are feasible and will be of in-estimable value in assessing the carcinogenic hazard of these drugs to man.

10. Summary

The chemical carcinogens comprise a large number of nonviral, nonradioactive low molecular-weight compounds capable of inducing neoplasms in a wide range of tissues in many animal species. These carcinogens encompass an extreme range of structures and include synthetic and naturally occurring or-ganic compounds and a number of inorganic compounds. While no common structural feature is evident, the active forms of the chemical carcinogens, usually formed meta-bolically, appear to be reactive electrophiles. These active forms attack nucleophilic centers in nucleic acids and proteins in vivo to yield covalently bound derivatives; where tested, electrophiles derived from carcino-genic agents are mutagenic. However, the molecular mechanism(s) of action of the chemical carcinogens are essentially un-known. Our knowledge of the metabolism of chemical carcinogens and of the means by which they induce tumors is not yet of significant predictive value in assessing the possible carcinogenicity of a chemical.

Much effort has been devoted to the de-velopment of tests for the detection of car-cinogenic activity of chemicals and to the interpretations of the results of these tests with respect to the risk for humans exposed to these chemicals. No generally applicable rapid test for carcinogenic activity is known. Lifetime tests of high dosage levels of chemicals in rats, mice, and hamsters appear to be the best procedures available. Many aspects of these tests require careful consideration with regard to such factors as positive and negative controls, uniformity of test animals, composition of diets, routes of administration, and dosage during pregnancy and infancy. Even with test groups of hundreds of animals, these tests are at best statistically capable of demonstrating increases of tumor incidence of not less than a few percent. Human tumor incidences well below this level from the use of a chemical would be catastrophic. The finding that a chemical is carcinogenic clearly calls for great prudence in its use in the human environment. The failure to detect carcinogenicity similarly calls for caution in the use of a chemical, because of the relative insensitivity of carcinogenicity tests and the uncertainties in the extrapolation of the results of animal tests to the human species.

Few data of value appear to exist on the carcinogenicity of the various drugs of abuse. Priorities should be established, and the most important of these drugs should be placed under test as soon as possible. Since the human experiments with these drugs are well under way, retrospective and prospective studies on the incidences of neoplasms in humans who have subjected and will subject themselves to these compounds should be instigated. Statistically adequate studies of this nature will be of inestimable value in assessing the carcinogenic hazard of the drugs of abuse.

References

Arcos, J., M. F. Argus, and G. Wolf (1968). *Chemical Induction of Cancer*, New York: Academic Press, vol. 1, part 2.

Clayson D. B. (1962). *Chemical Carcinogenesis*. Boston: Little, Brown.

Della Porta, G., and B. Terracini (1969). *Progr. Exp. Tumor Res.* 11:334.

FAO/WHO Expert Committee on Food Additives (1961). *Fifth Report. Evaluation of the Carcinogenic Hazards of Food Additives.* Geneva: World Health Organization, Technical Report Series No. 220.

Food Protection Committee, Food and Nutrition Board, National Academy of Sciences-National Research Council (1959). *Problems in the Evaluation of Carcinogenic Hazard from Use of Food Additives.* Washington, D.C.: National Academy of Sciences-National Research Council, Publication No. 749.

Grasso, P., and L. Golberg (1966). *Food Cosmet. Toxicol.* 4:297.

Higginson, J. (1969). *Canad. Cancer Conf.* 8:40.

Hueper, W. C., and W. D. Conway (1964). *Chemical Carcinogenesis and Cancers.* Springfield, Ill.: Thomas.

Klein, G. (1969). *Fed. Proc.* 28:1739.

Magee, P. N., and J. M. Barnes (1967). *Advan. Cancer Res.* 10:163.

Mantel, N., and W. R. Bryan (1961). *J Nat. Cancer Inst.* 27:455.

Miller, E. C., and J. A. Miller (1966). *Pharmacol. Rev.* 18:805.

Miller, J. A., and E. C. Miller (1965). *Cancer Res.* 25:1292.

——— (1969). In E. D. Bergmann and B. Pullman, eds., *Physico-Chemical Mechanisms of Carcinogenesis*, Jerusalem: Israel Academy of Sciences and Humanities, pp. 237–261.

Oettle, A. G. (1964). *J. Nat. Cancer Inst.* 33:383.

Toth, B. (1968). *Cancer Res.* 28:727.

Weisburger, J. H., and E. K. Weisburger (1968). In H. Busch, ed., *Methods in Cancer Research*. New York: Academic Press, vol. 1, pp. 307–398.

WHO Scientific Group (1969). *Principles for the Testing and Evaluation of Drugs for Carcinogenicity*. Geneva: World Health Organization, Technical Report Series No. 426.

6 Teratogenic Hazards

H. Kalter

The threat of teratogenesis posed by our continued and increasing exposure to man-made chemical substances pervading our environment is real. The problem is to estimate the nature and extent of the threat, so that apprehensions may be justified or fears allayed, and to develop appropriate action to curtail the use of dangerous substances or continue enjoying the benefits of safer ones.

The potential teratogenicity of chemicals may be gauged by administering them to appropriate test animals to determine whether under various conditions they may cause prenatal damage; and by surveying human populations to detect geographical or temporal aggregations of unusual types or frequencies of congenital malformations. Neither of these avenues can ensure success in preventing or in the early detection of congenital malformations produced in human populations by external agents, but together they may perhaps be quite efficient for the purpose.

1. Definition

Before briefly reviewing what is presently known of the teratogenic effects of psychoactive drugs in mammals, the definition of the term *congenital malformations* should be clarified. As used here in application to experimental animals, the term means gross structural abnormalities of prenatal origin present at or near birth and recognizable with the unaided senses or detectable by conventional methods of examination. Other definitions have been suggested, especially with reference to human subjects, which would include histological, metabolic, and even molecular defects; but for various reasons these are considered by the author to be impractical or erroneous [Kalter 1968].

2. Literature Review

The teratogenic and reproductive effects of quite a large number of psychoactive drugs have been investigated in laboratory mammals.

The results of many of these studies are summarized in the table on pp. 96–109, which should be consulted for references to specific substances.

Probably none of the psychoactive drugs or the so-called drugs of abuse has received as much publicity or has been so feared as LSD. The controversy over its potential harmfulness has reached into the levels of research, where a number of investigators reported it to be teratogenic while others reported it to be nonteratogenic. Various studies with rats were negative (see table) ; the word "abnormalities" in the title of Alexander et al.'s [1967] paper is misleading since, although a few offspring were still-born, no congenital malformations were reported.

Three LSD experiments have been made with mice. Auerbach and Rugowski [1967] reported a relatively high frequency of brain defects in offspring examined at an early stage of gestation ; Hanaway [1969] found apparent abnormalities only of the lens ; and DiPaolo et al. [1968] noted facial anomalies, which also occurred in controls, but at a lower percentage. Geber's [1967] work with hamsters is somewhat difficult to evaluate since the data were not clearly presented ; some malformed embryos were noted, but these results were unsupported by DiPaolo et al.'s [1968] hamster study. Some other hallucinogens, such as α-methyltryptamine, 2-bromo LSD, and mescaline, were reported to be teratogenic, but psilocin was not. Marihuana resin or extract was not terato-genic in mice, but it produced small to moderate frequencies of various malformations in rats, rabbits, and hamsters.

Amphetamines produced cardiac and other malformations in mice in some studies, but they seemed to be without effect in others. Various barbiturates apparently produced no or very few anomalies, except in one study.

The effects of numerous tranquilizers on reproductive functions, including terato-genesis, have been reported. The pheno-thiazine-derivative prochlorperazine was found teratogenic in some cases but not in others ; and chlorpromazine and related sub-stances were apparently ineffective. The Rauwolfia products reserpine and deserpidine produced no malformations except in two studies. Other tranquilizers found nonterato-genic in all but scattered instances were meprobamate, chlordiazepoxide, valnoct-amide, trifluperidol, haloperidol, fluphenazine, and flupenthixol.

The hypnotics glutethimide, methaqualone, and ethinamate produced no or relatively low frequencies of malformations. The anti-depressants imipramine, pipradol, methyl-phenidate, and pemoline were nonterato-genic except for a few possible sporadic instances, as were a large number of MAO-inhibiting antidepressants tested. Finally, morphine and nitrous oxide were teratogenic.

3. Problems in Interpretation

It cannot be emphasized too strongly that these experimental results are difficult to interpret so far as human beings are con-cerned. The data are sparse and fragmentary ; the species and strains of animals used were varied ; the numerous experimental conditions employed were diverse. That the results were sometimes contradictory is therefore not sur-prising. But of greater moment is that even had these studies been conducted under ideal and uniform conditions, as these were con-ceived of until recently, it would still be difficult to apply their results directly to human beings ; since facts and ideas have only relatively of late been uncovered or con-sidered that are important for teratology testing—such as the significance of the relation between the administered dose of a substance and its plasma levels and those of its active metabolites, for understanding species variation in drug response ; and the prevalence of various types of metabolic interactions and their importance for estimating the possible prenatal consequences of human exposure to environmental agents and contaminants. Taking such factors into account may make it possible to design more meaningful teratology-testing procedures.

4. Pitfalls

Before these methods are summarized the following should be stated. Individuals planning how the possible teratogenic effects of drugs may be detected in human beings should be aware of some lessons learned from experimental teratology about the pitfalls involved in interpreting their observations, whether positive or negative.

Many conditions must be met in order for agents to produce malformations. Some of these concern dose, mode of administration, gestation period, genotype, metabolic transformation and interaction, and various other less obvious parameters. For example, teratogenic agents malform only at a certain dose range, below which development is apparently undisturbed and above which embryonic or even maternal death results. The route by which an agent enters the body may sometimes determine whether it has an effect or not, or its degree of effect. Most agents are teratogenic only during the developmentally labile early period of gestation, when the embryo is being shaped and embryonic organs and tissues are first being formed. In human beings this period roughly extends from the end of the first week of pregnancy to the twelfth week. Vast differences in frequency, type, and severity of malformations may be owing to genetic factors, which may be of both embryonic and parental origin. Innocuous substances may be metabolically transformed into teratogenic ones; and the action of teratogens may be modified by concomitant events and experiences, or by chronic or intermittent rather than transient

exposure. Finally animal studies indicate that many other situations may influence the effectiveness of teratogens, including maternal nutritional, physiological, and disease states; socioeconomic circumstances and cultural practices; demographic patterns; and temporal and seasonal factors.

Thus, only when a set of facilitating conditions exists will a potentially teratogenic agent be enabled to manifest its effects: only when factors including effective dose, susceptible genotype, and responsive developmental period conjoin will the prenatal organism be irreversibly damaged. It is to be deduced, therefore, that establishing the teratogenicity of a substance for human beings will not be straightforward because, fortunately, all instances of exposure of pregnant women to it will not lead to deformity, since in some cases one or another of the necessary ingredients will be lacking.

There are still other difficulties. Thus, if defects are produced by a teratogenic substance the connection between the agent and its consequences may not easily be recognized, because one and the same agent may produce numerous types of defects, singly or combined; and any one type of defect may be caused by various agents. Further complications may be introduced by the fact that rare induced defects may be indistinguishable from more common sporadic defects.

Therefore it is reasonable to conjecture that if thalidomide had not caused a syndrome of malformations that was previously quite unusual, but had merely increased the frequency of an already rather prevalent defect, the relation between agent and malformation might have been much more slowly realized or possibly not realized yet. Finally, there is no doubt that only a fraction of the pregnant women who took thalidomide had defective children, and that in all the others some necessary conditions were missing.

Table 1. Teratogenic Hazards of Drugs of Abuse

Drug	Author(s)	Species	Stock, strain, or breed	Dose (mg/kg/day)	Route of administration[1]
Amphetamine	Bovet-Nitti and Bovet 1959	Rat	?	10	im
Amphetamine sulfate	Yasuda et al. 1965	Mouse	ICR-JCL	50	po
Barbital Na	Champakamalini and Rao 1967	Rat	Wistar	200	sc
Barbital Na	Persaud 1965	Rat	Potsdam	25–100	ip
Barbital Na	Persaud and Henderson 1969	Mouse	Rockefeller	65–330	ip
Barbital Na	Persaud and Henderson 1969	Rabbit	?	50, 200	iv
Chlordiazepoxide	Takano et al. 1963	Mouse	Japanese stock	?	ip
Chlordiazepoxide	Zbinden et al. 1961	Rat	CFN	20, 80	po
Chlorpromazine	Brock and Kreybig 1964	Rat	Wistar, BDII	10	ip
Chlorpromazine	Bovet-Nitti and Bovet 1959	Rat	?	20	im
Chlorpromazine	Chambon 1955	Rat	Commentry	30	sc
Chlorpromazine	Courrier and Marois 1953	Rat	?	10	sc
Chlorpromazine	Goldman and Yakovac 1964	Rat	Sprague-Dawley	2	im
Chlorpromazine	Hoffeld and Webster 1965	Rat	Sprague-Dawley	6	sc
Chlorpromazine	Hoffeld et al. 1967, 1968	Rat	Sprague-Dawley	6	sc
Chlorpromazine	Jewett and Norton 1966	Rat	Sprague-Dawley	6	sc
Chlorpromazine	Murai 1966	Rat	?	6	sc
Chlorpromazine	Murphree et al. 1962	Rat	Sprague-Dawley	5	sc
Chlorpromazine	Ordy et al. 1963, 1966	Mouse	C57BL/10	4, 16	po
Chlorpromazine	Roizin et al. 1959	Rat	?	12.5	sc
Chlorpromazine	Werboff and Kesner 1963	Rat	Sprague-Dawley	6	sc
Chlorpromazine	West 1964	Rat	?	30	?
Deserpidine	Tuchmann-Duplessis and Mercier-Parot 1961	Rat	Wistar	0.3, 0.45	? a

Day(s) of gestation treated[2]	Time offspring observed[3]	Effects		Comments
		Malformations	Other	
5	Term	None	None	
Throughout	19	None attributable to treatment	Fetal death	
9–20	21	None mentioned	Reduced fertility, fetal death, reduced fetal weight	
3, 4, 5, 8, or 12	?	None attributable to treatment	None	
2–7	19	60%, CNS,[4] limb, etc.	Fetal death	
1–10 or 10	?	None	None	
10	18	None mentioned		
Throughout	Term	None		
4	13	38%, CNS, etc., in BDII; not increased in Wistar		
5	Term	None mentioned	Abortion, fetal death	
For 3 days during 6–13	Term	None	Abortion, stillbirth, reduced fetal size	
8–15	Several days after treatment	None mentioned		
10	20	None		
5–8, 11–14, or 17–20	Postnatal	None mentioned	Behavior affected by early and midgestation treatment	
5–8, 11–14, or 17–20	Postnatal	None mentioned	Behavioral changes	Different test used than by Hoffeld and Webster 1965
4–7	Term and postnatal	None apparently found	Stillbirth, altered behavior, transient weight decrease	
5–8 or 17–20	Postnatal	None mentioned	Behavioral changes after early treatment	
Throughout	Term and postnatal	None mentioned	Reduced postnatal survival	
Throughout	Term and postnatal	None mentioned	Reduced litter size and fetal weight; reduced postnatal survival; liver and serum biochemical changes; behavioral changes	
Months	Term	None mentioned	Reduced litter size, stillbirth	
5–8, 11–14, or 17–20	Postnatal	None mentioned		
Throughout	20	None mentioned	Fetal death	
6–16	20 or term	6%, limb, tail, etc.	Abortion, fetal death, reduced fetal size	Effects produced by higher dosage only

Table 1. Teratogenic Hazards of Drugs of Abuse (continued)

Drug	Author(s)	Species	Stock, strain, or breed	Dose (mg/kg/day)	Route of administration[1]
Dexamphetamine sulfate	Nora et al. 1965	Mouse	A/J	50	ip
Dexamphetamine sulfate	Nora et al. 1968	Mouse	A/J, C57BL/6	50	ip
Dexamphetamine sulfate	Paget 1965	Rabbit	N.Z. White	up to 10	?
Ethinamate	Takano et al. 1963	Mouse	Japanese colony	400	ip
Flupenthixol	Spieth and Lorenz 1967	Rat	?	1–3	po
Fluphenazine	Spieth and Lorenz 1967	Rat	?	2	po
Glutethimide	McColl et al. 1963	Rat	Sprague-Dawley	(0.4%, in feed)	po
Glutethimide	McColl et al. 1967	Rabbit	Mixed	150	po
Glutethimide	Takano et al. 1963	Mouse	Japanese colony	100, 300	po, ip
Glutethimide	Tuchmann-Duplessis and Mercier-Parot 1963a	Rat	Wistar	50–500	po
Glutethimide	Tuchmann-Duplessis and Mercier-Parot 1963a	Mouse	Swiss albino	50–500	po
Glutethimide	Tuchmann-Duplessis and Mercier-Parot 1963a,b	Rabbit	Commercial	100–400	parenteral, po
Haloperidol	Tuchmann-Duplessis and Mercier-Parot 1967	Rat	Wistar	2.5–10	parenteral, po
Haloperidol	Vichi 1969	Rat	Wistar	0.1–4	im
Haloperidol	Vichi 1969	Mouse	Swiss	0.05–0.4	im
Harmaline HCl	Poulson and Robson 1963	Mouse	Guy's Hospital	0.4, 0.8	sc
Heptylhydrazine	Poulson and Robson 1963	Mouse	Guy's Hospital	0.5	sc

Day(s) of gestation treated[2]	Time offspring observed[3]	Effects		Comments
		Malformations	Other	
9	17–18	12%, cardiac; increased frequency of defects also occurring in controls	Fetal death	
9	17–18	11–13%, cardiac	Fetal death	Strain-specific cardiac defects
?	?	None		
10	8	4%, ?	Fetal death	
From 9 days before mating, throughout	Term	None		
From 9 days before mating, throughout	Term	None		
From 3 days before mating, throughout	Term	?% (low), axial skeleton	Stillbirth	
8–16	29 or term	None	None	
8–14 or 10	18	16%, ?	Fetal death	Only ip route effective
1–14 or 6–14	Near term	None	Reduced fertility	
6–14	Near term	None	Reduced fertility, fetal death	
6–12 or 8–14	20–26	None	Reduced fertility, fetal death	
1–12, 6–12, or 8–14	18, 20, and term	None	Retarded implantation	
Various, during week 2	21	None attributable to treatment		
Various, during week 2	19	Up to 53%, cleft palate, etc.	Fetal death	
1–6, 6–11, or 11–16	14, 18	None		
1–6, 6–11, or 11–16	14, 18	None		

Table 1. Teratogenic Hazards of Drugs of Abuse (continued)

Drug	Author(s)	Species	Stock, strain, or breed	Dose (mg/kg/day)	Route of administration[1]
Hexobarbital	Persaud 1965	Rat	Potsdam	50, 100	ip
HP 1275	Spector 1960	Rat	Wistar	(0.1–0.5 mg/ml, in drinking water)	po
HP 1275	Spector 1960	Mouse	?	(0.1–0.5 mg/ml, in drinking water)	po
HP 1325	Poulson and Robson 1963	Mouse	Guy's Hospital	2, 5	sc, po
Imipramine	Harper et al. 1965	Rat	Sprague-Dawley	5, 15	po
Imipramine	Harper et al. 1965	Mouse	Outbred	10–150	sc, po
Imipramine	Harper et al. 1965	Rabbit	N.Z. White	5–30	sc, po
Imipramine	Robson and Sullivan 1963	Rabbit	?	5–30	sc
Imipramine HCl imipramine-*N*-oxide HCl	Larsen 1963	Rabibt	Danish White	15, 25	sc
Iproclizide	Lauro et al. 1966	Rat	Chester Beatty	60, 120	po
Iproniazid	Poulson et al. 1960	Mouse	?	5–10	sc
Iproniazid	Poulson and Robson 1963	Mouse	Guy's Hospital	5–10	sc
Iproniazid	Werboff et al. 1961a	Rat	Sprague-Dawley	10–50	ip
Iproniazid	Werboff et al. 1961b	Rat	Sprague-Dawley	2–8	ip
Isocarboxazid	Takano et al. 1963	Mouse	Japanese stock	100	ip
Isocarboxazid	Werboff et al. 1961b	Rat	Sprague-Dawley	1–4	ip
LSD (Sandoz)	Alexander et al. 1967	Rat	Wistar	0.005	sc
Delysid (Sandoz) lot 65002	Auerbach and Rugowski 1967	Mouse	C57BL/6; C3H; BALB/c; and hybrid	ca. 0.04	ip

Day(s) of gestation treated[2]	Time offspring observed[3]	Effects — Malformations	Effects — Other	Comments
3, 4, 5, 8, or 12	?	None attributable to treatment	None	
Throughout	?	None	Reduced fertility	
Throughout	?	None	Reduced fertility	
1–6, 4–7, 6–11, or 11–16	14, 18	None	Implantation apparently prevented	
From 60 days before breeding, throughout	Term and weaning	None	Reduced litter size; reduced survival to weaning	No dose-response relation to postnatal survival
6–17	18	None attributable to treatment		
7–17	28–30	7%. CNS, kidney, etc.	Fetal death, reduced fetal weight	
1–13, 1–17 or 1–20	20, 29	?%, 3 grossly malformed	Fetal death	
3–18	Term, near term	2%, tail, kidney		
2—6, 7–11, or 12–16; or 7,8, or 9	Near term	None	Fetal death	.
1–6, 3–8, 6—11, or 11–16	7, 9, 12, 17	None mentioned	Implantation perhaps prevented	
1–6, 4–7, 6–11, or 11–16	9, 13, 18	None	Implantation apparently prevented	
8–14	Postnatal	None mentioned	Reduced litter size and birth weight, stillbirth, postnatal death	
5–8, 11–14, or 17–20	Postnatal	None mentioned	Fetal death, pregnancy interruption, reduced number weaned, behavioral changes	No dose-response relation
10	18	None mentioned	Fetal death	
5–8, 11–14, or 17–20	Postnatal	None mentioned	Behavioral changes	
4, 7, 8, 10, 13, or 16	Term	None	Reduced litter size; still-birth	
7, 8, 9, or 10	12	44%, CNS, etc., after day 7 or 8 treatment		Poor dose-response relation, 10% malformations in controls. (Malformations difficult to diagnose in early gestation)

Table 1. Teratogenic Hazards of Drugs of Abuse (continued)

Drug	Author(s)	Species	Stock, strain, or breed	Dose (mg/kg/day)	Route of administration[1]
Delysid (Sandoz) lot 65002	DiPaolo et al. 1968	Mouse	A/Cum, NIH	(0.016–1.2 mg, total/mouse)	ip
Delysid (Sandoz) lot 65002	DiPaolo et al. 1968	Hamster	NIH	0.08–2.5	ip
Delysid (Sandoz) lot 65002	Warkany and Takacs 1967	Rat	Wistar	0.0016–0.4	ip, po
LSD	Fabro and Sieber 1968	Rabbit	N.Z. White	0.02 or 0.1	po
2-Bromo-LSD	Geber 1967	Hamster	Lakeview	0.002–0.41	sc
LSD	Geber 1967	Hamster	Lakeview	0.0008–0.25	ip
LSD-25	Hanaway 1969	Mouse	Swiss-Webster	0.0125	ip
LSD	West 1962	Rat	?	1	ip
Marihuana extract, 2 geographic samples	Geber and Schramm 1969	Hamster	Lakeview	25–300	sc
Marihuana extract, 2 geographic samples	Geber and Schramm 1969	Rabbit	N.Z. White	130–500	sc
Marihuana resin	Persaud and Ellington 1967	Rat	?	4.2	ip
Marihuana resin	Persaud and Ellington 1967	Mouse	?	16	ip
Meprobamate	Bertrand 1960	Rat	Wistar	100, 250, 500	po
Meprobamate	Brar 1969	Mouse	Charles River	180–280	po
Meprobamate	Caldwell and Spille 1964	Rat	Wistar	32, 64, 128	po
Meprobamate	Clavert 1963	Mouse	Mixed	200, 400	sc
Meprobamate	Clavert 1963	Rabbit	Mixed	100–400	sc, po
Meprobamate	Hoffeld and Webster 1965	Rat	Sprague-Dawley	60	sc
Meprobamate	Hoffeld et al. 1967, 1968	Rat	Sprague-Dawley	60	sc
Meprobamate	Kletzkin et al. 1965	Rat	?	60	sc
Meprobamate	Murai 1966	Rat	?	60	sc
Meprobamate	Nishikawa 1963	Mouse	dd	100–750	sc
Meprobamate	Werboff and Kesner 1963	Rat	Sprague-Dawley	60	sc

Day(s) of gestation treated[2]	Time offspring observed[3]	Effects		Comments
		Malformations	Other	
7, 8, 9, or 10; or multiple	11 or 14	19%, facial, in A/Cum; none in NIH		3% facial defects in A/Cum controls
6, 7, or 8; or 7, 8, and 9	14	None attributable to treatment		
4, 5, 7, 8, or 9; or 7–12	21 or term	None attributable to treatment		
4–7, 7–9, or 8–12	23	None		
8	12	8%, CNS	Fetal death	No dose-response relation for malformations
8	12	6%, CNS	Fetal death	No dose-response relation for malformations
4, 5, 6, 7, 8, or 9	18	None external; 67%, lens, after day 6 or later treatment		
Throughout	?	Apparently none		
6, 7, or 8	12 or 13	3–9%, CNS, limb, umbilical hernia		
7–10	16 or 17	5–33%, CNS, limb, umbilical hernia	Fetal death at highest dosages	Samples different in degree of embryotoxicity
1–6	20	?% (high), limb, umbilical hernia	Fetal death, reduced fetal size	
6 or 1–6	?	None	Reduced fertility	
Throughout	24	None	Fetal death	
From 4 months before mating, throughout	Term or postnatal	None	None	
Throughout	Postnatal	None mentioned	None	
6–12	16	None attributable to treatment	None mentioned	
6–10, 10–14, 15–19, or 8–19	20 or 28	None attributable to treatment	Fetal death	
5–8, 11–14, or 17–20	Postnatal	None mentioned	Reduced offspring weight	
5–8, 11–14, or 17–20	Postnatal	None mentioned	Behavior changes	Different test used than by Hoffeld and Webster 1965
5–9, 10–14, or 14–18	Postnatal	None mentioned	None	
5–8, or 17–20	Postnatal	None mentioned	Behavioral changes	
8, 10, 12, or 14	19	Up to 44%, limbs, etc.	Fetal death	
5–8, 11–14, or 17–20	Postnatal	None mentioned	Behavioral changes	

Table 1. Teratogenic Hazards of Drugs of Abuse (continued)

Drug	Author(s)	Species	Stock, strain, or breed	Dose (mg/kg/day)	Route of administra- tion[1]
Mescaline	Geber 1967	Hamster	Lakeview	0.45–3.25	sc
Methaqualone	Bough et al. 1963	Rat	?	25–100	po
Methaqualone	Bough et al. 1963	Rabbit	N.Z. White, California	100–400	po
Methaqualone	McColl et al. 1963	Rat	Sprague-Dawley	(0.8%, in diet)	po
Methaqualone	McColl et al. 1967	Rabbit	Mixed	100	po
Methaqualone	Szirmai 1966	Rat	Wistar	200	ip
Methaqualone	Takano et al. 1963	Mouse	Japanese stock	150	ip
Methylphenidate	Takano et al. 1963	Mouse	Japanese colony	200	ip
α-Methyltryptamine	Yakovleva and Sorokina 1966	Rat	?	5–40	?
MO 911	Poulson and Robson 1963	Mouse	Guy's Hospital	2	sc
Morphine sulfate	Harpel and Gautieri 1968	Mouse	CF–1	100–500	sc
Nialamide	Poulson and Robson 1963	Mouse	Guy's Hospital	4	sc
Nialamide	Tuchmann- Duplessis and Mercier-Parot 1961b	Rat	Wistar	80	po
Nitromethaqualone	Szirmai 1966	Rat	Wistar	300	ip
Nitrous oxide	Fink et al. 1967	Rat	Sprague-Dawley	45–50%	Inhalation
Pemoline	Takano et al. 1963	Mouse	Japanese colony	10	ip
Pentobarbital Na	Goldman and Yakovac 1964	Rat	Sprague-Dawley	40	im
Pentobarbital Na	Setälä and Nyyssönen 1964	Mouse	RA	ca. 50–60	ip
Phenelzine	Poulson and Robson 1964	Mouse	Guy's Hospital	25	sc
Phenelzine derivatives	Poulson and Robson 1964	Mouse	Guy's Hospital	5–250	sc, po
Phenelzine derivatives WL 27	Poulson and Robson 1964	Rabbit	Guy's Hospital	10, 20	sc

Day(s) of gestation treated[2]	Time offspring observed[3]	Effects		Comments
		Malformations	Other	
8	12	17%, CNS	Fetal death	No dose-response relation for malformations
1–20	21	4%, cleft palate, etc.	Fetal death	Only highest dosages effective
8–15, 8–16, or 1–29	Near term	None attributable to treatment		
From 3 days before mating, throughout	Term	None	Stillbirth	
8–16	29 or term	None		
4	13	2%, ?		
10	18	7%, ?	Fetal death	
10	18	None mentioned	Fetal death	
1, 2, or 3 days during 4–13; or 2–21 or 3–18	?	ca. 5–8%, skeleton, etc.		
1–6 or 11–16	14, 18	None		
9 or 10	19	6%, CNS, day 9; 24%, axial skeleton; day 10	Fetal death	
1–6, 6–11, or 11–16	14, term	None	Implantation apparently prevented	
For 2 or 4 months before breeding, throughout	Term	None		
4	13	None		
9–11, 9–13, or 9–15	21	Up to 42%, skeleton	Fetal death	
10	18	None mentioned	Fetal death	
10	20	None	None	
1–4, or 1–15	Term	?%, head, limb	Reduced fertility, stillbirth	Data not presented
1–6	14	None mentioned	Fetal death, implantation probably prevented	Antifertility effect probably not due to MAO inhibition
1–3, 1–6, 6–11, or 11–16	14, 18	None	Implantation probably prevented	Antifertility effect probably not due to MAO inhibition
4–6 or 7–11	30	1/4, head, limbs		

Table 1. Teratogenic Hazards of Drugs of Abuse (continued)

Drug	Author(s)	Species	Stock, strain, or breed	Dose (mg/kg/day)	Route of administration[1]
Phenobarbital	McColl et al. 1963	Rat	Sprague-Dawley	(0.16%, in feed)	po
Phenobarbital	McColl et al. 1967	Rabbit	Mixed	50	po
Phenobarbital	Murai 1966	Rat	?	5	sc
Phenobarbital	Olivecrona 1964	Mouse	NMRI	1–4	ip
Pipradol	Takano et al. 1963	Mouse	Japanese colony	?	ip
Prochlorperazine	Roizin et al. 1966	Rat	Sprague-Dawley	10	iv
Prochlorperazine	Roux 1959	Rat	Wistar	ca. 10–80	parenteral, po
Prochlorperazine	Roux 1959	Mouse	?	ca. 40	po
Prochlorperazine	Takano et al. 1963	Mouse	Japanese stock	100	ip
Prochlorperazine	Vichi 1969	Rat	Wistar	2–10	im
Prochlorperazine	Vichi 1969	Mouse	Swiss	0.2–1	im
Promazine	Murphree et al. 1962	Rat	Sprague-Dawley	5	sc
Psilocin	Rolsten 1967	Mouse	C57BL/10	25	po
Reserpine	Arnaud 1963	Rabbit	?	ca. 0.1	parenteral
Reserpine	Bovet-Nitti and Bovet 1959	Rat	?	0.5	im
Reserpine	Gaunt et al. 1954	Rat	?	0.05	sc
Reserpine	Goldman and Yakovac 1965	Rat	Sprague-Dawley	0.1–1.5	im
Reserpine	Hoffeld and Webster 1965	Rat	Sprague-Dawley	0.1	sc
Reserpine	Hoffeld et al. 1967, 1968	Rat	Sprague-Dawley	0.1	sc
Reserpine	Jewett and Norton 1966	Rat	Sprague-Dawley	0.1	sc
Reserpine	Kehl et al. 1956	Rabbit	?	0.15–0.2	im po
Reserpine	Murai 1966	Rat	?	0.1	sc
Reserpine	Tuchmann-Duplessis and Mercier-Parot 1956	Rat	Wistar	ca. 0.25	sc
Reserpine	Werboff et al. 1961	Rat	Sprague-Dawley	0.1	ip
Reserpine	Werboff and Kesner 1963	Rat	Sprague-Dawley	0.1	sc

Day(s) of gestation treated[2]	Time offspring observed[3]	Effects		Comments
		Malformations	Other	
From 3 days before mating, throughout	Term	None	Reduced litter size	
8–16	29 or term	?%, skeleton, cardiac	Fetal death	
5–8 or 17–20	Postnatal	None mentioned	Behavioral changes, after earlier treatment	
During 5–14	18	None	Reduced fertility	
10	118	None mentioned		
Various	?	?%, eye		
Various	?	Total, 3%, CNS, etc.; 12%, cleft palate, day 13	Fetal death, abortion	
Various	?	?% (low), CNS, etc.	Fetal death	
10	18	None	Fetal death	
13 or 12–14	21	None attributable to treatment	Reduced litter size	
13 or 12–14	19	39%, cleft palate	Fetal death	
Throughout	Term and postnatal	None mentioned		
Throughout	Term	None mentioned		
1–30, 11–30, or 21–30	Term	None mentioned		
5	Term	None mentioned	Abortion, fetal death	
Continuous up to 21 weeks	Term	None mentioned	Reduced litter size and offspring weight	
9 or 10	20	Total, 4%, CNS, eye, etc.	Fetal death	
5–8, 11–14, or 17–20	Postnatal	None mentioned		
5–8, 11–14, or 17–20	Postnatal	None mentioned	Behavioral changes	Different test used than by Hoffeld and Webster 1965
4–7	Term and postnatal	None, apparently		
2–13, 9–19, or 20–27	Term	None mentioned	Implantation prevented, fetal death	
5–8 or 17–20	Postnatal	None mentioned	Behavioral changes, after early treatment	
1–10, 3–12, or 6–12	20 or term	None	Abortion	
8–14	Postnatal	None mentioned	Fetal death, behavioral changes	
5–8, 11–14, or 17–20	Postnatal	None mentioned		

Table 1. Teratogenic Hazards of Drugs of Abuse (continued)

Drug	Author(s)	Species	Stock, strain, of breed	Dose (mg/kg/day)	Route of administration[1]
Reserpine	West 1962, 1964	Rat	?	0.1–1	ip
Thiopental	Persaud 1965	Rat	Potsdam	50, 100	ip
Thiopental Na	Tanimura et al. 1967	Mouse	ICR-JCL	25–100	ip
Thioridizine	Murphree et al. 1962	Rat	Sprague-Dawley	5	sc
Tranylcypromine	Poulson and Robson 1963	Mouse	Guy's Hospital	0.1, 0.2	sc
Trifluperidol	Vichi 1969	Rat	Swiss	0.05–0.8	im
Valnoctamide	Tuchmann-Duplessis and Mercier-Parot 1965	Rat	Wistar	100–300	po
Valnoctamide	Tuchmann-Duplessis and Mercier-Parot 1965	Mouse	Swiss albino	100–400	po
Valnoctamide	Tuchmann-Duplessis and Mercier-Parot 1965	Rabbit	?	100–400	po

[1] im, intramuscular; ip, intraperitoneal; iv, intravenous; po, oral; sc, subcutaneous
[2] Day following that on which sexes put together, or day vaginal plugs or sperm in vaginal smear noted, called day 1 of gestation; where possible other systems were converted to this one. In some cases the system of denoting gestation time was not stated

Day(s) of gestation treated[2]	Time offspring observed[3]	Effects		Comments
		Malformations	Other	
Throughout	20	None mentioned	Fetal death	
3, 4, 5, 8, or 12	?	None attributable to treatment	None	
12	19	None	Fetal death, reduced fetal weight	
Throughout	Term and postnatal	None mentioned		
1–6, 4–7, 6–11, or 11–16	14, 18	None		
9–11 or 10–13	19	Up to 91%, cleft palate		
1–12, 6–12, or 7–9	Near term	None		
1–12, 6–12, or 6–8	Near term	None attributable to treatment		
6–8, 6–9, 6–12, or 7–9	Near term	None attributable to treatment		

[3] Time during gestation, at near term, or postnatal
[4] Central nervous system

5. Recommendations

It is recommended that before being released for public use all drugs and other substances to which the public may be exposed be tested for possible teratogenic effects in animals. For this purpose, the following protocol should be followed.

First of all, agents to be tested must be pure and stable, and when necessary they should simulate the products to which human beings are currently exposed. The dosages used should be based on the amount necessary to produce serum levels comparable to the ranges found in human beings after exposure to typical quantities of these substances. Multiples of this amount up to the maternal LD_{50} should be administered to determine the lowest dosage causing 100 percent fetal death, the highest causing no increased fetal mortality, and dosages between those two levels possibly producing significant frequencies of malformation. West [1964] tested over 40 drugs and found by charting the relation between fetal and maternal mortality that they fell into three categories: those giving a horizontal line, i.e., killing pregnant animals before being lethal to fetuses; those giving a steep line, i.e., killing all fetuses before being lethal to pregnant animals; and those giving a gentle slope, i.e., not killing pregnant animals and lethal only to some fetuses. It is of course in the last category that worrisome teratogenic drugs may be found. Wilson [1968] noted that of 27 drugs for which data were available, 63 percent killed all fetuses at one-eighth, or greater than, the maternal LD_{50} dosage, and 74 percent killed all fetuses at one-sixteenth, or more than, this dosage.

In order to establish the substance's dosage-serum level relations, half life, and fetal-tissue concentrations, as well as for testing its teratogenicity, it should be administered intravenously. Other parenteral routes are permissible, but they may be less favorable.

If oral administration is necessary at some stage of the testing, the substance should be given via gastric tube in an inert carrier. In the latter case food and water should be withheld for an hour before administration of the substance.

Treatment should consist of administering the substance as few times as possible to evoke teratogenicity. Ideally a single dose should be given. If this proves ineffective it must be repeated, but at no greater than daily intervals, and at lesser intervals if feasible. One purpose of this procedure is to minimize the possibility of inducing hepatic microsomal or other enzymes facilitating metabolism of the substance, by overexposure to it.

The substance should be administered, at discrete times, over the entire organogenetic period of prenatal life, since substances failing to affect development at some of these times may do so at others. At least two mammalian species should be used, and they should be chosen on the basis of similarity to human beings in pharmacokinetic and metabolic responses to the substance.

Standardized procedures should be used for animal breeding, housing, handling, feeding, etc.; for examining fetuses for congenital malformations; for defining time during pregnancy and nomenclature of congenital malformations; etc. Numbers of pregnant animals and offspring must be adequate for satisfactory statistical analysis. The study should be done again after a suitable period to establish repeatability. Appropriate controls must be collected contemporaneously with the experimental groups.

6. Summary

Quite a few teratological studies have been made in mammals with a wide variety of psychoactive drugs. This work has indicated that such drugs can cause structural abnormalities in embryos, and cautions us that similar phenomena are possible in human beings. In order to guard against such possibilities it is necessary to determine the teratogenic potential of substances by the best available procedures. A brief idea of what such tests should comprise is outlined in this chapter.

References

Alexander, G. J., B. E. Miles, G. M. Gold, and B. R. Alexander (1967). *Science* 157:459.

Arnaud, G. (1963). *C.R. Soc. Biol.* 157:1585.

Auerbach, R., and J. A. Rugowski (1967). *Science* 157:1325.

Bertrand, M. (1960). *C.R. Soc. Biol.* 154:2309.

Bough, R. G., M. R. Gurd, J. E. Hall, and B. Lessel (1963). *Nature* 200:656.

Bovet-Nitti, F., and D. Bovet (1959). *Proc. Soc. Exp. Biol. Med.* 100:555.

Brar, B. S. (1969). *Arch. Int. Pharmacodyn.* 177:416.

Brock, N., and T. Kreybig (1964). *Naunyn Schmiedeberg Arch. Exp. Path.* 249:117.

Caldwell, M. B., and D. F. Spille (1964). *Nature* 202:832.

Chambon, Y. (1955). *Ann. Endocr.* 16:912.

Champakamalini, A. V., and M. A. Rao (1967) *Curr. Sci.* 36:3

Clavert, J. (1963). *C.R. Soc. Biol.* 157:1481.

Courrier, R., and M. Marois (1953). *C.R. Soc. Biol.* 147:1922.

DiPaolo, J. A., H. M. Givelber, and H. Erwin (1968). *Nature* 220:490.

Fabro, S., and S. M. Sieber (1968). *Lancet* 1:639.

Fink, B. R., T. H. Shepard, and R. J. Blandau (1967). *Nature* 214:146.

Gaunt, R., A. A. Renzi, N. Antonchak, G. J. Miller, and M. Gilman (1954). *Ann. N.Y. Acad. Sci.* 59:22.

Geber, W. F. (1967). *Science* 158:265.

——, and L. C. Schramm (1969). *Toxic. Appl. Pharmacol.* 14:276.

Goldman, A. S., and W. C. Yakovac (1964). *Arch. Env. Health* 8:648.

——, and W. C. Yakovac (1965). *Proc. Soc. Exp. Biol. Med.* 118:857.

Hanaway, J. K. (1969). *Science* 164:574.

Harpel, H. S., Jr., and R. F. Gautieri (1968). *J. Pharmaceut. Sci.* 57:1590.

Harper, K. H., A. K. Palmer, and R. E. Davies (1965). *Arzneimittelforschung* 15:1218.

Hoffeld, D. R., and R. L. Webster (1965). *Nature* 205:1070.

——, R. L. Webster, and J. McNew (1967). *Nature* 215:182.

——, J. McNew, and R. L. Webster (1968). *Nature* 218:357.

Jewett, R. E., and S. Norton (1966). *Exp. Neur.* 14:33.

Kalter, H. (1968). *Teratology of the Central Nervous System.* Chicago: University of Chicago Press.

Kehl, R., A. Audibert, G. Gage, and J. Amarger (1956). *C.R. Soc. Biol.* 150:2196.

Kletzkin, M., H. Wojciechowski, and S. Margolin (1966). *Nature* 210:1290.

Larsen, V. (1963). *Acta Pharmacol.* 20:186.

Lauro, V., C. Giornelli, and A. Fanelli (1966). (1966). *Arch. Ostet. Ginec.* 71:153.

McColl, J. D., M. Globus, and S. Robinson (1963). *Experientia* 19:183.

——, S. Robinson, and M. Globus (1967). *Toxic. Appl. Pharmacol.* 10:244.

Murai, N. (1966). *Tohoku J. Exp. Med.* 89:265.

Murphree, O. D., B. L. Monroe, and L. D. Seager (1962). *J. Neuropsychiat.* 3:295.

Nishikawa, M. (1963). *Acta Anat. Nippon.* 38:258.

Nora, J. J., R. J. Sommerville, and F. C. Fraser (1968). *Teratology* 1:413.

——, D. G. Trasler, and F. C. Fraser (1965). *Lancet* 2:1021.

Olivecrona, H. (1964). *Acta Anat.* 58:217.

Ordy, J. M., A. Latanick, R. Johnson, and L. C. Massopust (1963). *Proc. Soc. Exp. Biol. Med.* 113:833.

——, T. Samorajski, R. L. Collins, and C. Rolsten (1966). *J. Pharmacol. Exp. Ther.* 151:110.

Paget, G. E. (1965). *Lancet* 2:1129.

Persaud, T. V. N. (1965). *Acta Biol. Med. Germ.* 14:89.

——, and A. C. Ellington (1967). *Lancet* 2:1306.

——, and A. C. Ellington (1968). *Lancet* 2:406.

——, and W. M. Henderson, (1969). *Arzneimittelforschung* 19:1309.

Poulson, E., M. Botros, and J. M. Robson (1960). *Science* 131:1101.

Poulson, E., and J. M. Robson (1963). *J. Endocrinol.* 27:147.

———, (1964). *J. Endocrinol.* 30:205.

Robson, J. M., and F. M. Sullivan (1963). *Lancet* 1:638.

Roizin, L., M. Lazar, and G. Gold (1966). *Fed. Proc.* 25:353 (abst.).

———, C. True, and M. Knight (1959). *Res. Publ. Ass. Nerv. Ment. Dis.* 37:285.

Rolsten, C. (1967). *Anat. Rec.* 157:311 (abst.).

Roux, C. (1959). *Arch. Fr. Pédiat.* 16:968.

Setälä, K., and O. Nyyssönen (1964). *Naturwissenschaften* 51:413.

Spector, W. G. (1960). *Nature* 187:514.

Spieth, K., and D. Lorenz (1967). *Naunyn Schmiedeberg Arch. Exp. Path.* 257:316.

Szirmai, E. A. (1966). *Aertztl. Forsch.* 20:47.

Takano, K., T. Tanimura, and H. Nishimura (1963). *Proc. Cong. Anom. Res. Ass. Jap.* 3:2 (abst.).

Tanimura, T., Y. Owaki, and H. Nishimura (1967). *Okaj. Folia Anat. Jap.* 43:219.

Tuchmann-Duplessis, H., and L. Mercier-Parot (1956). *C.R. Acad. Sci.* 243:410.

——— (1961a). *C.R. Soc. Biol.* 155:2291.

——— (1961b). *C.R. Acad. Sci.* 253:712.

——— (1963a). *C.R. Acad. Sci.* 256:1841.

——— (1963b). *C.R. Soc. Biol.* 157:5.

——— (1965). *C.R. Soc. Biol.* 159:6.

——— (1967). *C.R. Acad. Sci.* 264:114.

Vichi, F. (1969) Neuroleptic Drugs in Experimental Teratogenesis. In A. Bertelli and L. Donati, eds., *Teratology. Proceedings of a Symposium.* Amsterdam: Excerpta Med. Found., 87 pp.

Warkany, J., and E. Takacs (1968). *Science* 159:731.

Werboff, J., J. S. Gottlieb, E. L. Dembicki, and J. Havlena (1961a). *Exp. Neur.* 3:542.

Werboff, J., J. S. Gottlieb, J. Havlena, and T. J. Word (1961b). *Pediatrics* 27:318.

Werboff, J., and R. Kesner (1963). *Nature* 197:106.

West, G. B. (1962). *J. Pharm. Pharmacol.* 14:828.

———, (1964). *J. Pharm. Pharmacol.* 16:63.

Wilson, J. G. (1968). Introduction: Problems of Teratogenic Testing. In B. R. Fink, ed., *Toxicity of Anesthetics.* Baltimore: Williams and Wilkins, 259 pp.

Yakovleva, A. I., and M. N. Sorokina (1966). *Farmakol. Toksik.* 29:224.

Yasuda, M., F. Ariyuki, and H. Nishimura (1965). *Okaj. Folia Anat. Jap.* 41:227.

Zbinden, G., R. E. Bagdon, E. F. Keith, R. D. Phillips, and L. O. Randall (1961). *Toxic Appl. Pharmacol.* 3:619.

Recent Relevant Publications

Aeppli, L. (1969). Teratologische Studien mit Imipramin an Ratte und Kaninchen. *Arzneimittel. Forsch.* 19:1617–1640.

Alexander, G. J., G. M. Gold, B. E. Miles, and R. B. Alexander (1970). Lysergic acid diethylamide intake in pregnancy: Fetal damage in rats. *J. Pharmacol. Exp. Ther.* 173:48–59.

Auerbach, R. (1970). LSD: Teratogenicity in mice. *Science* 170:558.

Bertelli, A., P. E. Polani, R. Spector, M. J. Seller, H. Tuchmann-Duplessis, and L. Mercier-Parot (1968). Retentissement d'un neuroleptique, l'halopéridol, sur la gestation et le développement prénatal des rongeurs. *Arzneimittel. Forsch.* 18:1420–1424.

Brunaud, M. (1969). Effect of meprobamate: Acepromethazine combination on pregnancy, fetal morphology and post-natal development. *Boll. Chimicofarm.* 108:560–575.

Brunaud, M., J. Navarro, J. Salle, and G. Siou (1970). Pharmacological, toxicological, and teratological studies on dipotassium-7-chloro-3-carboxy-1,3-dihydro-2,2-dihydroxy-5-phenyl-2H-1,4-benzodiaze-pine-chloro-azepate (dipotassium chlorazepate, 4306CB), a new tranquillizer. *Arzneimittel. Forsch.* 20:123–124.

Cohen, A., and J. C. Pernot (1968). Réponse des surrénales foetales du rat á une agression dans différentes conditions experiméntales; effet du nembutal. *C.R. Soc. Biol.* 162:1675–1681.

Jacobs, R. M. (1970). The effect of central nervous system depressants, general anesthetics and muscle relaxants on palate closure in two strains of mice. *Anat. Rec.* 166:323 (abst.).

Kato, T., L. F. Jarvik, L. Roizin, and E. Moralishvili (1970). Chromosome studies in pregnant rhesus macaque given LSD-25. *Dis. Nerv. Syst.* 31:245–250.

Roux, C., R. Dupuis, and M. Aubry (1970). LSD: No teratogenic action in rats, mice, and hamsters. *Science* 169:588–589.

Vernadakis, A., and C. V. H. Clark (1970). Effects of prenatal administration of psychotropic drugs to rats on brain butyrylcholinesterase activity at birth. *Brain Res.* 12:460–.

Walker, B. E. (1969). Relation of embryonic movements to formation of cleft palate. *Teratology* 2:272 (abst.).

7 Genetic Hazards Due to Environmental Mutagens

J. F. Crow

The significance of genetic damage lies in the harmful effects that it has on future generations. Unfortunately, there is hardly ever any overt manifestation of genetic change in the individual in which it occurs. It will instead be visited on his descendants, and by the time it appears the damage is done and cannot be rectified.

1. What is Genetic Damage?

By genetic damage, I mean all kinds of changes in the hereditary material—the genes and chromosomes of the cell. There is also replicating material outside the cell nucleus, but it contains only a small part of the total genetic information and is quite probably redundant. Therefore, it is not likely that extranuclear damage is nearly as important as that to the chromosomes.

It is convenient to divide the genetic changes into chromosome aberrations and mutations. Chromosome aberrations involve gross changes in the chromosomes, many of which are directly observable by microscopic examination. In the strict sense, mutation means a change in the individual gene, but it is often impossible to distinguish between a changed gene and a chromosomal change that is too small to be visible with the microscope.

Among the cytogenetic changes, it is convenient to distinguish two broad categories. The first is change in the distribution of whole chromosomes during cell division, so that a cell receives too many or too few chromosomes. If the cell has one or more extra whole sets of chromosomes, it is *polyploid*. If it has one or more extra chromosomes, it is *polysomic*. Thus, a cell with the normal diploid complement, except that one chromosome is represented three times instead of two, is *trisomic*. The opposite of this condition, a cell in which one chromosome is represented only once rather than twice, is *monosomic*. The usual result of a polyploid, polysomic, or monosomic zygote is embryonic or fetal death. The exceptions are trisomics for three of the smaller chromosomes, which survive the prenatal period but which have multiple anomalies. Mongolism, the mildest of these, is the result of trisomy for the smallest chromosome. Abnormal numbers of X chromosomes lead to relatively minor abnormalities, usually associated with impaired sexual development.

The second category of chromosome aberrations involves chromosome breakage. Chromosomes that get broken may simply rejoin, in which case there is no permanent effect. If there are two or more breaks, various kinds of rearrangements are possible, with consequences that are to a large extent predictable from simple mechanical considerations. For example, if the rearrangement is such as to leave a chromosome with two spindle attachments, this is quite likely to lead to the chromosome being pulled two directions at once when the cell divides; or a chromosome fragment with no spindle attachment may simply get lost.

Many such rearrangements lead to cell death, with purely local consequences. The hazard to future generations is much greater if the rearrangement is such as to leave the total amount of chromosomal material intact, but simply to rearrange the parts in a way that is consistent with normal mechanical cell behavior during mitosis. For example, a reciprocal exchange of parts between two nonhomologous chromosomes produces a *translocation*. The consequences of this phenomenon can be devastating, because at meiosis the rearranged cell produces a large fraction (up to 50 percent or more) of gametes that are unbalanced in chromosome content. The embryo developing from an unbalanced gamete then dies prenatally or, if the imbalance is less, may survive but with multiple anomalies, the severity of which is roughly related to the degree of imbalance in chromosomal material.

There are also more subtle changes. For example, some abnormal chromosomes have a tendency to break or to get out of phase in reduplication [Shaw 1968]. It should also be mentioned that simply finding broken chromosome cells without clear evidence of rejoining does not prove permanent genetic damage. This, among other things, makes the current LSD data hard to interpret.

A point mutation may be as small as the substitution, gain, or loss of a single pyrimidine or purine in the DNA, or it may involve several bases. Ordinarily by any phenotypic criterion it will not be possible to distinguish between rearrangements, gains, or losses of small bits of chromosome material, and point mutations. Both conditions will follow the rules of Mendelian inheritance, and both can produce a wide variety of diseases and abnormalities.

Finally, it should be emphasized that genetic change can occur in cells throughout the body. From our standpoint, we are concerned with those that occur in the sperm or egg cells or in cells that are directly ancestral to them. Only if the change occurs in such *germ* cells can it be transmitted to future generations, so for the most part we can ignore changes in other or *somatic* cells. I might add that, although somatic mutations are not what we ordinarily worry about, it may well be that special tests for individual somatic cells with chromosome aberrations and mutations will be the best way to discover an increased mutation rate. By making the individual body cell the unit, instead of the zygote from which a mutant individual arises, there is an enormous amplification of cell numbers and a corresponding increase in the efficiency of the search for rare changes.

2. Mutations and Chromosome Aberrations Are Generally Harmful

The most important generalization about

mutations and chromosome aberrations is that their effect is harmful. There may also be mutants whose effects are so slight as to be effectively neutral; but since these have little effect one way or another, and are ordinarily not detected, they do not affect this argument one way or the other.

That the great majority of new mutants are harmful, or at best neutral, is both an empirical observation and a direct consequence of the theory of natural selection. An enormous number of mutant phenotypes have been studied in a large number of plants and animals, and finding one that is beneficial is indeed a rarity. When a beneficial mutant does arise, it will increase by natural selection so that it becomes the prevailing type. In this case any change from this type will now be mutant and harmful, relative to the former mutant which has now become the standard.

Needless to say, the environment does not stay constant and there must be almost continuous change in the relative harmfulness of different genes. A gene that caused an impairment in some body function might be lethal in a primitive environment, but only a nuisance in a society with a high living standard and sophisticated medical care. Furthermore, at many gene loci there is not any such thing as the "normal" gene; there are a number of types that are nearly the same or that produce favorable effects in special combinations. But none of these complications changes the general principle: those genes that are now a normal part of the population are there because, on the average, they are favorable. Random changes are mostly harmful for the same reason that a *random* tube replacement in a TV set is likely to make it worse.

3. What Kinds of Phenotypic Effects Are Produced?

The most important fact to emphasize is that there is no single effect derived from gene mutation. Since every part of the body and every chemical process in it is influenced by the genes in one way or another, we should not be surprised to discover that the range of effects produced by changes in the genetic material is wide.

At one extreme are very severe effects. Some normal genes are completely essential, so that a mutation that destroys or changes this function is incompatible with life. Such lethal mutations may cause death in very early embryonic stages, so early as not to be detected at all, or the change may be somewhat later so that there is a miscarriage. Or the death may be in infancy, or in childhood or even late in adult life.

There may be physical abnormalities or diseases. McKusick [1968] lists roughly 1,500 genetic diseases that appear to have a simple Mendelian inheritance. Some of these may not be genetic, but despite this the list is far more likely to be too small than too large, because many remain to be discovered. Most of these are individually rare, but collectively they amount to something like 1 percent of all live births, more if one includes conditions of more doubtful, but probably genetic, etiology.

At the other extreme are genes with very mild effects. Presumably, these grade into those with still milder effects, so small as to be imperceptible. It is clear that the effect of an increased mutation rate is not so much the occurrence of novel or bizarre types, but an increase of a whole host of ailments and weaknesses of varying severity, all of which are already present. For the most part, the effect is statistical rather than specific.

The evidence for these statements comes from a number of sources, mostly not from man. The most extensive studies have been on Drosophila, where it has been shown repeatedly that by far the most frequent class of mutant is one causing a slight decrease in survival and fertility. Supporting evidence in man comes, in addition to study of individual Mendelian traits, from the effects of consanguineous marriages. These marriages bring out mutants which occurred sometime in the past but which have remained hidden. For the most part the increased death and disease rate in children of consanguineous marriages comes not from specific genetic diseases, but from the ordinary causes of death. Presumably what is inherited is a general weakening that makes the person more likely to succumb to what he might otherwise have survived.

From the standpoint of the social burden, mental retardation and mental disease are extremely costly, whether measured in terms of actual dollars or in terms of human misery. An unknown but probably large part of severe mental retardation is genetic; chromosome anomalies constitute a substantial fraction of the total number. So almost certainly, one consequence of an increased mutation rate would be an increase in the number of mentally retarded. There would probably also be a general decrease in average intelligence, caused mainly by individually small effects; this is harder to be sure of. Supporting evidence comes from the lower intelligence scores from children of consanguineous marriages [Schull and Neel 1965].

4. How Would the Effects of Genetic Damage Be Distributed in Time?

The effects of errors in chromosome distribution would, for the most part, exert their total effect in the generation immediately following the event. If, because of a mistake made in some preceding cell division, an egg or sperm carries an abnormal number of chromosomes, the embryo that develops after fertilization will usually die before birth. If the extra chromosome is the one causing mongolism, then this disease will develop. It will usually last only one generation because persons with mongolism reproduce only with great rarity; the main exceptions

would be XXX and XYY types, which are fertile. If the chromosome mistake takes place some time during very early embryonic development, only part of the cells in the body would be affected. The severity of damage would depend on how large a fraction of cells this is and what parts of the body are affected. It would be transmitted to another generation only if the abnormal cells include some germ cells. In general, effects of errors in chromosome numbers have their major impact in the first generation and very little after that.

Translocations and some other rearrangements may have effects that last longer. A person with a normal amount of chromosome material but with the chromosomes rearranged is ordinarily normal. But at meiosis this person produces a high proportion of gametes with an unbalanced chromosome amount. The results are just like those mentioned in the paragraph above, except that the range of abnormalities is very broad, as would be expected, since the unbalance can involve little or much of the chromosome material. Furthermore, among the gametes produced by the person carrying the rearrangement will be some rearranged chromosomes, so that half of the normal children will be just like the parent. Then they too have a high probability of embryonic death and congenital defects in their children. This continues generation after generation until the strain dies out. If the rearrangement is such that all the unbalanced combinations lead to embryonic death, the translocation may simply cause an apparent partial sterility or high abortion rate. In general the effects of chromosome rearrangements may persist for several generations. The abnormalities may even skip a generation if all the eggs or sperms happen to receive only balanced chromosomes.

When we consider point mutations, the main consideration is whether the mutation is dominant or recessive. If the mutant is dominant, it is sufficient for either the egg or sperm to carry the mutant in order that the child show the mutant phenotype. If the condition is recessive, both the egg and the sperm must carry the mutant gene. This means that the kinetics of dominant and recessive mutants are greatly different.

The dominant trait appears in the generation immediately after the mutation event and continues to appear every generation until the mutant strain dies out. The time required for the extinction of the mutant gene depends, in addition to pure chance, on the severity of the effect. If the mutant causes a large depression of survival or fertility, the mutant strain persists only a few generations; with complete sterility, the mutant persists for only one generation.

A recessive mutant, on the other hand, may remain hidden in the population for many generations before it is expressed. It is expressed only when it is inherited from both parents. This can happen if the parents are consanguineous and if both parents have descended from an ancestor who carried the mutant gene. It may also happen if a person carrying the mutant gene marries a person carrying a pre-existing or independently arising mutant of the same kind. Both events have a low probability for most recessive genes, the first because consanguineous marriage is rare and the second because most harmful recessive genes are rare.

As a result it may be many generations before a recessive mutation is expressed. Indeed, it is likely that many, probably most, recessive mutants are never expressed. If Drosophila is a good guide, most recessive mutants are not completely recessive, but rather cause a very mild impairment in single dose. If this impairment is such as to decrease the probability of survival and fertility by even a few percent, it is enough to ensure

that most of the time the mutant is eliminated in this way before it ever has a chance to meet its counterpart in another gamete. If this is a correct interpretation, the effect of induced recessive mutants is a slight weakening that appears in the first generation after the mutation occurs and is gradually lost from the population, with a half-life of perhaps 20 to 40 generations.

Again using Drosophila as a guide, the most numerous class of mutants are by far those that cause only a slight impairment in function. They are somewhat more harmful in double dose than in single dose, but not a great deal more so. They too are probably eliminated by single dose effects before they have a chance to become homozygous. If this is generally correct, the kinetics are very much like those of recessive genes. They cause a small, nonspecific decrease in viability.

I should point out that mutations also occur spontaneously. So we have in the present population a collection of mutant genes that arose by mutation in the past. This "load" of mutations is responsible for a certain and unknown fraction of the current burden of disease, abnormality, mental retardation, and generally reduced health and vigor. Unless the induced mutation rate is enormous, the increase in disability from one generation of enhanced mutation is a small part of the accumulated load.

In summary, the genetic damage ranges from very severe and lethal effects to those that are very mild. The more severe the effect—more specifically, the greater the reduction in the probability of reproduction—the sooner the mutant is eliminated from the population. Those mutants with mild effects may persist for many generations, weakening each one slightly. Those recessive genes that happen to occur in double dose may do this at any time in the future, perhaps dozens or hundreds of generations later.

5. Which Is Worse, Many Mild Mutants or a Few Severe Ones?

We might be tempted to ignore the mutants with mild effects, and perhaps we should regard these as less important than those causing severe disease or mental retardation. The social burden of one mentally retarded child can indeed be enormous.

On the other hand there are two considerations that I think keep us from being able to dismiss mild mutants as unimportant. One is that, as mentioned before, these mutants are probably much more numerous than severe ones. The evidence from Drosophila is that these mutants are 10, 20, or more times as frequent as drastic mutants. The evidence in man is much weaker, coming mainly from studies of consanguineous marriages; but there is also every reason to think on *a priori* grounds that man is the same in this regard.

The second consideration is one emphasized by Muller [1950]. This is that, in a population of stable size, every mutant gene on the average will persist until it is eliminated. This happens through what Muller called a "genetic death," the premature death or equivalent in reduced fertility of one individual.

Another way of saying this is that if a mutant causes a 1 percent risk of death it will remain in the population for an average of 100 generations. It will therefore affect 100 persons. One hundred persons exposed to a 1 percent risk of death causes the same number of deaths as one person exposed to 100 percent risk. So, if we take a long term view and keep this system of mutation cost accounting, mild and severe mutants are equivalent. For this reason, we cannot, I think, ignore the effects of mild mutants.

There is ground for endless debate as to the appropriateness of this argument. Some system for eliminating several mutants at once could reduce the number of "genetic deaths" per mutant, and many such systems have been suggested. Furthermore, human misery may have only a rather indirect relationship to genetic deaths. How many early miscarriages equals one child with hemophilia? How many years of decreased adult life expectancy equals one congenital malformation? How do we compare mental and physical disease? How much concern should we have for disease and disability in the far future when the environment and the state of human knowledge are likely to be totally different? Are these mild mutants not the kind that are most easily compensated for by a good environment?

When the time comes for cost-benefit calculations, the quantifying of the genetic risk will be exceedingly difficult. All the considerations that I have mentioned, plus many that I have not, make it almost impossible to reach any effective overall measure. But I would emphasize that if we make assessments based only on dominant mutants and cytological effects in the immediate progeny, we will be ignoring less easily detected effects that may be more frequent and in the long run possibly more important.

6. Two Kinds of Fears with Drugs

The considerations that I have discussed so far would apply to any environmental mutagen. The fears are mainly those associated with a statistical increase in the amount of disease, death, and frustration in future generations. I have regarded it mainly as a population problem.

The population concern is mainly one of averages: the object is to keep the overall rate of mutation as low as possible. It does not matter very much what the spatial distribution of the mutagen is; it is the total number of mutations that matters. These are the kinds of considerations that are primary in the setting of maximum permissible radiation doses.

With drugs there is a potential risk of another

kind, one that is more important to the individual than to the population. If it should turn out that some drug that is used by a very small number of persons is very highly mutagenic, this may cause only a very small change in the total load of deleterious genes in the population. But the risk of cytogenetic effects and dominant mutations may be high enough to constitute a risk to the person because of his personal interest in the welfare of his own children and grandchildren.

So, it seems to me, there are two related but separable problems in mutation protection policy. We want to keep the overall mutation rate low, by detecting mutagenic drugs and keeping the population average exposure as low as feasible. Any benefit should be carefully weighed against the risk. At the same time, with drugs that are used by only a minority there may be a need to protect the person's own interest in his children, even if the number is small enough to make very little difference in the average.

References

McKusick, V. A. (1968). *Mendelian Inheritance in Man*. Baltimore: Johns Hopkins Press.

Muller, H. J. (1950). *Amer. J. Human Genet.* 2:111–176.

Schull, W. J., and J. V. Neel (1965). *The Effects of Inbreeding on Japanese Children*. New York: Harper and Row.

Shaw, Margery W. (1968). *Symposium on Human Cytogenetics*, Knoxville: University of Tennessee Press, pp. 5–11.

8 Structure–Activity Considerations in Potential Mutagenicity

E. Freese

1. Consequences of Alterations in the Genetic Material

An alteration of the genetic material of a cell may be lethal to the cell or it may cause a mutation, i.e., a change in the amount or kind of hereditary information. This distinction becomes meaningful only for replicating cells. Lethal alterations prevent indefinite cell multiplication, whereas mutations give rise to genotypically altered cells that can continue to duplicate. If an agent induces large chromosome aberrations, a small percentage of them can be cytologically detected under the light microscope. By a recombination analysis of many mutants, the relative extent of mutations along the DNA information strand can be determined and large alterations can be separated from point mutations. Most point mutations are changed only in one or few DNA bases, i.e., their extent is smaller than the genetic information determining a functional property, which is contained in a stretch of about 1,000 or more DNA bases.

Phenotypically, a mutation may lead to morphological changes or to altered biochemical requirements. In a diploid organism, a recessive mutation becomes expressed either when the dominant gene is located in a functionally inactive chromosome or when the mutation occurs in homozygous form in some later generation. Mutants are usually recessive when they have lost the ability to produce one or more enzymes owing to a point mutation or a deletion of some genetic material. Internal deletions come about by the exchange of information within a chromosome whereas end deletions occur either by the removal of a chromosomal piece or by the translocation of two chromosomes. Dominant lethal mutations can be defined only in multicellular organisms where cells can multiply many times before a developmental crisis occurs as the result of a developmental mutation [Srb et al. 1965]. It often requires elaborate cytological or genetic studies before dominant lethal mutations can be distinguished from the lethal effect of chromosome breaks. Chromosome breaks per se do not constitute mutations because they usually lead to the death of the cell or all of its early progeny owing to the loss of some vital information often as result of the breakage-fusion-bridge cycle. Only if broken chromosomes interact in such a way that new chromosomes are formed, which have each one centromere, which can duplicate accurately, and with which the altered cell can multiply indefinitely, a mutation has been formed; this mutation is usually extended in size. Point mutations in which only one or few DNA bases have been changed arise by different mechanisms.

The effect of different genetic alterations of individual cells on the whole organism depends on the stage of development and the type of cell affected. This is summarized in Table 1. Alterations that are lethal to a cell or *all* of its progeny are relatively harmless if they occur in gonal or germ cells, because no live progeny is then produced, or in fertilized cells very early in development (up to the blastula stage), because a dead cell can be easily replaced by a live one which just has to duplicate once more. Lethal effects are of less importance for organisms late in development or in the adult state, because for each dead cell many similarly differentiated live cells are available. Only early in development, at or after gastrulation, can lethal effects lead to teratogenic changes if the few determined cells leading to the development of a particular organ are affected. In contrast, point or extended mutations that occur in gonal or germ cells are usually harmful to the progeny irrespective of the stage of development; they can produce fetal death, congenital malformations, and metabolic or neurological diseases. Furthermore, dominant mutations can affect even somatic cells at any stage of development: in developing tissue they can

Table 1. Phenotypic Effect of Lethal or Mutagenic Alterations of Individual Cells on a Multicellular Organism

Cell Stage in Development	Dead Cell	Mutated Cell	
		Dominant E.g., loss of repressor by deletion; effect of extra chromosome; translocation in germinal cells	Recessive E.g., point mutation, deletion, or cryptic aberration (translocation)
Somatic Cells			
Very early development (to blastula)	—	Abnormal development (teratogenic)	—
Early development (from gastrula on)	Abnormal development (teratogenic)	same	—
Late development to adult	—	Neoplastic	—
Germinal Cells	—	Lethal (fetal death), or other phenotypic effects such as malformation, metabolic or neurological disease, mongoloids, Turner's syndrome. Expressed in next and all following generations	Lethal or other phenotypic effects. Expressed in next or any later generation when dominant information is in functionally inactive chromosome region; or expressed in later generation when in homozygous form
Germ Cells	—	Lethal, malformation, metabolic, or neurological disease. Expressed in next and all following surviving generations	same

induce teratogenic effects [Kalter, Chapter 6; Kalter 1968]; in cells that grow or can be induced to grow, agents which induce extended mutations apparently can also induce neoplastic changes (cancer, leukemia, myeloma) [Miller, Chapter 5; Miller and Miller 1969].

2. Chemical Causes of Chromosome Alterations

Most reactions which alter the hereditary information in a cell seem to be caused by a chemical or enzymic attack on DNA itself. The major exception to this rule is the effect of colchicine and certain alkaloids, which inhibit spindle formation and cause the production of polyploids; at low concentrations, they occasionally produce aneuploids in which only few chromosomes are added or deleted [Kihlman 1966]. Agents that alter DNA itself produce either mutagenic or inactivating DNA alterations [Freese and Freese 1966]. Mutagenic DNA alterations are minor alterations of the DNA bases which do not prevent DNA duplication, but which cause, occasionally or always, a change in the base sequence of DNA. Such DNA alterations are induced by base analogs (for example 2-aminopurine, and 5-bromouracil), which are incorporated into DNA or by the chemical alterations of DNA bases (such as the deamination of adenine or cytosine by nitrous acid, the hydroxylamination of cytosine by hydroxylamine, the alkylation of guanine by alkylating agents), or by the intercalation of acridine dyes between DNA bases. Mutagenic DNA alterations give rise to point mutations.

In contrast, inactivating DNA alterations have more drastic effects on DNA since they inhibit the duplication of DNA across the altered site. Such alterations arise when a DNA base is removed or the DNA backbone is broken as a consequence of treatment by alkylating agents, radical-producing agents, or base analogs which inhibit the duplication of DNA.

Many inactivating DNA alterations can be repaired by special cellular enzymes. Different organisms differ in the extent and the specificity of repair mechanisms. DNA alterations that have not been repaired lead to chromosome breaks which are usually lethal to the cell. If more than one inactivating DNA alteration or chromatid break occurs within a cell, and if the altered sites can undergo exchanges and restitution—which seem to be blocked or delayed after infection with certain viruses, for example measles—large heritable chromosome aberrations such as deletions, translocations, and inversions can be produced. When examined in a suitable test system, most, if not all, agents which induce inactivating DNA alterations or chromosome breaks in vivo have also been found to induce mutations, to liberate latent viruses, and to cause neoplastic changes or teratogenic effects.

Most compounds affecting DNA produce both mutagenic and inactivating DNA alterations, but the relative frequency of these two effects differs up to one million-fold for different compounds. A mutagenic test system which is very sensitive for one compound (e.g., transition-type point mutations) may therefore reveal no mutations with another compound that produces only other types of mutations (e.g., large chromosome alterations). There is also no correlation between toxic and mutagenic effects because some highly mutagenic compounds, e.g., certain base analogs, are barely toxic, whereas some highly toxic compounds, such as cyanide, are not mutagenic.

3. Potential Mutagenic Hazard of Drugs of Abuse

For most drugs of abuse no mutagenic tests have been undertaken. It is known that morphine and scopolamine induce chromosome breaks in plants [Oehlkers 1953]. LSD apparently binds to DNA [Wagner 1969]. Some antidepressant hydrazines, which are not

A. Scopolamine

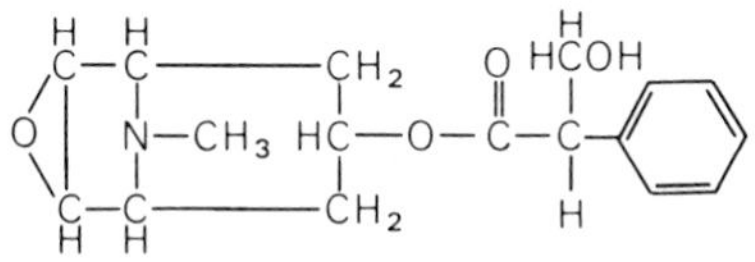

Scopolamine is an expoxide which may alkylate DNA. It also has an ester group which may be reactive. It might induce both point mutations and large chromosome aberrations. This is potentially the most effective mutagen among the drugs considered here.

B. Meprobamate

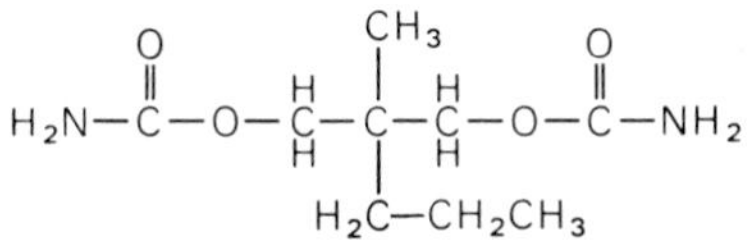

Meprobamate is a carbamate. Certain carbamates, such as urethan, are enzymatically converted to N-hydroxycarbamates or other compounds which produce radicals and which are known to induce inactivating DNA alterations or chromosome aberrations, but not point mutations [Freese 1967]. Whether meprobamate is mutagenic depends therefore on the specific enzyme content of the organism.

C. Phenolic Compounds

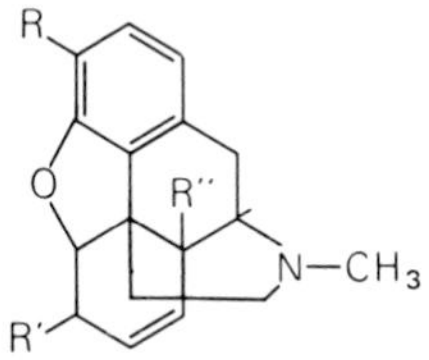

some R＝OH

Codeine, hydrocodone, hydromorphone, morphine, and tetrahydrocannabinol contain phenolic groups. Some phenols [Levan and Tjio 1948] and in particular morphine [Oehlkers 1953] have been found to produce chromosome breaks in plants at a low frequency [Levan and Tjio 1948], probably by formation of free radicals and peroxides [Freese et al. 1967].

D. Hydroxylamine Intermediates

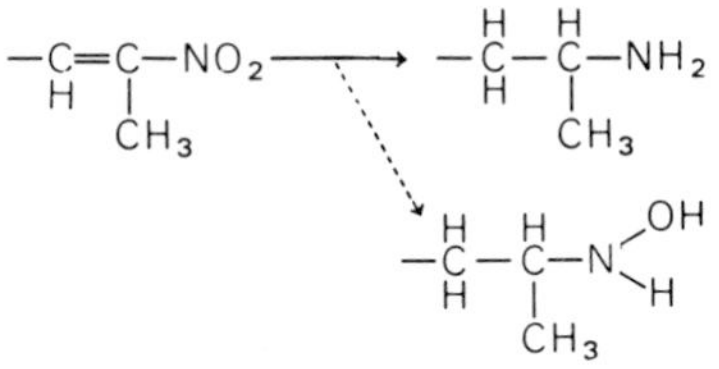

STP, MDA, and mescaline are chemically prepared by reduction of nitro compounds [Shulgin, Chapter 1]. If not purified, the preparation may contain some hydroxylamine resulting from incomplete reduction. Hydroxylamines are efficient chromosome-breaking and mutagenic agents [Freese et al. 1967].

E. Benzaldehyde

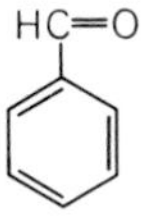

HC＝O

Benzaldehyde can form radicals and thereby may induce inactivating DNA alterations and chromosome aberrations, but not point mutations. It would probably be a very weak mutagen.

technically included among drugs of abuse, in-activate-transforming DNA [Freese et al. 1968]. But apart from LSD, for which results are un-clear [Moorhead et al., Chapter 11], no tests seem to have been made in mammalian systems. We can deduce from the mutagenic test results of other compounds that certain chemical groups can alter DNA and induce mutations. Among the drugs of abuse, several com-pounds carry such chemical groups and are potential mutagens. However, since most chemicals undergo many metabolic changes in vivo, the mutagenic effect can be activated or inactivated by enzymes. Consequently, all drugs should be screened for their muta-genicity in mammalian systems if reasonable assurance for the absence of genetic effects is desired.

4. Summary

Judging from known mutagens, certain chem-ical groups are prone to induce mutations. Such groups are present in some drugs of abuse, which are therefore potential mutagens. They include scopolamine (epoxide), benz-aldehyde, meprobamate (carbamate), and the phenols morphine, codeine, etc. In addition, hydroxylamine contaminants stemming from the chemical preparation of STP, MDA, and mescaline might induce mutations. But most chemicals undergo so many metabolic changes in vivo that all drugs should be screened for their mutagenicity in mammalian systems if reasonable assurance about the absence of genetic effects is desired.

References

Freese, E. and E. B. Freese (1966). *Radiat. Res. Suppl.* 6:97.

Freese, E., S. Sklarow, and E. B. Freese (1968). *Mutat. Res.* 5:343.

Freese, E. B. (1967). *Mol. Gen. Genet.* 100:150.

J. Gerson, H. Taber, H. Rhaese, and E. Freese (1967). *Mutat. Res.* 4:517.

Kalter, H. (1968). *Teratology of the Central Nervous System.* Chicago: University of Chicago Press.

Kihlman, B. A. (1966). *Actions of Chemicals on Dividing Cells.* Englewood Cliffs, N.J.: Prentice-Hall.

Levan, A. and J. H. Tjio (1948). *Hereditas* 34:453.

Miller, J. A. and Miller, E. C. (1969). In E.D. Bergmann and B. Pullman, eds., *Physico-Chemical Mechanisms of Carcinogenesis.* Vol. 1, pp. 237–261. Jerusalem Symposia in Quantum Chemistry and Biochemistry.

Oehlkers, F. (1953). *Heredity* 6 (Suppl.):95.

Srb, A. M., Owen, R. D., and Edgar, R. S. (1965). *General Genetics,* San Francisco: Freeman, 2nd edition.

Wagner, T. E. (1969). *Nature* 5:1170.

III. Methods for Mutagenicity Testing

9 Microbial Methods for Mutagenicity Testing

F. J. de Serres

1. General Concepts

Man's chemical environment is becoming increasingly complex. Every year an increasing number of new man-made chemicals is put into widespread distribution in such forms as food additives, drugs, industrial compounds cosmetics, insecticides, and herbicides. There is always the danger that some of these may have undetected, long-term genetic effects. For this reason it is desirable to develop relatively simple tests for mutagenicity that will determine whether a given chemical can produce gene mutations at a significantly higher frequency than that which occurs spontaneously.

For the results of mutagenicity tests to be applicable to man, it is important to test not only the original compound but also its metabolic breakdown products. Mammalian test systems, such as human cells in culture, in which such assays could be performed directly, are still in the exploratory stages. At the present time, the best assays for the detection of gene mutations are based on microbial test systems.

Mutagenicity tests usually involve direct treatment of the microbial cells with the mutagen for varying periods of time, removal of the mutagen by washing and/or neutralization, and then inoculation of the treated cells into growth medium for assay. Such treatment usually limits the evaluation to the original compound. Evaluation of both the original compound and its metabolic breakdown products can be made with the host-mediated assay [Legator, Chapter 12; Gabridge and Legator 1969]. In this assay the microbial test system is injected into mammals that have been treated with a chemical, either by direct feeding or by intraperitoneal or intravenous injection. After a period of incubation varying from a few hours to several days, the microbial cells are removed, washed, and placed in various growth media for evaluation. These experiments have been done primarily with mice and rats, but in theory it is possible to use a wide variety of mammalian hosts. Where little is known about the metabolic fate of a particular compound it might be advisable to use a variety of mammalian hosts.

The microbial test systems that are now most suitable for the detection of gene mutations are found in bacteria and fungi. They range from test systems capable of detecting a particular type of genetic alteration to those capable of detecting a broad spectrum of genetic alteration. Some currently available ones are particularly well suited for routine screening programs. However, the simple ones that make use of a spot test give only very limited information. Those that give the most complete information have somewhat more complicated technical procedures and may require a series of genetic tests. Developmental work is being done to simplify the more complicated tests and also to develop new, simplified test systems. The characteristics of some of the most promising ones are summarized in Table I.

2. Characteristics of Various Microbial Test Systems for Mutagenicity

2.1. C Gene of the Histidine Operon of *Salmonella typhimurium*

Alterations in aminotransferase (C gene) mutants in the histidine operon have been identified on the basis of specific revertibility tests after treatment with chemical mutagens [Ames and Whitfield 1966; Whitfield et al, 1966]. Nonsense, missense, and frameshift mutants are known. Each mutant reverts as a result of a particular type of genetic alteration. By selection of mutants that revert at high frequencies after treatment, a tester set can be developed which is capable of detecting and identifying the mutagenic activity of both strong and weak mutagens.

A suspension of each mutant in the tester set is spread over the surface of minimal medium supplemented with a trace of histidine (0.2 µmole per ml) so that the background lawn can grow slightly and so that any inhibition by the compounds to be tested can be seen. The chemicals to be tested are dissolved in distilled water, and a drop of each is placed at spaced intervals around the periphery of each plate. After 2 days of incubation at 37° C, mutagenic activity is indicated by the presence of a ring of revertant colonies around the spot where a chemical was added. Weak mutagems will produce only a few revertants and strong mutagens will produce many revertants. The type of genetic alteration produced by each chemical is indicated by the particular mutants in the tester set which are induced to revert. This test system is well adapted for routine screening of chemicals for mutagenic activity. The major disadvantage is that it is a reverse-mutation system which can detect only *particular types of genetic alterations*.

2.2. Early Genes in the Purine Biosynthetic Pathway in *Saccharomyces cerevisiae*

In yeast there are two recessive genes, *ad-1* and *ad-2*, which give a requirement for adenine and which cause the accumulation of a red pigment. When a haploid red clone is plated on YEP medium (1% yeast extract, 2% bactopeptone, and 8% glucose +1.5% agar), some of the colonies differ in color from the original red [Roman 1956]. Both white and pale pink types are found which retain their phenotype on transfer and plating. In addition, as red colonies continue to grow on solid medium, they form white and pale pink papillae from which stable mutant types can also be obtained.

Genetic analysis has shown that some of the white or pale pink variants are due to reversion of the ad-1 or ad-2 allele to adenine independence. But when a stable ad-1 or ad-2 allele was used, then all of the white or pale pink colonies were found to result from mutation in one of 5 genes controlling earlier

Table 1. Characteristics of Different Microbial Assay Systems for Mutagenicity

	Genetic Effect				Ploidy			Meta-bolic Stage		Character-ization of the Mutants		Stage of Deve-lopment		General Utility	
	Genic		Chromosomal		Haploid	Diploid	Heterokaryon								
	Forward mutation (Number of loci)	Reverse Mutation	Somatic Recombination	Interstitial Deletions	n	2n	n+n	Dividing	Nondividing	Phenotypic	Identification at the molecular level	Complete	Developmental Work Required	Simple Test	Complicated Test
Prokaryotes 1. C gene of histidine operon *Salmonella typhimurium* Eukaryotes	0	+	0	0	+	0	0	+	+	+	+	+	0	+	0
2. Early genes in purine biosynthetic pathway *Saccharomyces cerevisiae*	+(5) +(1→5)	0 0	0 +	0 0?	+ 0	0 +	0 0	0 0	+ +	+ +	0 0	+ +	0 0	0 0	+ +
3. Tester set of *ad-3B* mutants *Neurospora crassa*	0	+	0	0	+	0	0	0	+	+	+	+	0	0	+
4. Canavanine resistance *Neurospora crassa*	+(2)	0	0	0	+	0	0	0	+	+	0	0	+	+	0
5. 4-Methyl tryptophane resistance *Neurospora crassa*	+(1) +(1)	0 0	0 0	0 +	+ 0	0 0	0 +	0 0	+ +	+ +	0 0	+ 0	0 +	+ +	0 0
6. 2-Thioxanthine resistance *Aspergillus nidulans*	+(8)	0	0	0	+	0	0	0	+	+	0	+	0	0	+
7. Recessive lethals over entire genome *Neurospora crassa*	+(>2000)	0	0	+	0	0	+	0	+	0	0	+	0	+	0
8. *ad-3* region *Neurospora crassa*	+(2) +(2)	0 0	0 0	0 +	+ 0	0 0	0 +	+ +	+ +	+ +	+ +	+ +	0 0	0 0	+ +

steps in purine biosynthesis: ad-3, ad-4, ad-5, ad-6, or ad-7. The mutant genes in the pale pink colonies were found to be intermediate alleles at these same loci.

To screen for mutagenicity a suspension of cells of a stable ad-1 or ad-2 mutant in sterile water is treated for the same time period with varying concentrations of the chemical. The treated cells, as well as untreated controls, are plated on the surface of YEP agar and the plates are screened for the presence of white and pale pink colonies among the red colonies. The presence of a higher frequency of such variants than is present in the plating of the untreated control indicates mutagenic activity. The genotypes of the white and pale pink variants can be determined in crosses with the appropriate tester strains to determine the spectrum of induced genetic alterations.

This is a forward-mutation system and presumably is capable of detecting any type of genetic alteration which will produce gene mutation by intragenic alteration.

2.3. Tester Set of *ad-3B* Mutants in *Neurospora crassa*

The genetic alterations in a series of nitrous-acid induced ad-3B mutants of *Neurospora crassa* were identified on the basis of specific revertibility after treatment with chemical mutagens [Malling 1966; Malling and de Serres 1968]. A tester set has been developed consisting of 8 mutants which revert at high frequency after treatment. Four mutants revert only by base-pair substitutions; 2 by AT → GC and the other 2 by GC → AT. Two mutants revert only by base-pair insertion or deletion, and 2 mutants revert only spontaneously.

The tester set is used to test for mutagenic activity and for specificity of this activity. Suspensions of each mutant strain are treated for a constant period of time with varying concentrations of the chemical. The treated suspensions and untreated controls are plated in minimal medium supplemented with 2 mg/ml of adenine to permit minimal back-

ground growth. After 7 to 9 days incubation at 30°C the number of revertant colonies are counted. A higher frequency of revertant colonies in the treated series than in the untreated control indicates mutagenic activity. Specificity is indicated when only those strains requiring the same type of genetic alteration to revert are affected. Strong mutagens will produce a high frequency of reversion, weak mutagens a low frequency.

This method is useful for rapid screening tests for mutagenicity. However, because it screens for particular types of genetic alterations, a negative test does not mean that the compound is not mutagenic. It is possible for a chemical to produce genetic alterations which would not be detected by any of the 8 strains in this tester set.

2.4. Canavanine Resistance in *Neurospora crassa*

In *Neurospora crassa* wild type strains are usually sensitive to the amino acid canavanine [Horowitz and Srb 1948] and there are two nonallelic genes that cover sensitivity, namely, r and s [Lockhart and Garner, 1955]. Treated spores of a sensitive wild type strain are plated onto media containing canavanine to detect mutations for resistance. Mutants of the type rS are also sensitive, but Rs is resistant, with strains of genotype RS intermediate in sensitivity.

Sensitive strains have been used to detect mutagenic activity of chemicals [Smith and Srb 1951] by plating spores treated with the chemical as well as untreated control spores in medium containing canavanine to detect mutations for resistance. The mutation rs to Rs (resistance) results from reverse-mutation rather than forward-mutation. Thus the spectrum of genetic alterations detectable with with this system is expected to be limited. Although this test system provides a relatively simple test for mutagenicity, a negative result does not necessarily indicate a lack of mutagenic activity.

2.5. Resistance to 4-Methyltryptophan in *Neurospora crassa*

Neurospora has at least two systems which enable it to accumulate amino acids and to concentrate them up to 100 times the level present in the surrounding medium. The mtr+ locus controls the uptake system which preferentially takes up the aromatic amino acids [Lester 1966; Stadler 1966]. However, other amino acids can be concentrated by this system as well as certain amino acid analogs. As these amino acid analogs are concentrated by the cell, synthesis of the normal amino acid is stopped as growth is inhibited. Strains resistant to the effect of the amino acid analog 4-methyltryptophan (4MT) result from mutation at the mtr locus (mtr+ → mtr); the mtr mutants are recessive to the wild type allele.

To use this system to determine the mutagenicity of chemicals, treated conidia (and untreated controls) are plated out in the presence of 4-MT. At high concentrations of this analog growth of mtr+ conidia is greatly inhibited and the only colonies formed are those resulting from mutations to resistance (mtr). Mutagenicity is indicated by a higher frequency of colonies (mtr mutants) in the treated series than in the control series.

This is a forward-mutation system which is capable of detecting any type of genetic alteration resulting in the inactivation (partial or complete) of the mtr+ allele by intragenic alteration. By using a heterokaryon heterozygous at the mtr locus, the system can be made to detect extragenic mutations where the mtr+ locus is inactivated by chromosome deletion. Thus the production of recessive lethal mutations at this locus both by gene mutation and by chromosome breakage and deletion can be detected. This is a simple test system which can be used for routine screening and which is capable of detecting a broad spectrum of genetic damage. There is not as yet any simple way to distinguish the recessive lethal mutations resulting from gene mutations from those resulting from chromosome deletion. Thus, although a heterokaryon heterozygous for mtr is theoretically capable of detecting all types of genetic damage, no characterization of the mtr mutants is possible.

2.6. 2-Thioxanthine Resistance in *Aspergillus nidulans*

In *Aspergillus nidulans* 2-thioxanthine produces an effect on conidial pigmentation. Green-conidiating wild type strains conidiate yellow on 2-thioxanthine, but certain mutant strains which are resistant to 2-thioxanthine conidiate green. Resistance results from mutation at one of eight gene loci [Alderson and Scazzocchio 1967]. The resistant mutants have been phenotypically characterized as lacking the enzyme xanthine dehydrogenase (XDH), and being unable to grow on hypoxanthine as a sole source of nitrogen. Failure to grow on certain other sole nitrogen sources divides the XDH mutants into 3 classes: (1) hx mutants which fail to grow on hypoxanthine (2 genes); (2) uaY mutants which also lack urate oxidase activity and fail to grow on hypoxanthine or uric acid (1 gene); and (3) cnx mutants which also lack nitrate reductase activity and fail to grow on hypoxanthine or nitrate (5 genes).

To use this test system to assay for mutagenicity, conidia from a haploid wild type are treated with different concentrations of the chemical for the same time period and treated conidia (as well as untreated controls) are plated out in medium containing 2-thioxanthine to give about 200 colonies per plate. After 3 or 4 days of incubation at 37°C, the platings are examined for green colonies which are resistant. These resistant colonies are picked and plated to establish pure strains. Conidia from the mutant strains are then tested for growth on 5 different supplemented media to determine their growth requirements. In this way each mutant is assigned to one of eight different loci.

This is a forward-mutation test system that

is capable of detecting any genetic alteration at these eight loci leading to a loss of XDH activity. Because the system utilizes a haploid strain, the analysis is limited to those mutations which result from intragenic alterations. Chromosome deletions would not be recovered since they are haplolethal. This system is especially well suited for routine screening since the steps for mutant purification and identification are relatively simple.

2.7. Recessive Lethal Mutations over the Entire Genome in *Neurospora crassa*

By using a two-component heterokaryon of Neurospora with each component marked with the appropriate biochemical and morphological markers, it is possible to determine the frequency of recessive lethal mutations occurring over the entire genome [Atwood 1949]. The heterokaryon has an arginine (arg-6) requirement in component I, and a methionine (meth-7) requirement and a morphological marker amycelial (amyc) in component II. Recessive lethal mutations induced in component II are propagated indefinitely because of the presence of the normal alleles in component I. A two-component heterokaryon of this type produces three types of colonies: one heterokaryotic type containing at least one nucleus of each genotype, and two homokaryotic types containing only nuclei of component I genotype or component II genotype. By plating on minimal medium only the heterokaryotic conidia will grow; by plating on minimal medium supplemented with arginine or methionine the homokaryotic conidia can grow. If no recessive lethal mutation is present in the meth-amyc nucleus, this component forms a tiny morphologically distinct colony on minimal + methionine. If a recessive lethal mutation has been induced only morphologically normal (large) colonies are found.

The frequency of heterokaryotic colonies which do not produce the tiny amyc colonies on plating gives a minimal estimate of the re-

cessive lethal frequency, since lethal mutations occurring in treated conidia with more than one meth-amyc nucleus are not detected. However, since the average number of nuclei per conidium is about 2.3, it seems likely that the majority of the recessive lethal mutations are detected.

To test for mutagenicity with this test system, conidia of the heterokaryon are treated and are plated on minimal medium. A random sample of about 100 to 150 colonies are isolated and subcultured. Conidia from each isolate are then plated to screen for the presence of amyc colonies on minimal medium supplemented with methionine. Plates containing normal but no amycelial colonies are scored as lethals. Mutagenicity is indicated by a higher frequency of lethals in the treated series than the untreated controls.

This is a forward-mutation system capable, in theory, of detecting any type of genetic alteration which results in the inactivation of any of the genes in the genome. Homology tests of recessive lethal mutations in general [Atwood and Mukai 1953] show that they consist of both gene mutations and chromosome deletions that may cover more than one locus. This test system provides a simple assay for mutagenicity which tests for an effect on a very large number of genes. It is not possible to further characterize the recessive lethal mutants obtained.

2.8. ad-3 Mutants of *Neurospora crassa*

Mutation of two genes in the purine biosynthetic pathway, ad-3A and ad-3B, results not only in a requirement for adenine but the accumulation of a reddish purple pigment in the vacuoles of the mycelium. Because the ad-3 mutants are phenotypically distinguishable from the wild type on the basis of this pigment accumulation, it has been possible to develop a direct method for their recovery [de Serres and Kølmark 1958]. The spectrum of ad-3 mutants recovered with this method ranges from nonleaky mutants having a complete requirement for adenine to leaky mutants with only partial requirements. Mutants at the ad-3B locus show allelic complementation and have a linear complementation map with 17 complons [de Serres et al. 1967]. A correlation has been found between complementation pattern and genetic alteration at the molecular level [Malling and de Serres 1967, 1968], so that the heterokaryon test for allelic complementation can be used to obtain presumptive evidence of the spectrum of genetic alterations at the molecular level.

By using a two-component heterokaryon, heterozygous at both the ad-3A and ad-3B loci, it is possible to obtain not only those recessive mutations resulting from intragenic alteration but also those resulting from chromosome deletion [de Serres and Osterbind 1962]. Thus with this test system it is possible to study forward-mutation resulting from a wide variety of genetic alterations.

To assay for mutagenicity, the conidia from the two-component heterokaryon are treated with varying concentrations of a chemical for a constant period of time and the treated conidia are incubated in 10 L liquid medium made viscous with 0.15 percent agar in 12 L Florence flasks for 7 days in the dark at 30°C. The contents of each jug are analyzed for the presence of ad-3 mutants by pouring 1,500 ml aliquots into large white photographic developing trays and scanning for the presence of small reddish purple colonies among the white background colonies; 10 ml samples of the background colonies are reserved for direct counts to estimate the total number of colonies per flask. The purple colonies are subcultured and plated out to make them homokaryotic for the adenine requirement, and a subculture of this homokaryotic derivative is put into stock culture. A series of genetic tests is then performed to determine genotype and allelic complementation and to distinguish the point mutations from the chromosome deletions.

The ad-3 test system undoubtedly provides the most sophisticated microbial test for mutagenicity. The ability to obtain precise quantitative data makes it possible to obtain dose-response curves not only for the induction of ad-3 mutants in general but also for each of the subclasses of point mutations and chromosome deletions. In addition it is possible to obtain presumptive evidence of the spectrum of genetic alterations, resulting in point mutations at the molecular level.

This test system provides a genetic analysis "in depth" of the spectrum of mutation resulting in the production of recessive lethal mutations at two specific loci in the genome of Neurospora.

3. Selection of Assay Systems for Screening Programs

For the results of any screening tests for mutagenicity on drugs of abuse to be applicable to man, they should be able to detect both point mutations and chromosome deletions because in diploid cells, as we have in man, recessive lethal mutations result from both of these types of genetic alteration. The problem with most microbial assay systems is that they are haploid and that they can detect only point mutations, chromosome deletions being haploid lethal. There is no diploid microbial assay capable of detecting both types of recessive lethal mutations.

The two-component heterokaryons of Neurospora come closest to a diploid assay system, and they are capable of detecting both types of recessive lethal mutations. The simplest test with this system is to assay for recessive lethal mutations occurring over the entire genome. The only drawback to this particular assay is that it is not possible to characterize the recessive lethal mutations which are induced with any simple test. But if this test system were used as a primary screen in any large-scale testing program, compounds giving a positive result in the initial

Table 2. Genetic Composition of Each Component of Heterokaryon 12, a Two-Component Heterokaryon Used in Forward Mutation Experiments

Linkage Group	Genotype of Each Component	
	Component I (strain number 74-OR60-29A)	Component II (strain number 74-OR31-16A)
I	A, hist-2, ad-3A, ad-3B, nic-2	A, al-2
III	ad-2	—
IV	—	cot
V	inos	—
VI	—	pan-2

Genetic markers are as follows: A: mating type; hist-2: histidine-requiring; ad-3A, ad-3B, ad-2 :adenine-requiring; nic-2: niacin-requiring; al-2 : albino mycelium and conidia; cot: temperature-sensitive colonial (slower growth the higher the temperature); inos: inositol-requiring; pan-2 : pantothenate-requiring.

screen could be used in a second experiment to induce recessive lethal mutations with the ad-3 test system, where it is possible to characterize them. Furthermore with careful selection of a two-component heterokaryon, such as the one indicated in Table 2, both recessive lethal analyses can be made with the same system. With heterokaryon 12, recessive lethal mutations occurring over the entire genome can be screened by first plating conidia on minimal medium; single-colony isolates are then made of the heterokaryotic colonies, and these are transferred to test tubes containing minimal agar slants. When the cultures have conidiated, they are plated on minimal medium supplemented with calcium pantothenate, and the plates are incubated at 35°C. If no recessive lethal mutation has been induced in component II tiny, dense colonies (cot) will be formed among the large sparse colonies (cot$^+$); if a recessive lethal mutation has been induced anywhere in the genome of component II, the tiny, dense colonies will be absent. The cot marker makes possible a simple visual test for the detection of a recessive lethal muta- tion anywhere in the genome of component II of this heterokaryon. Since heterokaryon 12 is also heterozygous for the ad-3 genes ad-3A and ad-3B, heterokaryotic conidia from this strain can be screened for ad-3 mutations with the direct method [de Serres and Kølmark 1958] as described in a previous section.

By utilizing a Neurospora two-component heterokaryon as the test organism in the host-mediated assay of Legator [Gabridge and Legator 1969], tests can be made not only of the original compound but also of its metabolic breakdown products. In the host-mediated assay the chemical can be fed to the animal or injected either subcutaneously, intravenously, or intraperitoneally. Asexual spores from the Neurospora two-component heterokaryon are then injected into the peritoneal cavity and left there for various periods of time [Legator and Malling 1971]. In this way the spores are exposed not only to the original compound but also to any metabolic breakdown products. The spores are then removed and screened for recessive lethal mutations induced either over the genome or in the ad-3 region.

In summary, the data obtained in such screening tests using the Neurospora assay system, especially in conjunction with in vivo mammalian tests, should be directly applicable to man. Neurospora is an eukaryotic organism; the two-component heterokaryon effectively mimics a diploid cell; and the host-mediated assay makes it possible not only to test the original compound for mutagenicity but also its metabolic breakdown products.

4. Summary

A number of test systems have been developed with either bacteria or fungi which are capable of detecting the genetic damage produced by mutagenic chemicals. The test systems range from those capable of detecting particular kinds of genetic alterations to those capable of detecting a broad spectrum of genetic alteration. The test systems include both forward and reverse mutation assays. With *Neurospora crassa* two test systems exist that permit a thorough evaluation of a chemical for microbial mutagenicity. The first assay permits one to detect a broad spectrum of genetic alterations (point mutation or chromosome deletion) resulting in recessive lethal mutations over the entire genome. In the second assay the recessive lethal mutations occurring at two specific loci in the ad-3 region are obtained for a thorough characterization by a series of simple genetic tests. These tests distinguish point mutations from chromosome deletions and permit a presumptive identification of the genetic alterations which produce point mutations at the molecular level. By using Neurospora as the test organism in the host-mediated assay, tests can be made not only on the original chemical compound but also on its metabolic breakdown products.

References

Alderson, T. and C. Scazzocchio (1967). *Mutat. Res.* 4:567–577.

Ames, B. N., and H. J. Whitfield, Jr. (1966). *Cold Spring Harbor Symp. Quant. Biol.* 31:221–225.

Atwood, K. C. (1949). *Biol. Bull.* 97:254–255.

———, and F. Mukai (1953). *Proc. Nat. Acad. Sci.* 39:1027–1035.

de Serres, F. J., and H. G. Kølmark (1958). *Nature* 182:1249–1250.

de Serres, F. J., and R. S. Osterbind (1962). *Genetics* 47:793–796.

de Serres, F. J., H. E. Brockman, W. E. Barnett, and H. G. Kølmark (1967). *Mutat. Res.* 4:415–424.

Gabridge, M. G., and M. S. Legator (1969). *Proc. Soc. Exp. Biol. Med.* 130:831–834.

Horowitz, N. H., and A. M. Srb (1948). *J. Biol. Chem.* 174:371–387.

Legator, M. S., and H. V. Malling (1971). In A. Hollaender, ed., *Enviromental Chemical Mutagens*, New York: Plenum Press.

Lester, G. (1966). *J. Bacteriol.* 91:677–684.

Lockhart, W. R., and H. R. Garner (1955). *Genetics* 40:721–725.

Malling, H. V. (1966). *Mutat. Res.* 3:470–476.

———, and F. J. de Serres (1967). *Mutat. Res.* 4:425–440.

——— (1968). *Mutat. Res.* 5:359–371.

Roman, H. (1956). *Compt. Rend. Trav. Lab. Carlsberg Ser. Physiol.* 26:299–314.

Smith, H. H., and A. M. Srb (1951). *Science* 114:490–492.

Stadler, D. (1966). *Genetics* 54:677–685.

Whitfield, H. J., Jr., R. G. Martin, and B. N. Ames (1966). *J. Mol. Biol.* 21:335–355.

10 Drosophila Methods for Mutagenicity Testing

J. F. Crow and S. Abrahamson

The fruit fly, *Drosophila melanogaster*, is the organism in which both radiation-induced and chemically-induced mutations were first demonstrated. In both cases, the success depended on techniques, first developed by H. J. Muller, for efficient and unambiguous detection of new mutations. These methods, with some refinements and improvements, still constitute the basic mutation-detecting system in Drosophila.

For precision of mutation detection and for the capacity to resolve these mutations into specific kinds of chemical changes, the microbial systems [DeSerres chapter 9] are superior. The enormous numbers that can be scored and the great multiplication in efficiency that comes with such mutation-selecting systems cannot be matched in Drosophila. On the other hand, from some standpoints Drosophila techniques are more efficient than corresponding tests in the mouse. Furthermore, Drosophila offers efficient tests for translocations and for chromosome loss. So Drosophila, we think, has a role in the testing of environmental agents that may cause genetic damage.

We shall discuss here only those systems which seem particularly useful. They are the classical test for X-linked recessive lethals, tests for translocations, and systems for detecting the loss of a chromosome or chromosome fragment. Other available tests include tests for lethal mosaics, autosomal lethal tests, tests for recessive visible mutants on the X-chromosome or at selected autosomal loci, dominant lethal tests, detachment of attached X-chromosomes, mutations accumulated over many generations of chronic treatment, and tests for mutants with minor viability effects.

A recent review of Drosophila techniques, particularly applicable to screening for chemical mutagens, has been prepared by Abrahamson and Lewis [1970]. An earlier comprehensive review of Drosophila methodologies is found in a paper by Muller and

Oster [1963]. Both of these papers contain extensive bibliographies.

In this article we mainly summarize the 1970 review of Abrahamson and Lewis, to which the reader is referred for full details.

1. Tests for X-Linked Recessive Lethal Mutations

The method, essentially the same as first developed by Muller, requires two generations, and more if any ambiguous cases require retesting. It detects recessive lethal mutations arising in either sex. Under ordinary circumstances one tests males because it is then certain that any lethal mutant transmitted in a sperm arose during the lifetime of the male; otherwise he would be dead. With females this fact is not clear, but with minor modifications of the system, the time of mutation in the female can be rendered equally unambiguous.

The fly to be tested, in this case, a male, is treated by whatever method is appropriate to the chemical—usually by feeding or by injections into the abdominal cavity. The treated males are mated to females that carry special X-chromosomes. The most frequently used chromosome, termed *Muller-5* or *Basc*, carries the recessive gene for apricot eye color and the small duplication that causes the dominant Bar-shaped eye. This chromosome also has a complicated inversion within an inversion, the effect of which is virtually to remove all recombination when the X-chromosome is heterozygous. The F_1 females are allowed to mate with the males emerging in the same culture and are then placed in individual vials. Each vial then constitutes a test of one X-chromosome from the sperm produced by the treated male. If this chromosome carries a recessive lethal mutant there will be no males except those with apricot-Bar eyes, since those with normal eyes would have been killed by the lethal chromosome.

This method lends itself to routine organization and rapid scoring, for it is quick and simple to examine a culture for the absence of normal-eyed males. In the Wisconsin laboratory, a staff of two or three people can analyze 5 to 10,000 chromosomes per month. An advantage of the system is its ability to detect all kinds of recessive mutants that produce a lethal effect and that are located anywhere along the X-chromosome. These may range from single base changes to small deletions and rearrangements. The capacity to detect both nucleotide changes and chromosome breaks is important, for the chemical being tested may do only one or the other.

The biggest weakness of the system is that one fly culture provides one item of data, so the test is necessarily quite expensive. To detect a doubling of the spontaneous rate would require thousands of tests. There are other pitfalls for the unwary, for example, a troublesome tendency in the Muller-5 strain to accumulate extra Y-chromosomes, which leads to secondary nondisjunction, which in turn causes some lethal chromosomes to be missed. Another problem is that lethal chromosomes may occur in clusters if the mutation event occurred several generations prior to meiosis, and this phenomenon complicates the statistical analysis. For a discussion of these and other problems and the proper precautions, see Abrahamson and Lewis [1970].

Similar test systems are available for autosomes, but they are not so clean, since there is always some uncertainty with autosomal recessives as to whether the lethal chromosome was actually induced by the treatment or was inherited from an earlier generation. This ambiguity does not obtain for X-linked loci, as mentioned earlier.

2. Tests for Chromosome Rearrangements

Since translocations are an important part of inherited human cytogenetic abnormalities, this is a class of event that should be looked for when chemicals are screened. The most widely used test makes use of changed linkage relationships resulting from translocations. This procedure takes advantage of the absence of crossing-over in Drosophila males.

Treated males are crossed to females that have recessive marker genes on each of the autosomes. Then the progeny males are crossed individually to the same multiply-marked strain. Translocations are detected by linkages between the previously independent marker genes. Translocations involving the X-chromosome can be included by using females with attached X-chromosomes.

This system is objective and usually the interpretation of any culture is unambiguous. The weakness is that it is inefficient for large-scale tests because, as with the X-linked lethal test, a whole culture of flies is required to assay one gamete for the presence or absence of a translocation. The test requires 2 generations, or more if any retesting is needed; thus a complete test requires a minimum of 4 to 6 weeks.

There are also tests for chromosome re-arrangements that require only one generation and in which each fly is a test of a gamete. These tests make use of the phenomenon of position effect. The most efficient is the "transvection" test [Lewis 1954]. The mutant bithorax in transposition with the mutant ultrabithorax is very sensitive to rearrangements that alter the pairing relations of chromosome number 3. Thus, an exaggerated bithorax phenotype signals a re-arrangement in chromosome 3; it may be a translocation or inversion, or something more complicated.

The increased efficiency that comes by re-ducing the time to one generation and making each fly constitute a test of one gamete is enormous. The disadvantage is that the phenotypic change is not very constant, and considerable experience is required to recog-nize the sometimes subtle morphological changes. However, in the hands of an expert, this is a very efficient way of detecting trans-missible chromosome rearrangements.

3. Tests for Nondisjunction and Chromosome Loss

There are several systems for detecting non-disjunction. One of the simplest and best is the direct search for exceptions to the ordinary rules of X-linked inheritance. A more elegant system that detects nondisjunction, loss of either the X or Y, and loss of parts of the Y through chromosome breakage, is also available. A female with appropriate gene markers on her X chromosomes is mated to a treated male that has dominant marker genes on both the X and Y chromosomes. Those on the Y are genes normally on the X, but which have been put on the Y by translocation. Since both the X and Y are labeled, the loss of either can be detected. Also, since the Y chromosome is marked at both ends, a deletion that removes either marker can be detected. Similarly, if the male transmits both an X and a Y, this can be detected. Thus the system can detect any of these changes. It is an efficient system, since each fly is a test for a gamete. One investigator can easily screen 5,000 gametes per day for chromo-some loss or nondisjunction. It should, however, be emphasized that considerable skill is required to manage stocks and the tests.

4. Recent Examples of the Use of These Methods in Drug Tests

We might mention that three of the four systems that we have discussed have recently been used for testing drugs. Experiments by Browning [1968], Vann [1969], and Markowitz et al. [1969] agree in showing a slight increase in the frequency of recessive lethals from a high concentration of ingested LSD. On the other hand, there is no evidence for chromosome loss (Browning), nor for heritable chromosome rearrangements by the bithorax system (Markowitz et al.).

5. Summary and Recommendations

Drosophila tests for recessive mutations are intermediate in sensitivity between microbial and mouse systems. In addition to the classical tests for X-linked lethal mutations, there are efficient tests for rearrangements and for chromosome loss.

We believe that these Drosophila tests have a useful place in an overall drug testing program. Lacking the sensitivity of the micro-organism tests, Drosophila systems are not as suitable for preliminary screening of large numbers of chemicals. But when more thorough tests are indicated, in addition to in vivo mammalian systems, Drosophila tests can provide useful information at moderate expense.

References

Abrahamson, S., and E. B. Lewis (1971). The detection of mutations in *Drosophila melanogaster*. In A. Hollaender, ed., *Environmental Chemical Mutagens*, New York: Plenum Press.

Browning, L. S. (1968). *Science* 161:1022.

Lewis, E. B. (1954). *Amer. Natur.* 88:225.

Markowitz, E. H., G. E. Brosseau, and E. Markowitz (1969). *Mutat. Res.* 8:337.

Muller, H. J., and I. I. Oster (1963). Some mutational techniques in Drosophila. In W. J. Burdette, ed., *Methodology in Basic Genetics*, San Francisco: Holden-Day.

Vann, E. (1969). *Nature* 223:95.

11   Cytogenetic Methods for Mutagenicity Testing

P. S. Moorhead, L. F. Jarvik, and M. M. Cohen

1. Chromosomal Damage Induced by Drugs of Abuse—Survey of the Literature

In the preparation of this review over one hundred references were thoroughly examined. Unfortunately, many proved to be only statements of opinion, editorial or otherwise. Two major questions were considered: first, which of these drugs, when used by man, cause chromosomal damage? and second, what is the relationship between chromosome damage and subsequent morbidity or teratogenicity?

The chief problems encountered in attempting to evaluate the findings on chromosome damage reported to date were lack of adequate numbers of subjects in the drug and control groups; insufficient knowledge of pertinent exogenous events such as exposure to radiation, viral infection, chemicals, food additives, and other pharmacological agents for drug groups as well as controls; lack of information on the composition of preparations bought illicitly by drug users (e.g. contaminants, dose, etc.) and, therefore, questionable applicability of findings obtained from users of such "street" supplies to users of pure compounds; finally, the possibility of large individual differences in susceptibility to the chromosome-breaking action of various agents.

With regard to the eventual consequences of chromosome damage to the individual and his progeny we lack vital data on the fate of cells having suffered chromosomal damage. If chromosome damage results in cell death, and only a relatively small proportion of cells have suffered such damage, then there are probably no serious consequences for either the individual or his offspring. If the proportion of cells with lethal chromosome damage is large, then the consequences may be serious in terms of individual morbidity and mortality, but there will be no transmissible damage to future generations. By contrast, survival of cells having sustained chromosomal damage represents a threat to future generations as well as the affected individual. Such damaged cells may be sequestered, and years later they may initiate the formation of abnormal clones with the development of malignant neoplasia. Likewise, damaged gonadal cells may transmit the chromosomal damage to future generations and produce congenital abnormalities. In the last-mentioned respect, certain types of chromosomal damage are more serious than others. Ring chromosomes, for example, are known to be transmissible from one generation to the next and to produce visible phenotypic as well as chromosomal abnormalities. Small acentric fragments, by contrast, are unstable and tend to be lost upon subsequent cell division. Yet, the deletion may be dysgenic for future generations even if not grossly detectable.

It is with considerations such as those described above in mind that the literature was reviewed.

Since the literature is most extensive with regard to LSD, that drug is listed separately. Studies have further been divided into human studies in vivo and in vitro, and animal studies.

1.1. LSD and Chromosomes

1.1.1. In Vivo Human Studies

There are ten reports comparing chromosome findings in leukocyte cultures taken from persons after exposure to LSD and from unexposed controls (Table 1). Six of these studies concern chromosomes of drug users, with ignorance of factors such as dose or doses of LSD taken, or purity of compound. Further, nearly all of these users employed other drugs as well. Users showed higher percentages of breaks than controls in all but one of the studies [Loughman et al. 1967]. Since many drugs, known and unknown, were taken by these users either before or at the same time as LSD, all we can conclude from these studies is that persons using drugs of abuse show higher percent-

ages of chromosome breaks than do other persons. A causal relationship cannot be deduced from these correlations, inasmuch as diet, exposure to infection, and general living conditions, as well as drug intake, generally differ between users and controls.

Findings with regard to major structural abnormalities parallel those of breaks, where reported. Surprisingly, dicentrics, ring chromosomes, and exchange figures were seen in some of the controls as well as in some users.

In another study, which appeared in print after Table 1 had been completed [Judd et al. 1969], three groups of subjects were compared: heavy users of LSD (9 continuous users), formerly heavy users who discontinued use of LSD at least 15 months prior to the chromosome examination (8 former users), and persons who had never used LSD (8 drug-free controls). The results of this single-blind experiment (persons examining the chromosomes were unaware of the subjects' drug history) failed to show significant differences in percent of chromosome breaks among the three groups. Indeed, the continued users showed the lowest percentage of breaks (0.32%) and the former users the highest (1.80%), the drug-free controls having an intermediate value (0.72%). Moreover, the authors did not find the frequency of chromosome abnormalities to be related to any of the following variables: total number of times LSD was ingested; total amount of LSD ingested; length of time LSD was used; or length of time since last dose. This single-blind study with a well-controlled experimental design did not support the finding that LSD causes an increase in chromosomal aberrations over and above that which can be found in a normal control population.

There are reports also on five groups of persons examined after medical administration of LSD (Table 1), and three of these reports [Bender and Siva Sankar 1968; Sparkes et al. 1968; and Tjio et al. 1969]

Table 1. Reports on Leukocyte Cultures Taken from Persons After Exposure to LSD and from Unexposed Controls

Subjects Exposed to LSD

Author	Year	Number of Subjects	Age Range in Years	Source of Subjects	Number of Metaphases	Mean % Breaks
Irwin & Egozcue	1967	8	—	volunteers from users	1,600	23.6
Loughman et al.	1967	8	—	clients, welfare agency	697	0
Cohen et al.	1967	18	19–52	—	4,292	13.2
		4	2 mo.–5.5 yr.	—	1,000	11.9
Bender & Sankar	1968	5	7–11	schizophrenic patients	50	<2.0
Egozcue et al.	1968	46	17–43	—	9,140	18.8
		4	1–18 mo.	—	800	21.5
Sparkes et al.	1968	4	19–24	schizophrenic and other psychiatric patients	937	2.2
		4	28–45	psychoneurotic patients	914	1.5
Nielsen et al.	1968	5	29–48	patients	358	1.7
Abbo et al.	1968	9	24–57	patients	266	8.3
Valenti	1969	10	15–25	patients	894	10.0
Tjio et al.	1969	8	—	normal volunteers	1,646	2.8

Subjects Not Exposed to LSD (Controls)

Author	Year	Number of Subjects[3]	Age Range in Years	Source of Subjects	Number of Metaphases	Mean % Breaks
Irwin & Egozcue	1967	8	—	volunteers	1,600	10.3
Loughman et al.	1967	19	—	—	673	0.4
Cohen et al.	1967	12	22–55	drug-free	2,674	3.8
Bender & Sankar	1968	5	Children	schizophrenic	50	<2.0
Egozcue et al.	1968	14	17–30	drug-free	2,800	9.0
Sparkes et al.	1968	4	21–50	hospital volunteers	950	1.6
Nielsen et al.	1968	40	17–59	30 patients 10 hospital personnel	1,312	0.4
Abbo et al.	1968	32	24–59	—	1,022	3.5
Valenti	1969					
Tjio et al.	1969	2	—	normal	—	2.7

[1] Major structural abnormalities include dicentrics, multiradials, ring chromosomes, etc.
[2] M.A. = Medical Administration; D.U. = Drug User; I.U. = In Utero
[3] Other drugs used (see text)

Range % Breaks	Number of Major Structural Abnormalities	Mean % Gaps	Dose Range in μg[2]	Duration	Interval Between Last Dose and Culture
12.0–38.0	10	—	D.U. 200–2.800	4–200 doses	1–180 days
0	0	0.4	D.U. 100–4.000[3]	12–100 doses	1–22 days
5.3–25.1	17	—	D.U. 300–600[3]	2–300 doses	2–33 weeks
4.0–19.0	—	—	I.U. 50–600[3]	1–4 doses	1st–3rd trimester
—	—	—	M.A. 100–150	5.5–35 months	20–48 months
8.0–45.0	More than in controls	—	D.U. 100–2.800[3]	—	1–360 days
9.5–28.0	—	—	I.U. 150–500[3]	2nd trimester	—
0.9–3.4	4	3.6	D.U. 250–1.000[3]	5–24 months	0.2–6 months
0.4–2.5	2	4.9	M.A 250–500[3]	12–48 months	1–60 months
0–6.9	0	15.9	M.A. 50–300	3–39 months	6–38 months
3.3–13.3	0	—	M.A. 200–800, total[3]	—	9–39 months
0–20.8	36	—	D.U. 250–25,000, total[3]	3–24 months	7–215 days
2.0–3.8	—	—	M.A. 300–4,800, total	1–26 doses	67–443 days

Range % Breaks	Number of Major Structural Abnormalities	Mean % Gaps
7.0–16.5	4	—
—	1	0.6
2.0–5.5	0	—
—	—	—
6.0–16.5	observed	—
0.8–2.6	1	6.4
0–?	0	9.1
0–?	0	—
—	—	—

Table 2. Chromosome Abnormalities Before and After In Vivo Exposure of Human Subjects to LSD

Author	Hungerford et al. 1968		Tjio et al. 1969		
Number and Source of Subjects	4 patients with behavior problems	3 controls matched to patients	21 patients with alcoholism or neurosis	11 patients with alcoholism or neurosis	5 users from NIH study
Dose Range in Micrograms	180–200 per treatment	180–200 per treatment	250–450 once	50 once	1 µg/kg before first post-treatment 2 µg/kg before fourth post-treatment

Abnormalities

I. Pretreatment					
A. Mean % Breaks	1	—	4.4	4.1	3.3
B. Number of Major Structural Abnormalities	0	—	27	0	—
II. Post-treatment					
A. Mean % Breaks (during)					
1. 1 week	4.0	2.0			
2. 1–2 weeks	4.4	0.7			
3. 1–4 weeks (after)	3.3	1.0			
4. 1–6 months	1.1	—			
B. Number of Major Structural Abnormalities (during)					
1. 1 week	3	0			
2. 1–2 weeks	3	0			
3. 1–4 weeks (after)	0	0			
4. 1–6 months	1	—			
C. Mean % Breaks					
1. 1–10 days			4.2	9.3	
a. 30 min.					3.3
b. 1 day					2.8
c. 2 days					3.4
2. 1–33 days			(3.4 in 8 subjects)[1]		
a. 30 min.					2.9
b. 1 day					2.4
c. 2 days					5.7
D. Number of Major Structural Abnormalities					
1. 1–10 days			4	40	
a. 30 min.					—
b. 1 day					—
c. 2 days					—
2. 1–33 days			—	—	
a. 30 min.					—
b. 1 day					—
c. 2 days					—

[1] Taken from both groups of patients with alcoholism or neurosis.

failed to find an increase in breaks or structural abnormalities even though large doses of the pure compound were administered. Incidentally, additional drugs had been used as well by the subjects of two of these studies. The other two groups did manifest an increase in breaks [Abbo et al. 1968; and Nielsen et al. 1968]; and in one of them apparently LSD alone had been used.

None of the above-mentioned studies fulfills what would generally be regarded as minimal criteria of a scientifically acceptable research design. These criteria include chromosome analyses before exposure to LSD of persons known not to have been exposed to other drugs, to radiation, or to viral infection during a specified preceding interval, and of controls matched for as many variables as possible other than exposure to LSD; administration of pure drug in known dosages; chromosome analyses at specified intervals during and following drug administration; and adequate numbers of subjects in both groups.

There are, however, two studies approaching fulfillment of these criteria (Table 2). The first of these [Hungerford et al 1968], concerns three patients on whom blood cultures were set up one hour before LSD administration (for a fourth patient only post-treatment values could be obtained), to whom known doses of LSD were administered, for whom further blood cultures were set up during the course of LSD administration (which extended over a period of one month) and again one to six months after the last dose of drug had been injected. Three control subjects were matched to the patients according to age and sex, but they were otherwise not identified. Each of these controls had three leukocyte cultures for chromosome analysis, with a range of breaks from 0 to 3 percent (range of means 0.7–2.0%), without any consistent trend characterizing the three-week interval during which blood for chromosome analysis was taken.

The LSD subjects, by contrast, showed a range of breaks from 1 to 7 percent during the time of LSD administration, with a decrease in mean after the second post-treatment culture from 4.4 to 3.3 percent, compared to a pretreatment mean of 1.0 percent. One to six months after termination of LSD administration, the breaks had returned to a mean of 1.1 percent in the LSD group.

Hungerford and collaborators [1968] also observed a number of structural abnormalities (four dicentrics and one quadriradial) in 1,425 metaphases counted from three LSD subjects, but none in the 300 metaphases from the same subjects counted before LSD administration, and none in 900 metaphases of the three control subjects.

Aside from the paucity of subjects, interpretation of the result is complicated by the fact that each patient received another drug (chlorpromazine) together with LSD, at least once in the course of the study. Nonetheless, Hungerford and associates are probably justified in concluding that LSD produced a transient increase in chromosome breaks, the increase lasting less than one to six months.

The second study, by Tjio et al [1969], includes a far larger number of subjects (Table 2). Chromosome examinations were performed on 32 patients before and at least once after they were given pure LSD in a double-blind study. No statistically significant increase after LSD administration was noted either for the low-dose group (11 patients, one dose of LSD at 50 μg) or for the high-dose group (21 patients, one dose of LSD at between 250 and 450 μg). In the high-dose group the mean percentage of breaks before and after LSD was 4.39 and 4.16 percent, respectively, and in the low-dose group it was 4.05 and 9.26 percent, respectively. The combined total for both groups (32 patients) was somewhat lower before than after LSD (4.28 vs. 5.91%, respectively),

Table 3. Reports on Chromosomes from Human Leukocytes Cultured Without and With Added LSD (in vitro)

Without added LSD (in vitro)

Author	Year	Number of Subjects	Age Range in Years	Source of Subjects
Cohen et al.	1967a	6	—	—
Cohen et al.	1967b	6	—	—
Jarvik et al.	1968	11	22–61	normal volunteers, patients with psychiatric or neurologic diseases, and genetic counseling cases
Kato and Jarvik	1969	2	31–32	normal volunteers
Genest	1969	1	—	—

With added LSD (in vitro)

Author	Year	Number of Subjects	Age Range in Years	Source of Subjects	Final Concentration in Flask (in µg/ml)
Cohen et al.	1967a	6	—	—	0.001, 0.01, 0.1, 1.0, and 10.0
Cohen et al.	1967b	2	—	—	0.001, 0.01, 0.1, 1.0, and 10.0
Jarvik et al.	1968	8	22–61	normal volunteers, patients with psychiatric or neurologic diseases, and genetic counseling cases	0.01
Kato and Jarvik	1969	2	31–32	normal volunteers	0.001, 0.01, and 1.0
Genest	1969	1	—	—	0.1, 1.0, and 10.0

[1] Major structural abnormalities include dicentrics, multiradials, ring chromosomes, etc.

	Number of Metaphases	Mean % Breaks	Range % Breaks	Number of Major Structural Abnormalities[1]	Mean % Gaps
	1,680	3.9	—	—	—
	925	3.7	—	—	—
	720	4.7	0–9.0	1	6.0
				—	
	100	5.0	—	0	—
	26	15	—	(0?)	—

Time Exposed to LSD in Hours	Number of Metaphases	Mean % Breaks	Range % Breaks	Number of Major Abnormalities	Mean % Gaps
4, 24, and 48	7,735	13.0	7.7–17.5	observed number unspecified	—
4, 24, and 48	2,678	14.3	5.0–36.8	observed number unspecified	—
4	498	10.2	0–15.0	2	10.4
4 and 24	600	5.0	2.0–12.0	0	—
24	64	12.5	7.1–20.8	(0?)	—

but not significantly so. The large number of cells counted per sample (at least 200) lends strength to these observations.

Unfortunately, 31 of the 32 patients received one or more drugs during their hospitalization before the pre-LSD blood sample was drawn, and 7 of the 32 were receiving other drugs at the time that the blood sample was obtained. In addition, several of the patients had upper respiratory infections. The authors emphasize the fact that neither the 7 patients on other drugs (with two exceptions) nor the 4 patients with documented symptoms of viral infection (with one exception) showed unusually high chromosomal aberration rates in pre-LSD cultures. Equally noteworthy is the lack of statistically significant differences in chromosomal aberrations before and after LSD, when the comparison is restricted to those 7 patients who neither had an upper respiratory tract viral infection nor received any drug for a period of four weeks preceding the pre-LSD sample. However, in a group of eight patients with two, instead of one, post-LSD culture, only two failed to show a post-LSD increase and all, except for these two, showed a decrease on repeat post-LSD culture [Tjio et al. 1969, p. 851, Table 3]. Further, a small increase in chromosomal abnormalities was recorded for five LSD users after they had received known doses of pure LSD [Tjio et al. 1969], but this increase (2.81% to 3.57%) was statistically not significant.

It is not surprising that the data are not definitive when we bear in mind the great variability in chromosomal abnormalities seen not only from laboratory to laboratory and from person to person but even in the same person from day to day. The last point is well illustrated by Tjio et al. [1969], who report a monumental amount of data (over 27,000 cell counts) which includes chromosome examinations on two normal drug-free subjects on eight successive days for one subject and nine for the other. The percentage of chromosome aberrations varied between 1.48 and 3.38 percent for one subject and between 1.96 and 4.76 percent for the other subject.

With regard to human in vivo studies, we can concur with Tjio et al. that at the present time there is "no *definitive* evidence that LSD damages chromosomes of human white blood cells *in vivo* as studied in 72 hour cultures." We also concur with their conclusion that "further research in this complex field is obviously needed."

With regard to human prenatal exposure, 8 infants born to mothers who had taken LSD (Table 1)—as well as marijuana in the case of one study [Egozcue et al. 1968], and amphetamine, cocaine, and marijuana in the case of the other study [Cohen et al. 1967]—showed a relatively high frequency of breaks (range 4–28%). Break frequencies as high as 28 percent have been known to occur following upper respiratory or gastrointestinal symptoms, and a high frequency cannot be attributed—on the basis of available information—to LSD exposure years prior to leukocyte culture. For want of controls, conclusions are precluded at this time.

1.1.2. In Vitro Human Cell Studies

Of five in vitro human experiments, three reported an increase in breaks with LSD [Cohen et al. 1967a and 1967b; Jarvik et al. 1968] and two did not (Table 3). No dose-response curve could be derived by any of the investigators in a concentration high enough to show any effect apparently equaling in effectiveness the highest dose compatible with cell survival. Failure to obtain dose-response curves for LSD may be due to the fact that low enough doses have not been adequately tested, a concentration of 0.001 Mg/ml being effective. It is possible also [Freese, personal communication 1969] that inactivation occurs at higher concentrations, keeping the effective concentration at a constant level.

Cells from some subjects may be relatively resistant to the chromosome-breaking action of LSD and others may be susceptible (compare Kato and Jarvik 1969 with Jarvik et al. 1968 in Table 3).

Conclusions based on in vitro studies must be drawn with particular care since substances added to cells in culture are not subject to metabolic alteration, may affect various parameters such as pH, and are directly accessible to the cell. It is not unexpected, therefore, that many agents can cause chromosomal damage in culture, provided that they are added in sufficient amounts, at the right time, and to the right cells [Jarvik 1969]. Deprivation of essential amino acids may also induce chromosome damage [Freed and Schatz 1969].

A comparison of the efficiency of LSD in inducing chromosome damage is available [Jarvik et al. 1968]. In a concentration approximating the blood level of a heavy user, LSD doubled chromosome breaks over control values, and the same doubling occurred upon addition of ergonovine maleate, a commonly used oxytocic, and aspirin. The concentration of aspirin in the leukocyte cultures was equivalent to the blood level achieved after the ingestion of four aspirin tablets. By way of comparison, a doubling of breaks plus gaps was observed in cells cultured from fetuses which had been naturally infected in utero with rubella virus [Chang et al. 1966]. In contrast, streptonigrin, an anticancer agent, produced a seven-fold increase.

Conflicting results are not limited to LSD. So far, there are published data on few chromosome studies in aspirin use. Maurer et al. (1970) concluded that aspirin in vivo or in vitro produced no significant increases in chromosome damage. Examination of children admitted with acute aspirin toxicity did not show a higher frequency of chromosome aberrations than customary in that particular laboratory [Cohen, personal communication 1969]. It is possible that acute intoxication differs from chronic administration in terms of survival of affected cells— clarification certainly is needed.

Concerning in vitro human studies, further well-controlled experiments are essential. In addition, some indication will have to be obtained, possibly from animal studies, concerning the extent to which in vitro findings can be extrapolated to in vivo situations.

1.1.3. Animal Studies

Mice. Of two groups first reporting break frequencies in animals [Cohen and Mukherjee 1968; Skakkebaek et al. 1968], both looked at meiotic chromosomes in mice and both found a marked increase in abnormalities due to LSD despite the use of different concentrations of LSD (25 μg/kg and 1 μg/kg, respectively). Cohen and Mukherjee [1968] also examined bone marrow cells in mice and noted that LSD [25 μg/kg] nearly quadrupled the control breakage frequency (14.7 vs. 4.0%) with a marked increase also in structural abnormalities.

Jagiello and Polani [1969], by contrast, could not confirm abnormalities in meiotic chromosomes of mice as a result of LSD treatment.

Monkeys. In a pilot study [Kato et al. 1970], serial chromosome examinations were performed on six pregnant Rhesus monkeys. Four of the monkeys were given injections of LSD and two, serving as controls, saline solution. The two monkeys receiving the highest doses of LSD (0.5 to 1.0 mg/kg) showed an increase in breaks after LSD injection with a return to normal after several weeks or months. The temporary nature of the rise in chromosome breaks in these two

Table 4. Reports on Leukocyte Cultures Taken from Persons After Exposure to Psychiatric Drugs and from Unexposed Controls

Drug Exposed Subjects

Author	Number of Subjects	Age Range (in years)	Number of Metaphases	Mean % Breaks	Range % Breaks
Cohen et al. 1967	3	9–30	700	10.6	4.0–17.4
Cohen et al. 1969	6	26–54	533	2.8	1.3–4.0
	3	31–44	296	4.4	3.1–7.0
	3	29–52	297	3.0	1.0–4.1
	6	12–24	555	2.9	1.0–5.1
	4	46–57	303	3.0	0–9.1
	3	—	300	6.0	5.0–7.0
	3	—	300	2.3	1.0–3.0
	2	—	174	2.3	1.2–3.4
	3	—	300	3.0	1.0–5.0
	2	—	200	2.0	1.0–3.0
	3	—	300	2.0	1.0–3.0
	2	—	146	2.7	2.7–2.8
Nielsen et al. 1969	5	<50	299	1.0	not given
	8	50+	495	2.4	not given
	10	<50	736	3.5	not given
	5	50+	311	4.5	not given

Unexposed Controls

Author	Number of Subjects	Age Range (in years)	Number of Metaphases	Mean % Breaks	Range % Breaks
Cohen et al. 1967	12	22–55	2,674	3.8	2.0–5.5
Cohen et al. 1969	6	21–61	579	2.9	1.3–4.0
	6	14–19	473	2.5	1.4–4.7
	4	42–63	302	3.6	1.4–6.0
	3 } same sub- jects as above	—	300	5.0	4.0–6.0
	3	—	289	4.8	1.1–7.0
	3	—	233	0.9	0–1.2
	3	—	244	4.9	2.6–7.0
	3	—	266	1.9	1.5–2.0
	3	—	300	3.0	0–6.0
	2		166	2.4	2.0–3.0
Nielsen et al. 1969	30	<50	1,030	0.2	—
	11	50+	554	0.5	—

[1] Three major structural abnormalities were included, the only ones reported in all the cases listed on this table.

Name of Major Drug	Dose Range in mg/day	Duration	Other Drugs Taken
chlorpromazine	200	3 weeks– 1½ years	thioridazine diphenylhydramine opiates
chlorpromazine	100–400	1–24 months	*chloralhydrates
fluphenazine	100	3–6 months	***trihexphendyl
thiordiazine	100–200	4–12 months	
diazepam	10–60	36–72 months	vitamins
chlordiazepoxide	10–30	2–24 months	
chlordiazepoxide	30	1 week	
chlordiazepoxide	30	3 weeks	
chlordiazepoxide	30	5 weeks	
chlordiazepoxide	30	2 weeks	
chlordiazepoxide	30	4 weeks	
chlordiazepoxide	30	6 weeks	
chlordiazepoxide	30	8 weeks	
chlorpromazine	125–500 mg/day (highest)	0.5–161 months	
perphenazine	12–72 mg/day (highest)	1–108 months	orphenadrine

Drugs Taken

not specified

not specified
vitamins and antiepileptics
hydrochlorthiazide, K-Lyte digitalis vitamins
1 week ⎫
3 weeks ⎬ sequential samples
5 weeks ⎭

2 weeks ⎫
4 weeks ⎪ sequential samples
6 weeks ⎬
8 weeks ⎭

not specified
not specified

monkeys agrees with the findings of Hungerford and colleagues [1968] for humans. The doses used in these monkeys, however, were extremely high, and two other monkeys given LSD in doses of 0.125 to 0.250 mg/kg did not show a measurable increase in chromosome breaks 4 and 7 days, respectively, after the last dose of LSD. These lower doses were still sufficiently high to produce marked behavioral effects and exceed many-fold doses used in man. No major structural abnormalities were seen in any of the postdrug cultures, regardless of dose.

Of the six products of the pregnancy, two were stillborn and one died of pneumonia at the age of one month—all three of them offspring of mothers given LSD. The lone survivor of an LSD-treated mother did not show a significant increase in chromosome breaks and appeared normal. Nonetheless, the high mortality, prenatal and neonatal, for the offspring of LSD-mothers suggests the need for expanded, well-controlled studies, using animals living before and after impregnation under clearly defined laboratory conditions rather than animals shipped from Asia while pregnant.

Drosophila. Investigations of the mutagenic effects of drugs through the use of Drosophila and appropriate genetically marked stocks also provide assessment of chromosome breakage. Grace, Carlson, and Goodman [1968] failed to find any effect, whether of mutation or translocation, resulting from the injection of LSD into Drosophila males (1,100 and 500 μg/ml of a tartrate solution). The higher two doses were said to be equivalent to the introduction of one liter of the concentration into a human subject. No indication of translocation was obtained among 4,205 test progeny. Tobin and Tobin [1969] observed no increase in lethals in offspring derived from chromosomes exposed to LSD injected during the postmeiotic and meiotic stages of the male germ cells. Similarly, no

increase in lethal induction from larval feeding experiments was obtained.

These authors conclude that the investigation indicates that LSD is not a chemical mutagen but caution that the reaction between LSD and DNA is poorly understood and that a "relatively small number was included in the test sample."

The third study, involving intraperitoneal injection of LSD into Drosophila males [Browning 1968], did report a significant increase in recessive lethal mutations. However, the dose employed was extreme, being "highly toxic and partially sterilizing" (4,000 μg per gram body weight).

Isolated case reports. Isolated case reports have not been included in the tabulations. Recognizing the value of such reports in instances of repeated occurrence of well-defined syndromes, like thalidomide-induced phocomelia, isolated cases must be weighed carefully. Despite widespread use of a drug like LSD, these reports are limited to one case of leg deformity, one of hand malformation, two of leukemia, and a few other abnormalities, increased frequency of chromosome breaks in peripheral leukocytes of isolated cases—all without proper controls. These cases are not likely to contribute much to our knowledge in this area.

1.2. Marijuana

Only a single study was found, and that was in a letter to the authors. Martin [1969] could demonstrate no chromosome change (Table 5) in leukocytes or fibroblasts following in vitro treatment of cultures with cannabis (40–200 μg/ml).

1.3. Chlorpromazine (Thorazine)

1.3.1. In Vivo Human Studies

Cohen et al. [1967a and 1969] examined the chromosomes of nine patients who received the drug therapeutically. These investigators failed to find an increase in breaks compared to 18 controls, even though many of the patients had taken other drugs as well

Table 5. Reports on Chromosomes from Human Cell Lines Cultured Without and With Added Drugs (in vitro)

Without Added Drugs (in vitro)

Author	Year	Number of Metaphases	Mean% Breaks	Range % Breaks	Number of Major Structural Abnormalities[1]
Abdullah and Miller	1968	200	0.5	0–1	0
Cohen et al.	1969	—	0.8	—	—
Staiger	1969	602	6.6	4.0–10.0	3
		500	9.2	6.0–14.0	—
Martin	1969	—	—	—	—

With Added Drugs (in vitro)

Author	Year	Number of Metaphases	Mean % Breaks	Range % Breaks	Number of Major Structural Abnormalities[1]	Name of Drugs	Dose Range	Duration
Abdullah and Miller	1968	200	8.0	6.0–10.0	3	chlorpromazine	8×10^{-6} M	48 hours
Cohen et al.	1969	—	—	0–2.5	—	chlorpromazine	1, 10, and 100 µg/ml[2]	6, 24, and 48 hours
Staiger	1969	901	7.3	1.0–17.0	3	chlordiazepoxide	50–200 µg/ml	8 hours and 3 days
		800	6.8	4.0–13.0	4	diazepam	12.5–50 µg/ml	8 hours and 4 days
Martin	1969	—	No breaks found		—	cannabis	40–200 µg/ml	6–72 hours

[1] Major structural abnormalities include dicentrics, multiradials, ring chromosomes, etc.
[2] No mitoses observed with the doses of 1 mg and 10 mg/ml.

(Table 5). No predrug chromosome data are available.

Nielsen et al. [1969], by contrast, found a markedly higher frequency of breaks in 13 patients on chlorpromazine compared to 41 controls (Table 5).

1.3.2. In Vitro Human Studies
Abdullah and Miller [1968], using human diploid fibroblasts, reported a marked increase in chromosomal abnormalities following chlorpromazine treatment. Cohen et al. [1969] failed to demonstrate a similar effect in human leukocytes (Table 5).

1.4. Chlordiazepoxide (Librium)
1.4.1. 1. In Vivo Human Studies
Cohen et al. [1969] report sequential studies extending over an 8-week period, in 6 patients who were given the drug. Neither an increase in breaks, compared to 6 controls, nor the appearance of abnormal forms could be demonstrated by the investigators (Table 4). An additional 4 patients studied once also gave negative results.

1.4.2. In Vitro Human Studies
In vitro studies by Staiger [1969] on three human cell lines were also negative (Table 5), as was a study of hamsters [Schmid and Staiger 1969].

1.5. Other Drugs
Negative results have been reported for diazepam (Valium), fluphenazine (Prolixin, Permitil) and thioridazine (Mellaril) by Cohen et al. [1969], and for medazepam (Nobrium) by Schmid and Staiger [1969]. An increase in breaks has been attributed by Nielsen et al. [1969] to perphenazine (Trilafon, also an ingredient of Triavil) but all of the 15 patients receiving perphenazine also received orphenadrine (Disipal) (Table 4).

1.6. Summation
Although clearly inadequate in depth, the existing data are highly suggestive of LSD-induced chromosome damage when the drug is added in vitro. The best estimate is that under in vitro conditions LSD produces a doubling of chromosomal aberrations. The results of animal studies and in vivo human studies are contradictory. As an informed guess, the likelihood is that LSD does not do more than double the break frequency observed in persons who have not been exposed to LSD. Data for drugs other than LSD are scanty and very few investigations have been performed.

2. Cytogenetic Methodologies

2.1. Significance of Chromosomal Damage
Classical methods for determining muta-genicity in microbial systems and in Droso-phila have been discussed elsewhere (Chapters 9 and 10).

Methods for quantitative scoring of recip-rocal translocations induced in the gonads of treated male Drosophila are also simple and practical, depending upon the use of genetic-ally marked stocks and the scoring of progeny by phenotype. However, in man it is very difficult to determine mutation frequency, and yet a long list of chemicals exist which are known to be mutagenic from experimental studies using microorganisms, plants, and insects. Thus, a prime objective is to deter-mine which of these, as well as other agents in our environment, are capable of interacting with human genetic material so as to produce mutation. "Mutation" is here defined as "a change in the amount or kind of hereditary information" in the cell (Chapter 8).

Cytogenetic test systems depend on detec-tion of microscopically visible changes in the metaphase chromosomes, and these are classified according to morphology. Changes involving chromosome breakage can lead to loss or exchanges of extensive segments of the hereditary material. Effects other than breakage can also cause gains or losses, but of entire chromosomes (*nondisjunction*) or of sets of chromosomes (*polyploidy*). Subtoxic concentrations of the chemical agent being considered, which block the initiation or the completion of DNA synthesis or inhibit completion of anaphase separation, result in cell death, or its equivalent—failure to contribute genetically to later somatic or germ line cell generations. Cytologically, metaphase difficulties are reflected in interphase as multinucleated cells, and many of these cells are nonviable. Less severe effects upon the spindle contribute numerically altered cell products, cells with aneuploid numbers of chromosomes. All the major classes of chromosome-breaking agents—irradiation, chemicals, and viruses—can induce nondisjunctive effects and polyploidy. Nondisjunction occurs in meiosis, or in mitosis, and is the result of failure of spindle attachment or spindle movement so that both chromosomes of a pair are included within one daughter cell. This cell is then trisomic and the other daughter cell is monosomic for that chromosome.

Endoreduplication is the continued replication of the chromosomes in the face of failure of cell division and results in polyploidy, the presence of more than two haploid sets of chromosomes per cell. Polyploid cells, generally less favored than normal cells in terms of growth potential, are in themselves little cause for concern regarding somatic or germ cell mutation. However, marked increases in polyploids generally do accompany chromosome restructuring induced by radiation, chemicals, and viruses. Triploid and tetraploid fetuses very rarely survive to term of pregnancy, except where there is some evidence of cell mosaicism including normal, or nearly normal, cells.

Colchicine and other compounds can produce endoreduplication without inducing any chromosome breakage or rearrangement. A number of chemicals can induce polyploidy, but these are chemically quite unrelated to each other or to colchicine [Kihlman 1966, pp. 110–113]. The relative lipid solubility

seemed related to effectiveness for certain narcotic-like compounds, including ether and chloroform, but the mechanism of action must be quite different from that of colchicine itself, which is highly soluble in water [Levan and Östergren 1943; Steinegger and Levan 1947]. The possibility that ether or chloroform might constitute unrecognized genetic hazards seems remote as both are strongly mitodepressive and their effects upon the spindle are obtained only at concentrations which are close to the threshold of cell toxicity [Deysson 1968]. However, in this, as in so many other cases, very little is yet known regarding such effects on mammalian meiosis. Colcemid can induce very high frequencies of abnormal eggs in mice [Edwards 1961 as cited in Russell 1964]. Among the common solvents, benzene is known to be associated with increased incidence of chromosome breakage and with cancer [Tough and Court Brown 1965].

Aneuploidy in man does make up a small but significant proportion of all major birth malformations. These chromosomal disorders resulting from meiotic nondisjunction include G-trisomy (Down's syndrome or mongolism), 17-trisomy, D-trisomy, and various sex chromosome anomalies (XXX, XXY, XYY, XO, and mosaics of these). These abnormalities comprise an appreciable social burden at present, and the key factors underlying their incidence are not fully determined. The most common birth defect is the aneuploid condition of G-trisomy, and its incidence has for many years been known to be correlated directly with the age of the mother. Down's syndrome has been implicated with epidemics of infective hepatitis in Australia by Stoller and Collman [1965], but this is clearly not so in U.S. populations [Miller, 1970].

The presence of an abnormal chromosome created by rearrangement of segments among and within normal chromosomes would produce effects similar to those observed in the viable trisomies, but of course the degree of severity of effect will be roughly correlated with the amount of genetic material duplicated or deleted. Such "marker" chromosomes can result in a lethal or a viable mutant through the immediate consequences of a genetic deficiency and/or duplications of a series of genes, or through genetic imbalances produced during subsequent mitotic difficulties. Most extremely abnormal chromosomes, such as dicentrics, rings, or abnormally long chromosomes lead to cell death during divisions following the initial break event; but this does not necessarily occur to all the progeny. A fraction of the genetic restructuring may be propagated in mutant daughter cells which survive and proliferate. These cells with viable chromosomal mutations, whether of detectable size or not, constitute a source for concern within the context of potential hazards to human populations.

Chemical agents may have different modalities of damage to cellular DNA or to chromosome structure, and questions concerning this constitute an important area of fundamental research quite relevant to the problems of detection of potentially hazardous compounds. Some agents may be capable of inducing gene mutations without producing increases in visible chromosome breakage. Cattanach et al. [1968] relate that "Ethyl methanesulfonate (EMS) induces mutation in Habrobracon, Neurospora, bacteria, yeast, and bacteriophage; however, in maize and in barley breakage of chromosomes was not greatly increased, and the majority of point mutations produced were considered to be unassociated with small deletions." Cattanach et al. [1968] demonstrated that in the mouse EMS did produce high frequencies of chromosome breakage (dominant lethals and translocations) in postmeiotic germ cells.

Cytogenetic assessment, whether in germ cell or in somatic cell populations, therefore can be a measure of only a part of the total mutation which is originally present or induced. The production of chromosome breakage is not necessarily a measure of point mutation, however extensive circumstantial evidence exists which links chromosomal abnormalities with point mutations. Radiation clearly yields increases in both phenomena, and studies of chemicals in general support this association. Kihlman [1966] calls attention to the strong correlation between chromosome breakage—as studied in mammalian cells cultured and treated in vitro—and increased gene mutation in microorganisms or insects, for fourteen chemical agents so far studied in both ways (Table 6). In Drosophila, at least 20 percent of the sex-linked recessives have been considered to involve deletions or rearrangements [Slizynska and Slizynski 1947]; and dominant lethals are generally regarded as having a basis in chromosome breakage, being a mixed class of mutations [Russell 1962, 1694].

The small fraction of chromosomal mutations which are compatible with cell survival and propagation have obvious importance in vertical transmission through the germ cells, being capable of causing defects in various aspects of development in offspring resulting from fertilizations with such mutated gametes. Viable genetic deficiencies exert their effects primarily in the immediate progeny and therefore act as dominants (or *haplo-sufficient* mutations). Genetic duplications would act similarly and either may give rise to dominant lethals or semilethals. The terms *dominant lethal* and *lethal* properly mean mutants which causes the elimination or genetic death of the cell or individual, and the failure of eventual propagation [Chapter 13]. The designation *semilethal* implies a reduced likelihood of achieving effective sexual maturity and function in the case of the zygote and a reduced chance of contributing to the next cellular generation in the somatic cell population.

Semilethal implies a reduced likelihood of achieving the mean level of the population's usual reproductive success and survival for its progeny.

Such terminations of the genetic continuity through mutation can follow from cell death, individual death, or from various gross or subtle defects which interfere with normal function of the individual. Thus, a semilethal debilitates to some fractional degree and is eliminated, on the average, in a correspondingly greater number of generations the lesser is its effect in the individual [Muller 1950]. A general increase in developmental defects from lethals and semilethals could be difficult to demonstrate upon the background of ill-defined variability already present and involving any or all of the tissue systems. The certain clinical detection of such increments in the population might be impossible although it could inflict severe social costs and private distress [Chapter 7]. Therefore, whether at the gene or chromosomal level such defects may express themselves at any point—in the early blastula, where the social consequences would be nil; in the embryo, causing derangements of some essential pattern of development; or in juvenile and adult life. Perhaps our immediate concern should be directed only to factors which introduce increments upon the background level of aberrations, but we should not exclude the hope of reducing the "spontaneous" incidence itself.

Zygotes which are grossly abnormal in their chromosomes are largely eliminated by spontaneous abortion: about 70 percent of very early human abortuses (first 6 weeks) are detectably abnormal in chromosome content. Half of the abortuses surviving the first 10 weeks and 20 percent of those surviving 20 weeks are abnormal, consisting of triploids, trisomics, some tetraploids, and gross translocations [Boué, Boué, and Lazar 1967; Carr 1965, 1967a]. Carr [1967b] has shown that a

Table 6. Comparison Between Chromosome-Breaking and Mutagenic Effects of Chemicals in Plant and Animal Materials

| Compound | Chromosomal Aberrations | | Mutagenic Effect |
	Plant Root-tips	Mammalian Cells in Tissue Culture	
Adenine	+	+	+
2,6 Diaminopurine	−	+	+
Caffeine	+	±	+
8-Ethoxycaffeine	+	±	±
Purine riboside	−	+	+
Deoxyadenosine	+	+	No data
5-Fluorodeoxyuridine	+	+	No data
5-Bromodeoxyuridine	−	+	+
Cytosine arabinoside	−	+	No data
Maleic hydrazide	+	−	−
Azaserine	+	+	+
Streptonigrin	+	+	+
Mitomycin C	+	+	+
Hydroxylamine	±	+	+
Nitrogen mustard	+	+	+
Triethylenemelamine	+	+	+
Diepoxybutane	+	+	+

+ marked effect;
− no effect;
± effect very low, although just about significant.
Source: Bengt A. Kihlman, *Actions of Chemicals on Dividing Cells* © 1966. Reprinted by permission of Prentice-Hall, Inc., Englewood Cliffs, New Jersey.

very high proportion of the initial pregnancies following cessation of contraceptive hormonal administration result in spontaneous abortion, and that most abnormal abortuses are triploid. Information now being accumulated on frequencies of chromosomally abnormal offspring which reach full term in such cases will be of considerable interest.

Apart from death of the individual, cell death in itself may be of importance in teratology even though delayed for several cell generations; but this is likely to be so only where the tissue anlagen or the zygote consists of relatively small numbers of cells, as in the blastula or early embryo. Early exposure of the human embryo to an agent such as rubella virus results in severe dysgenesis and both cell death and mitotic inhibition are thought to be significant in this, while chromatid and chromosome aberrations are only minimally increased [Chang et al. 1966].

In human cells the loss of an entire G chromosome, the smallest of the complement, containing approximately 0.8 percent of the total cell DNA, is known to be compatible with cell viability in vitro. At the organism level a deletion of approximately half that size is compatible with life in the cri-du-chat syndrome—a severe maldevelopment caused by the presumed loss of a specific segment of chromosome 5. In chronic myelogenous leukemia, a detectable deletion involving an estimated 0.28 percent of the DNA [Rudkin 1965] not only permits cell survival but presumably endows the cell with its abnormal growth properties. If deletions of this same size are artificially distributed throughout the human karyotype, it can be estimated that less than 20 percent of all possible locations would permit cytological detection. For smaller, and presumedly therefore less often lethal deletions, the ratio between undetected and detected aberrations would be, of course, even larger. Thus, apart from the absolute size,

karyological considerations relating to position limit detection to only a fraction of the total aberrations present.

Abnormalities in blood cells of Japanese fishermen who were exposed to radioactive fallout and who were studied ten and eleven years afterward were nonrandomly represented in the smallest chromosome group, the G group [Ishihara and Kumatori 1967]. Whether this reflects preferential survival of less extensive terminal deletions, because of their small size, or a predisposition peculiar to one of these two pairs is not known.

A major risk in somatic cell mutations, besides the teratological one, is the possibility of neoplastic change. That chromosomal alteration plays any significant role in the initiation of cancer is not proved in spite of the high degree of association between chromosomal changes and various neoplastic conditions [Nowell 1965]. With the exception of a specific deletion of a G chromosome in chronic myelogenous leukemia, chromosome changes are nonspecific for particular types of tumors. However, there is considerable firm evidence of the clonal origin of tumors and one may view chromosomal breakage and rearrangements as providing a source of genetic plasticity which is essential to the series of evolutionary changes leading to greater autonomy which define tumor progression [Black 1968; Defendi and Lehman 1965; Moorhead and Weinstein 1966]. Chromosome breakage might also be important in the promotion of opportunities for the integration of viral DNA within the host cell genome which occurs in the early phase of viral transformation and tumorigenesis [Westphal and Dulbecco 1968]. The persistence of cells displaying chromosome damage long after the initial effect is not necessarily significant from the standpoint of an intrinsic risk from the dicentric or bizarre exchange that is easily detected; it is important as indication of persisting changes not seen and more likely to survive in any case. Under conditions of in vivo recruitment into cell division these cells must be considered as a risk in regard to neoplasia.

The quantitative determination of increases in incidence of chromosomal aberrations therefore are considered to be reliable, if not absolute indicators of the presence of a range of alterations of the genetic material beyond those actually observed. Substances inducing such increases in structural abnormalities certainly must be assumed to produce deletions, etc. which extend into the subvisible, if not the molecular range. Research indicating otherwise, that certain modes of length of aberration occur or that certain sizes are "forbidden" by the mechanics of breakage, might be possible through refinements of automated karyotypic analysis. Machine methods now being developed will undoubtedly permit greater resolution and statistical extensions of the number of cells which can be studied [Ruddle 1965; Mendelsohn, 1969].

2.2. Classification of Breakage Aberrations

Any systematic description of the various effects to be considered under chromosomal aberrations is encumbered by a necessary intermingling of morphological terminology with the physiological processes involved. These processes are DNA synthesis, chromosomal condensation, spindle action, cytokinesis, and the energy requirements underlying them. In brief, almost all effects observable involve either chromosome breakage or alterations in the number of chromosomes per cell. Numerical changes, in aneuploidy and polyploidy, have been discussed in the previous section, but there are two major hypotheses of chromosome breakage and unfortunately a variety of nomenclature systems for classification of the products of breakage. Other visible effects which fall outside the two major groupings include *pulverization* and *anomolous condensation* (despiraliza-

tion, etc.). These general phenomena may affect only a region of a chromosome, one chromosome, or many chromosomes. Their genetic consequences are unclear, but pulverization seems to involve disruption of normal DNA synthesis [Nichols et al. 1967].

The "breakage first" hypothesis assumes that in G1 of the cell's cycle the chromosome is continuous and is effectively single in its response to breaking agents. The break remains open for a brief time; during this period exchanges with other break products may occur and, if not, restitution occurs. In the "exchange" hypothesis of Revell [1955, 1959], the initial event is not a structural break but is an unstable state produced locally on a chromosome which may revert (heal) within a short time. The lesion may proceed to a secondary state which is stable and of longer duration, and thereafter genetic interchange becomes a possibility. All chromatid aberrations are thought to arise as the result of exchanges between and within sister chromatids. Thus an existing mechanism or property of the cell is invoked, the capacity to undergo exchange of material, as in normal crossing over at meiosis.

In the following resumes of aberration classifications certain assumptions as to mechanism of breakage are implied, based largely on the "breakage first" view. Since even the number of strands involved is not known and other basic facts concerning chromosome substructure are lacking at present, we can only present these with an emphasis on the observed morphology. Among the more widely used classification systems for scoring of metaphase aberrations are those described by Östergren and Wakonig [1954], Revell [1955, 1959]; Evans [1962]; and Court Brown et al. [1966]. (Evans' review is especially valuable).

In defining breakage for microscopic scoring, it is difficult to distinguish between a break which actually involves a physical discontinuity and a "gap." The gap is defined as an achromatic segment of the intact chromatid. If after the initial event there is no "healing," the result at metaphase would be an "open break," leading to elimination of an acentric fragment. During a period following irradiation most of the breaks undergo reunion with the result that the "pieces" remain in the same position, as can be determined from fractionated dose experiments. Evidence for healing or restitution of the original condition is more difficult to obtain in chemical or virus effect studies where the agent's action is broadly diffused in time and may show site preferences due to timing of DNA synthesis or a chemical affinity for differentiated regions (secondary constrictions, etc.). Some authors define the open or true break as involving displacement of the distal fragment, and others require nonalignment between the apparent pieces. Still others establish an arbitrary distance for the displacement. such as the width of a chromatid, regardless of alignment. The latter definition of an open break is arbitrary, but as a criterion it permits comparison of data obtained at different times or by different workers.

Secondary constrictions, which are normal features of the chromosomes and which are consistent in location, are not scored as gaps, of course. However, it should be noted that most secondary constrictions are sporadic in occurrence; on morphological grounds alone, they are indistinguishable from gaps [Ferguson-Smith et al. 1962; Palmer and Funderburk 1965].

In most studies of experimentally produced chromosome breakage, gaps are produced together with obvious breaks. Gaps are often entirely ignored, being considered as having no proportionate relation to the extent of actual genetic losses, as may be determined by comparative anaphase analysis of acentric fragments. Apparently no simple relation holds between the ratio of gaps to breaks in different materials [Conger 1967], and in the absence of a reconciliation of theories, an unambiguous definition of criteria actually used is essential.

One characteristic used to classify chromosome breakage is whether one or both chromatids are involved. If at the same site both chromatids are affected, the defect is termed *chromosome break*; if only one is so involved, it is termed a *chromatid break*. Whether or not the chromosome behaves as a single unit or double unit at the time of the initial insult that produces the break determines which kind of lesion results. This, in turn, is dependent upon the stage of the cell cycle at that time. If a cell is in the G1 phase of the cell cycle, before DNA synthesis (S), the chromosome is effectively single; if a break is produced at this time, the lesion itself is replicated appearing then in both chromatids after the S period, yielding a chromosome break at metaphase. If the insult occurs after S, during G2 or thereafter, the chromosome is a dual structure and a chromatid break is the usual result. Damage during the period of DNA synthesis produces a combination of both types of breakage observed in the same cell, depending on whether the individual chromosome had not started or had finished the synthesis of its DNA.

If the initial event affects both chromatids, after the chromosome is effectively doubled, this is often termed an *isochromatid break*. Such lesions are introduced in the chromatids, but each chromatid is affected at the same site. Either the track of an ionizing particle or a chemical which affects those sites which become vulnerable at the same time could produce this condition. The isochromatid break is distinguishable from a chromosome break only inferentially, by the fact that other lesions in the same cell or cell material are predominantly chromatid breaks.

The term *delayed isolocus break* has been

introduced by Östergren and Wakonig [1954].
These authors described a typical example as
a constriction or gap in one chromatid with a
break at the corresponding position on the
other. Such paired lesions may range from
only a weak constriction in one to an obvious
open break in the other, or any combination
of these. The authors describing this term
felt that a partial defect produced in the
chromosome when it is a single unit is repro-
duced in both chromatids at the isolocus
point during DNA synthesis, but various
mitotic forces and pressures subsequently
applied produce the morphologies observed.
Alternatively, this type of lesion might reflect
only slight differences in timing of DNA synthesis

If no restitution occurs, a structural mutation
must result, producing a simple terminal
deletion at least. If more than one break
occurs in a cell, a rejoining between the segments produced can yield intrachanges
(between parts of one chromosome) or
interchanges (between parts of different
chromosomes). Further subclassifications are
many and may indicate whether the exchange
was symmetrical or unsymmetrical, stable or
unstable [Court Brown et al, 1966], intra-
arm or interarm, etc. Symmetrical exchange
entails no mechanical difficulties at anaphase
and no genetic deficiencies. These are therefore stable and cells with such monocentric
"marker" chromosomes retain all of the
original genetic material. Unsymmetrical
exchanges (unstable) involve either mechanical difficulties, as with rings and
dicentrics, or the production of daughter
cells which are respectively deficient and
duplicated for a chromosome segment or
segments. The primary factor determining
whether a rearrangement or an open break
will result seems to be the retention by
the cell of its ability to synthesize protein
and/or DNA.

Certain useful advantages can be had from
anaphase aberration analysis which are not
possible in metaphase. Karl Sax [1941]
pioneered the development of cytogenetic
scoring as a means of quantitative assessment of genetic damage and anaphase
analysis of plant cells was extensively
employed. The advantages are a relatively
unambiguous scoring system, especially for
terminal deletions, and simplicity of technical
preparations. However, with mammalian cells
cultured in vitro as monolayers, considerable
time must be spent in locating sufficient
numbers of anaphases and there is somewhat
greater error in selection for the stage of
anaphase which permits distinction between
true chromosome bridges and pseudo-
chiasmata. For anaphase studies, colchicine,
hypotonic pretreatment, or trypsinization of
cells are unnecessary, which should eliminate
some sources of variability. Mammalian cells
growing in monolayers on coverglasses can
be fixed and stained in situ. The types of
aberrations that can be distinguished readily
at anaphase are *acentric fragment*, a paired
segment of chromatids left at the equator of
the dividing cell, from a simple break; *attached fragment*, a paired segment of
attached chromatids which are apart from the
main body of chromosomes but oriented in
line with them, seemingly attached by an
attenuated thread of chromatin; *chromosome bridge*, a length of chromatin linking both
chromosome groups as they approach the
poles, the result of asymmetrical rearrangement; and *pseudochiasma*, the adherence
(stickiness) of two chromatids or of two
chromosomes during separation, not involving
an exchange.

2.3. Technical Considerations

For study of mitotic metaphase chromosomes
of mammals the necessary cytological
methods are well developed and in wide
application [Moorhead and Nowell 1964].
These techniques require a dividing population, as occurs in the bone marrow, or a
population of cells induced to undergo

mitosis in ordinary cell culture or through the use of a mitogenic substance. Artificial arrest of cells at metaphase with drugs such as colchicine or colcemid is usually employed but is not essential. A means of flattening the cells to permit visualization of all the chromosomes is necessary and is obtainable either by squashing under a coverglass or by rapid evaporation of the fixative on the surface of a glass slide (air- and ignition-drying). Meiotic studies are feasible using essentially similar procedures, but they require more expertise and greater expenditure of detailed effort for obtaining significant numbers of satisfactory cells for study.

Short-term cultures of circulating lymphoblasts have proved to be the most valuable cell source for determination of chromosome damage suffered by humans as a result of accidental irradiation or long-term exposure to chemicals. While for leukemias the diagnostic value of such determinations is debatable, it is thought that the amount of radiation received may be assayed best through such determinations. This technique provides a convenient access to cells that were exposed in vivo and sampling can be performed repeatedly with little inconvenience or hazard to the subject. Only small volumes of blood are needed and circulating lymphoblasts of most laboratory animals may be studied in much the same fashion. Cells with damage may reside in the blood for years without undergoing mitosis, but upon cultivation in vitro and exposure to an introduced mitogen, these cells are stimulated to enter division and thereby reveal exchanges and other first-order types of aberrations. Introduction of the drug in vitro allows circumvention of metabolic factors where desired and removal of doubt as to the effective dosage reaching the cell. For in vitro studies, lymphoblasts from normal healthy subjects can be subjected to the chemical agent in the culture vessel.

Mass cultures of diploid human fibroblasts from embryonic tissues or from the skin of newborn or adult also can be used. Human fibroblasts and fibroblast cells from various animals retain their normal karyotype constitution during long, but eventually limited, periods of cell propagation. "Stock" or standardized diploid human cell lines can be monitored for possible contaminants or chromosome changes and widely distributed for use as test cells [Hayflick 1968]. Permanently established human cell lines are usually mixoploid and display persisting instability of their karyotypic patterns.

Besides circulating lymphocytes there are three prime sources of growing cells: bone marrow, testes and embryonic tissues. Bone marrow is perhaps the tissue of choice for cytogenetic determinations by a direct examination of chromosomes in a cell population normally undergoing continual mitotic activity. Sacrifice of the animal is most practical but not absolutely necessary. For sequential studies, on the same animals, of course, the lymphocyte culture would be preferable, but certain laboratory animals, as the rat, have proved difficult for use with blood cell cultures.

Spermatogonial cell populations can also provide direct preparations of actively dividing cells without any intervening cultivation in vitro being necessary. Embryonic tissue can be examined in direct preparation but short-term or long-term cell culture is more useful; even a brief period of culture greatly increases the yield of healthy dividing cells, the most important single factor in obtaining cytologically excellent material.

A consideration of the sources of variability and possibly introduced errors may place in perspective some of the discrepancies noted in the many published studies on effects of LSD. Much of this variability may be due to individual variation, in donor-cell response to phytohemagglutinin, or to serum or other factors of the culture medium. Culture conditions themselves may influence the proportion (and type?) of lymphocytes entering into mitosis. The exclusion of contamination with extraneous microorganisms, for example yeast or mycoplasma, demand consistent and patient care on the part of technicians. Many laboratories routinely monitor fibroblast cultures for passenger organisms such as these, but tests would not normally be performed on short-term blood cultures. Inadvertent mycoplasma infection of some types is capable of inducing high levels of chromosome breakage, presumedly by depletion of components of the medium [Paton et al. 1965; Aula and Nichols 1967]. Inadequate media could conceivably account for certain sporadic occasions of unexplained increases in untreated control values for breakage. Freed and Schatz [1969] demonstrated that the elimination of single amino acids from standard media induced marked increases in breakage in chromosomes of Chinese hamster cells. Kihlman [1966] notes that nonspecific factors such as pH or temperature can cause enhancements of chemically induced breakage values, but for mammalian chromosomes there are few such reports. Hampel and Levan [1964] treated human fibroblasts in vitro to low temperatures, thereby causing chromosome breaks and gaps, but other factors were apparently critical also, since replication of the effect was not always obtained.

Control cells for in vitro studies should be obtained from the same donor(s) if exogenous agents are added to cultures. If in vivo effects are being tested, it is preferable to study cells of the same subject sequentially, before and after drug administration. Control and treated individuals should be matched as closely as possible for obvious factors such as sex, age, race, and occupation. Cultures should of course be propagated and processed in parallel, utilizing the same lots of medium, trypsin, colcemide, fixative, stains, etc. and should be manipulated on the same days. Because of the possibility of near-toxic effects of chemicals, or unwanted viruses, upon chromosome morphology and on entry into mitosis, it may be valuable to add a known chromosome breaking agent, as a positive control.

Valid comparisons of data depend on internal consistency in methods during microscopic examination, that is, fixed criteria for the kinds of aberrations tallied. Reliable cytological scoring demands equal attention to each cell examined and to each parameter considered. This is necessary in the face of problems of observer fatigue and possible observer bias. Ideally, cultures should be randomized and referred to only by coded numbers assigned by others. Even in the same material, truly comparable opportunities for detection of chromosome aberrations obtain only in metaphase cells which are similar in degree of condensation and in cytological quality. For reasons not understood, chromosome preparations from bone marrow are generally of lower cytological quality than those from cultured fibroblasts or leukocytes, but in general these differences are not severe. Variation of quality necessitates the selection of usable metaphases, which is usually done under low-power optics.

Among the numerous published technical procedures for the making of preparations of mammalian chromosomes none is so exceptional as to urge its adoption as the unique method of choice [Chicago Conference, 1966; Geneva Conference, 1966]. Published data on control frequencies of breakage, and even for achromatic gaps, are fairly comparable [Evans et al. 1967]. Studies in which the techniques for preparing chromosomes for cytological examination have been systematically compared are few; Aula [1965] found no differences in detected aberrations in cell material prepared both by air-drying and squashing.

Buckton and Pike [1964] established that frequencies of aberrations scored in cultures from irradiated patients may vary according to time of fixation. Phytohemagglutinin-stimulated blood cultures harvested after 50 hours in vitro revealed a higher frequency of aberration than did those harvested at 72 hours. The elimination of a part of the unstable types of abnormalities seemed to have occurred since some cells had completed more than one mitosis in the 72-hour culture. As a realistic measure of the degree of reproducibility normally obtained, Evans [1967] notes differences in efficiencies of yield of radiation-induced aberrations, as determined in three laboratories, but states that the technical differences as to fixation time could well account for this phenomenon.

The time necessary for careful microscopic analysis is considerable and therefore many studies published are simply inadequate in numbers of cells examined per determination. Unwarranted extrapolations of the findings beyond the few subjects studied are discussed and cautioned against by Kruskal and Haberman [1968]. Statistical handling of the variability must be appropriate (see "Homogeneity of Variances" by Bartlett [1937] ; and see Gossett [1908] for tests of differences between means ; Fisher [1924] for variances of two populations ; Stevens [1942] for small samples).

With an appreciation of the limitations discussed in mind, experimental and practical screening procedures could be devised which should yield quantitative information on the interaction between potential mutagens and human genetic material. Other aspects of chromosome damage which might be explored concern effects on mitotic index, time of action of drugs, correlation of damage with concentration or length of exposure, types of chromosome damage which predominate, and the possibility of nonrandom localization of damage to specific regions or chromosome groups.

3. Recommended Guidelines

3.1. Screening for Genetic Hazards

There is an urgent need for hard facts on the chromosomal effects of LSD as well as of other drugs. Because of the present limited number of laboratories capable of performing chromosome investigations and the commitments of these laboratories to various lines of research, the necessary data can best be obtained by well-designed, well-controlled, blind, co-operative studies combining human cell in vitro experiments with both in vivo and in vitro studies in animals.

Cytogenetic determinations can be obtained on a variety of tissues from many common laboratory animals, and adaptations for screening purposes are clearly feasible. Combination with techniques such as the dominant lethal test and the host-mediated assay is highly desirable, and of particular importance is the examination of gonadal cells in animals. At present, for the assessment of the possible genetic risks to humans, using these methods in concert should provide the best available approach.

Cytogenetic evaluation is considered a practical and reasonably rapid technique, and although problems of variability exist, proper experimental design and sufficient resources ought to permit overcoming this disadvantage. Still, this cannot be relied upon alone, but must be supported by corroborative evidence from animal and microorganism assays specifically designed to test compounds for gene mutagenesis, teratogenesis, and carcinogenesis.

There is sufficient evidence of a relation between chromosome-breaking ability and the ability to induce neoplasia to warrant concern. However, to the organism, damaged cells are expendable, be they somatic or gametic. Perhaps only under rare co-conditions do cells with chromosomal abnormalities of the type produced by ergot derivatives, aspirin, caffeine [Kihlman and Levan 1949; Novick 1956; Zetterberg 1960], or transient viral infections, lead to carcinogenesis. Nonetheless there is a need to investigate whether compounds hitherto considered innocuous to man account for part of the unexplained neoplasia, fetal wastage, neonatal morbidity, and mortality. Conceivably, use of such compounds could result in a doubling of the "spontaneous" rate. Clearly our ignorance in these matters is considerable, and the possibilities represent more than speculative theory.

For drugs used in psychiatry the need for facts is perhaps even more urgent than it is for drugs of abuse, since such large numbers of patients are taking these drugs for prolonged periods of time. With regard to these drugs, human in vivo experiments should be pursued, being ancillary to initial screening procedures. Long-term follow-up studies will be required to answer questions concerning the possible sequestration of abnormal cells (with later cloning and induction of neoplasia), as well as possible teratogenic effects upon human progeny.

Practicality urges the determination of priorities concerning test screening—depending upon relevance, sensitivity, and costs. For the cytogenetic aspects of testing, an initial phase of screening is recommended which would include human leukocytes and human fibroblasts exposed to the drug in vitro, and animal cells from testicular tissue and bone marrow (and possibly circulating blood) exposed in vivo. These two baseline assessments should be regarded as a minimum for preliminary testing and of equal significance at this stage. They are quite complementary, the one providing the fact that the compound can or cannot interact with human genetic material, and the other, a greater relevance in the opportunity to examine gonadal tissues.

Logically, ancillary studies of those drugs or chemicals yielding positive findings should include extensions to other mammals, examination of fetal animal tissues, and studies on meiotic division and on blood culture cells from humans medically or socially exposed.

3.2. Research and Development of Methods

It is recommended that certain related research problems should receive attention and support, since advances in these areas could greatly extend the practicality or validity of cytogenetic assessment as a screening tool. These should include studies on mammalian meiosis, computer approaches to automation of karyotype analysis, studies on structural heterozygosis in man, and cellular growth phenomena such as response to mitogens. As Lederberg indicated in discussions in this conference, perhaps attempts should be made to devise lifetime exposure cytogenetic assay systems. Each exposure results in a shower of effects, the majority of which are eliminated but leave a small residue of potentially dangerous cells. Chronic exposure to chromosome-breaking compounds constitutes the condition of greatest concern. As Atwood has suggested (Chapter 15), an adaptation of the Curtis system for examination of anaphase aberrations in mouse liver after hepatectomy may be a useful means for such an assay. Peripheral blood cultures of cells from animals so exposed would likewise provide cells which have undergone little or no cell division, until provoked to do so at the will of the researchist.

Human cytogenetic studies in which scoring is restricted entirely to the easily detected aberrations (such as dicentrics) may provide an equally sensitive but more rapid, and therefore more economical, means for analysis of populations. Ishihara and Kumatori [1967] have systematically compared the use of such a simplified approach to the usual one involving a thorough karyotypic analysis, and they have concluded that the thresholds of detection in a group of persons known to have received irradiation were quite similar. Dicentrics and similar exchange markers occur very rarely (1/800 or less) in circulating leukocytes of control populations [Court Brown et al. 1967], and while occurring in greater frequency in cultured human diploid fibroblasts, they are still relatively rare (1/200 approx.). It is conceivable that dicentrics and other "unstables" have more significance in irradiation than they do in chemical or drug exposure, but there is no evidence to support this thesis. In any case, possibly reliable but more practical methods for cytogenetic screening can be devised and such questions should be pursued.

Screening procedures as developed for assessment of cytogenetic damage can, of course, be applied as well to the monitoring and testing of various environmental factors, such as pesticides, industrial chemicals, etc.; and a pooling of resources directed toward such problems would substantially reduce the effort and costs. (While not large, costs of such research are considerable, being estimated at $100 to $500 per 100-cell sample, depending upon the depth of analysis.) It would be most wasteful to fragment our efforts regarding genetic dangers among a variety of problems such as drug abuse, environmental pollutants, drug product standards, etc.

3.3. Fundamental Research

Less urgent, but of great importance, would be the support of fundamental research which might yield changes in our concepts concerning mutation and chromosome breakage. Progress in basic studies on the mechanisms of chromosome breakage, on chromosome substructure, and in the area of research termed *somatic cell genetics* could have clear and perhaps striking applications and significance. Perhaps only then could truly "definitive" test systems be devised for determining our course in terms of medical, eugenic, or social actions. In the meantime, we are morally forced to treat our suspicions as if they were proofs.

The generous assistance of Dr. T. Kato in the preparation and tabulation of the literature survey for Section 1, Chromosomal Damage Induced by Drugs of Abuse, is gratefully acknowledged.

Appreciation is expressed to Mrs. M. Yerzley for assisting in preparation of the bibliography and to Miss L. Bettner and Mrs. D. Catalano for typing of the tables.

References

Abbo, G., A. Norris, and H. Zellweger (1968). *Humangenetik* 6:253.

Abdullah, S., and O. J. Miller (1968). *Dis. Nerv. Syst.* 29:829.

Abelson, P. H. (1968). *Science* 159:1189.

Alexander, G. J., S. Machiz, and R. B. Alexander (1968). *Fed. Proc.* 27:220.

———, B. E. Miles, G. M. Gold and R. B. Alexander (1967). *Science* 157:459.

Anonymous (1967). *Lancet* 1:36.

Anonymous (1967). *Lancet* 2:504.

Anonymous (1967). *Brit. Med. J.* 4:124.

Anonymous (1969). *Brit. Med. J.* 2:775

Arena, J. M. (1964). *North Carolina Med. J.* pp. 210–211.

Auerbach, R., and J. A. Rugowski (1967). *Science* 157:1325.

Aula, P. (1965). *Annales Academiae Scientiarum Fennicae, Series A, IV,* 89:1.

———, and W. W. Nichols (1967). *J. Cell. Physiol.* 70:281.

Barron, F., M. E. Jarvik, and S. Bunnell, Jr. (1964). *Sci. Amer.* 210:3.

Bartlett, M. S. (1937). *Suppl. to J. Roy. Statist. Soc.* 4:137.

Bender, L., and D. V. Siva Sankar (1968). *Science* 159:749.

Bennet, G. (1968). *Brit. J. Psychiat.* 114:1219.

Black, P. H. (1968). *Ann. Rev. Microbiol.* 22 : 391.

Blumenfield, M., and L. Glickman (1968). *Psychiat. Digest* p. 23.

Boué, J. G., A. Boué, and P. Lazar (1967). *Annales de Genetique* 10 : 179.

Browning, L. S. (1968). *Science* 161 : 1022.

Buckton, K. E., and M. C. Pike (1964). *Nature* 202 : 714.

Caldwell, A. E. (1967). *Dis. Nerv. Syst.* 28 : 816.

Carakushansky, G., R. L. Neu, and L. I. Gardner (1969). *Lancet* 1 : 150.

Caratzali, A., and I. C. Roman (1969). *C.R. Acad. Sci.* (D) (Paris), 268 : 191.

Carr, D. H. (1965). *Obstet. Gynec.* 26 : 308.

———— (1967a). In K. Benirschke, ed., *Comparative Aspects of Reproductive Failure,* New York : Springer-Verlag.

———— (1967b). *Lancet* 2 : 830.

Cattanach, B. M., C. E. Pollard, and J. H. Isaacson (1968). *Mutat. Res.* 6 : 297.

Chang, T. H., P. S. Moorhead, J. G. Boué, S. A. Plotkin, and J. M. Hoskins (1966). *Proc. Soc. Exp. Biol. Med.* 122 : 236.

Chicago Conference (1966). Standardization in Human Cytogenetics. *Birth Defects: Original Article Series, II: 2,* New York : The National Foundation.

Cohen, M. M. (1969). Personal communication.

————, et al. (1967). *Med. Sci.* 65 and 67.

————, K. Hirschhorn, and W. A. Frosch (1967a). *New Eng. J. Med.* 277 : 1043.

————, K. Hirschhorn, and W. A. Frosch (1968). *New Eng. J. Med.* 278 : 222.

————, K. Hirschhorn, and W. A. Frosch, (1969). *J.A.M.A ,* 207 : 2425.

————, K. Hirschhorn, and S. Verbo (1968). *Pediat. Res.* 2 : 486.

————, M. J. Marinello, and N. Back (1967b). *Science* 155 : 1417.

————, and A. B. Mukherjee (1968). *Nature* 219 : 1072.

————, and M. W. Shaw (1965). *In Vitro* 1 : 50.

Conger, A. D. (1967). *Mutat. Res.* 4 : 449.

Court Brown, W. M. (1967). *Lancet* 3 : 1154.

————, P. A. Jacobs, K. E. Buckton, I. M. Tough, E. V. Kuenssber, and J. D. E. Knox (1966). *Eugenics Lab. Mem.* XLII.

Dahlberg, C. C. (1968). *Sandoz Panorama* pp. 23–27.

————, R. Mechaneck, and S. Feldstin (1968). *Amer. J. Psychiat.* 125 : 137.

Darlington, C. D., and A. Haque (1962). *Cytogenetics* 1 : 196.

Davoli, E. (1968). *Clin. Proc. Child. Hosp. D.C.,* 24 : 152.

Defendi, V., and J. M. Lehman (1965). *J. Cell Comp. Physiol.* 66 : 351.

Denson, R. (1968). *Canad. Med. Ass. J.* 98 : 609.

Deysson, Guy (1968). *Int. Rev. Cytol.* 24 : 99.

Dipaolo, J. A., and G. J. Alexander (1967). *Science* 158 : 522.

————, H. M. Givelber, and H. Erwin (1968). *Nature,* 220 : 490–491.

Dohner, V. A. (1968). *Science* 160 : 1061.

Editorial (1967). *New Eng. J. Med.* 277 : 1090.

Editorial (F. J. A., Jr.) (1967). *Med. Sci.* 17 and 65.

Editorial (1968). *J.A.M.A.* 204 : 259.

Editorial (1968). *Med. World News :* pp. 21–23.

Edwards, R. G. (1961). *Exp. Cell Res.* 24 : 615.

Eells, K. (1968). Listing compiled at California Institute of Technology.

Egozcue, J., S. Irwin, and C. A. Maruffo (1968). *J.A.M.A.* 204 : 122.

Ellinwood, E. H., Jr. (1968). *Int. J. Neuropsychiat.* 4 : 45.

Evans, H. J. (1962). *Int. Rev. Cytol.* 13 : 221.

Evans, H. J. (1967). In H. J. Evans, W. M. Court Brown, and A. S. McLean, eds., *Human Radiation Cytogenetics,* Amsterdam : North-Holland, pp. 20–36.

————, W. M. Court Brown, and A. S. McLean, eds. (1967). *Human Radiation Cytogenetics,* Amsterdam : North-Holland, 218 pp.

Fabro, S., and S. M. Sieber (1968). *Lancet* 1 : 639.

Ferguson-Smith, M. A., M. E. Ferguson-Smith, P. M. Ellis, and M. Dickson (1962). *Cytogenetics* 1 : 325.

Fischer, R. (1969). *Science* 163 : 1144.

Fisher, R. A. (1924). *Proceedings of the International Mathematical Congress,* Toronto, p. 805.

Fitzgerald, P. H. (1968). *New Eng. J. Med.* 278 : 1404.

———, and J. R. E. Dobson (1968). *Lancet* 1:1036.

Freed, J. J., and S. A. Schatz (1969). *Exp. Cell Res.* 55:393.

Freedman, D. X. (1968). *Arch. Gen. Psychiat.* 18:330.

Freese, E. (1969). Personal communication.

Friedrich, U., and J. Nielsen (1969). *Lancet* 2:435.

Garson, O. M., and M. K. Robson (1969). *Brit. Med. J.* 2:800.

Geber, W. F. (1967). *Science* 158:265.

Genest, P. (1969). *Laval Medical* 40:56.

Geneva Conference (1966). Standardization of Procedures for Chromosome Studies in Abortion. World Health Organization Group. *Cytogenetics* 5:361.

Gooch, P. C., and C. L. Fischer (1969). *Cytogenetics* 8:1.

Goodlin, R. C. (1968). *J.A.M.A.* 203:171.

Gossett, W. S. (1908). *Biometrika* 6:1.

Grace, D., E. A. Carlson, and P. Goodman (1968). *Science* 161:694.

Grossbard, L., D. Rosen, E. McGilvray, A. de Capoa, O. Miller, and A. Bank (1968). *J.A.M.A.* 205:791.

Hampel, K. E., and A. Levan (1964). *Hereditas* 51:315.

———, B. Kober, D. Rosch, H. Gerhartz, and K. H. Meining (1966). *Blood* 27:816.

Hanaway, J. K. (1969). *Science* 164:574.

Hayflick, L. (1968). In *Cell Cultures for Virus Vaccine Production,* National Cancer Institute Monograph 29:83.

Hecht, F., R. K. Beals, M. H. Lees, H. Jolly, and P. Roberts (1968). *Lancet* 2:1087.

Heddle, J. A. (1969). *Fed. Proc.* 28:1790.

Hirschhorn, K. (1969). *Hospital Practice,* 4:98.

———, and M. M. Cohen (1967). *Ann. Intern. Med.* 67:1109.

——— (1968). *Ann. N.Y. Acad. Sci.* 151:977.

Houston, B. K. (1969). *Amer. J. Psychiat.* 126:137.

Hungerford, D. A., K. M. Taylor, C. Shagass, G. U. LaBadie, G. B. Balaban, and G. R. Paton (1968). *J.A.M.A.* 206:2287.

Idanpaan-Heikkla, J., et al. (1969). *New Eng. J. Med.* 330.

———, and J. C. Schoolar (1969). *Science* 164:1295.

——— (1969). *Lancet* 1:221.

Irwin, S., and J. Egozcue (1967) *Science* 157:313.

——— (1968). *Science* 159:749.

Ishihara, T., and T. Kumatori (1967). In H. J. Evans, W. M. Court Brown, and A. S. McLean, eds., *Human Radiation Cytogenetics,* Amsterdam: North-Holland.

Jacobs, J. C., W. A. Blanc, A. de Capoa, et al. (1968). *Lancet* i:499–503.

Jacobson, C. B., and V. L. Magyar (1968). *Clin. Proc. Child. Hosp. D.C.* 24:153.

Jagiello, G., and P. E. Polani (1969). *Cytogenetics* 8:136.

Japundzic, M., B. Knezevic, V. Djordjevic-Camba, and I. Japundzic (1967). *Exp. Cell Res.* 48:163.

Jarvik, L. F. (1968). *Science* 162:621.

——— (1969). *Amer. J. Psychiat.* 126:633.

———, and T. Kato (1968). *Lancet* i:250.

———, T. Kato, B. Saunders, and E. Moralishvili (1968). In D. A. Efron, ed., *Psychopharmacology: A Review of Progress.* Washington D.C.: U.S. Dept. of Health, Education and Welfare, Public Health Service Publ. No. 1836, pp. 1247–1252.

Judd, L. L., W. W. Brandkamp, and W. H. McGlothlin (1969). *Amer. J. Psychiat.* 126:626.

Kalter, H. (1967). In P. E. Siegler and J. H. Moyer, eds., *Animal and Clinical Pharmacologic Techniques in Drug Evaluation,* Chicago: Year Book, vol. 2, pp. 123–129.

Kato, T., and L. F. Jarvik (1969). *Dis. Nerv. Syst.* 30:42.

———, L. F. Jarvik, L. Roizin, and E. Moralishvili (1970). *Dis. Nerv. Syst.* 31:245.

Kaufmann, B. N., and D. Schuler (1967). In P. E. Siegler and J. H. Moyer, eds., *Animal and Clinical Pharmacologic Techniques in Drug Evaluation,* Chicago: Year Book, vol. 2, pp. 113–122.

Kihlman, B. A. (1966). *Actions of Chemicals on Dividing Cells,* Englewood Cliffs, N.J.: Prentice-Hall, 260 pp.

Kihlman, B., and A. Levan (1949). *Hereditas* 36:134.

Kruskal, W. H., and S. Haberman (1968). *Science* 162:1508.

Kushner, V. P., and I. A. Khodosova (1967). *Tsitologiia* 9:442.

Legator, M. S., et al. (1969). *Science* 165:1139.

Levan, A., and G. Östergren (1943). *Hereditas* 29 : 381.

Loughman, W. D., T. W. Sargent, and D. M. Israelstam (1967). *Science* 158 : 508.

Louria, D. B. (1968). *New Eng. J. Med.* 278 : 435.

Lucas, G. J., and W. Lehrnbecher (1969). *New Eng. J. Med.* 281 : 1018.

MacKenzie, J. B., and G. E. Stone (1968). *Mammalian Chromosome Newsletter.*

Mahler, H. R., and M. B. Baylor (1967). *Proc. Nat. Acad. Sci. U.S.A.* 58 : 256.

Marshall, M. (1969). *Case Western Reserve— Medical Alumni Bulletin* 33 : 21.

Martin, P. A. (1969). *Lancet* 1 : 370.

Maurer, I., D. Weinstein, and H. Solomon (1970). *Science* 169 : 198–201.

Meletti, Paolo (1953). *Caryologia,* vol. 5, No. 3.

Melvin, J. B. (1967). *Exp. Cell Res.* 45 : 559.

Mendelsohn, M. L., D. H. Hungerford, B. H. Mayall, B. Perry, T. Conway, and J. M. S. Prewitt (1969). *Ann. N.Y. Acad. Sci.* 157 : 376.

Miller, O. J., et al. (unpublished). Genetic Predisposition of Chromosome Breakage in Albino Individuals with Bleeding Tendency and in Heterozygous Carriers.

Miller, R. W. (1970). In *Genetic Concepts and Neoplasia,* Twenty-third Annual Symposium on Fundamental Cancer Research. The University of Texas M. D. Anderson Hospital and Tumor Institute. Baltimore : Williams and Wilkins, pp. 78–84.

Millichap, J. G. (1968). *J.A.M.A.* 206 : 1527.

Molé-Bajer, J. (1967). *Chromosoma* 22 : 465.

Moorhead, P. S., and P. C. Nowell (1964). *Meth. Med. Res.* 10 : 310.

———, and D. Weinstein (1966). In W. H. Kirsten, ed., *Recent Results in Cancer Research: VI, Malignant Transformation by Viruses,* New York: Springer-Verlag, pp. 104–111.

Motulsky, A. G. (1967). In P. E. Siegler and J. H. Moyer, eds., *Animal and Clinical Pharmacologic Techniques in Drug Evaluation,* Chicago : Year Book, pp. 97–104.

Mueller, G. C., and K. Kajiwara (1966). *Biochem. Biophys. Acta* 119 : 557.

Muller, H. J. (1950). *Amer. J. Human Genetics* 2 : 111.

Myers, W. A. (1968). *Science* 160 : 1062.

Nagata, C., and O. Martensson (1968). *J. Theor. Biol.* 19 : 133.

Nichols, W. W., P. Aula, A. Levan, W. Heneen, and E. Norrby (1967). *J. Cell Biol.* 35 : 257.

Nielsen, J., U. Friedrich, E. Jacobsen, and T. Tsuboi (1968). *Brit. Med. J.* 2 : 801.

———, U. Friedrich, and T. Tsuboi (1968). *Nature* 218 : 488.

———, U. Friedrich, and T. Tsuboi (1969). *Brit. Med. J.* 3 : 634.

Nora, J. J. (1968). *J.A.M.A.* 203 : 1075 (Letter to the Journal).

———, A. H. Nora, R. J. Sommerville, R. M. Hill, and D. G. McNamara (1967). *J.A.M.A.* 202 : 1065.

Nosal, G. (1969). *Laval Medical* 40 : 48.

Novick, A. (1956). *Brookhaven Symp.* 8 : 201.

Nowell, P. C. (1965). *Progr. Exp. Tumor. Res.* 7 : 83.

Östergren, G., and T. Wakonig (1954). *Bot. Not.* pp. 351–375.

Ostertag, W., E. Duisberg, and M. Sturmann (1965). *Mutat. Res.* 2 : 293.

Palmer, C. G., and S. Funderburk (1965). *Cytogenetics* 4 : 261.

Palmer, K., S. Green, K. Petersen, and M. Legator (1969). *Mammalian Chromosome Newsletter,* 10 : 50.

Pavan, C. (1967). *Triangle, Sandoz Med. J.* 8 : 42.

Paton, G. R., J. P. Jacobs, and F. T. Perkins (1965). *Nature* 207 : 43.

Persaud, T. V. N., and A. C. Ellington (1968). *Lancet* 2 : 406.

——— (1968). *W.I. Med. J.* 17 : 232.

Pihl, A., and P. Eker (1966). *Biochem. Pharmacol.* 15 : 769.

Piper, W. N., and W. F. Bousquet (1968). *Biochem. Biophys. Res. Commun.* 33 : 602.

Rappaport, B. S. (1968). *New Eng. J. Med.* 278 : 222.

Revell, S. H. (1955). In Z. M. Bacq and P. Alexander, eds., *Proceedings of the Radiological Symposium at Liege,* London : Butterworth.

——— (1959). *Proc. Royal Soc. London* (Series B), 150 : 563.

Ruddle, F. H., and R. S. Ledley (1965). In G. Yerganian, ed., *The Chromosome, Structural and Functional Aspects, In Vitro* 1 : 21–25.

Rudkin, G. T. (1965). In C. J. Dawe, ed., *The Chromosome, Structural and Functional Aspects,* Annual Symposium, The Tissue Culture Association, Inc., *In Vitro* 1 : 12–20.

Rusk, H. A. (1968). *Med. World News,* p. 109.

Russell, L. B. (1962). In A. G. Steinberg and A. G. Bearn, eds., *Progress in Medical Genetics,* New York: Grune and Stratton, pp. 230–294.

—— (1964). In C. Pavan, C. Chagàs, O. Frota-Pessoa, and L. R. Caldas, eds., *Mammalian Cytogenetics and Related Problems in Radiobiology,* New York: Pergamon, pp. 61–86.

Sato, H., and E. Pergament (1968). *Lancet* 1:639.

Sax, K. (1941). *Cold Spring Harbor Symp. Quant. Biol.* 9:93.

Schmid, W., and G. R. Staiger (1969). *Mutat. Res.* 7:99.

Schmitt, J. A. (1968). *J.A.M.A.* 203:166.

Schwarz, C. J. (1968). *J. Nerv. Ment. Dis.* 146:174.

Sentein, P. (1967). *Chromosoma* 21:51.

Sharma, A. K., and A. K. Bal (1956). *Proceedings of the National Institute of Sciences of India,* 22B:57–68.

Sideropoulos, A. S., and D. M. Shankel (1968). *J. Bact.* 96:198.

Skakkebaek, N. E., J. Philip, and O. J. Rafaelsen (1968). *Science* 160:1246.

Slizynska, H., and B. M. Slizynski (1947). *Proc. Roy. Soc. Edinburgh* 62:234.

Smart, R. G., and K. Bateman (1968). *Canad. Med. Ass. J.* 99:805.

Smith, D. E., and A. J. Rose (1968). *Clin. Ped.* 7:317.

Sparkes, R. S., J. Melnyk, and L. P. Bozzetti (1968). *Science* 160:1343.

Staiger, G. R. (1969). *Mutat. Res.* 7:109.

Steinegger, E., and A. Levan (1947). *Hereditas* 33:385.

Stevens, W. L. (1942). *J. Genetics* 43:301.

Stoller, A., and R. D. Collman (1965). *Nature* 206:903.

Stone, D., E. Lamson, Y. S. Chang, and K. W. Pickering (1969). *Science* 164:568.

Timakov, V. D., A. G. Skavronskaya, and V. N. Pokrovskii (1966). *Fed. Proc.* (Transl. Suppl.), 25:913.

Tjio, J. H., W. N. Pahnke, and A. A. Kurland (1969). *J.A.M.A.* 210:849.

Tobin, J. M., and J. M. Tobin (1969). *Dis. Nerv. Syst.* 30:47 (Suppl.).

Tough, I. M., and W. M. Court Brown (1965) *Lancet* 1:684.

Tsuda, F., K. Abe, K. Kokubun, T. Hashimoto, and H. Nemoto (1963). *Lancet* 1:726.

Tuchmann-Duplessis, H. (1967). *Wien Med. Wschr.* 117:379.

Ungerleider, J. T., et al. (1968). *Amer. J. Psychiat.* 124:1483.

Valenti, C. (1969). In J. Zubin and C. Shagass, eds., *Neurobiological Aspects of Psychopathology,* New York: Grune and Stratton, pp. 275–280.

Voogd, C. E., and V. D. Vet P. (1969). *Experientia* 25:85.

Vrba, M. (1967). *Humangenetik* 4:371.

Wagner, T. E. (1969). *Nature* 222:1170.

Warkany, J., and E. Takacs (1968). *Science* 159:731.

Westphal, H., and R. Dulbecco (1968). *Proc. Nat. Acad. Sci.* 59:1158.

Whitmore, F. W. (1968). *Science* 162:1058.

Zellweger, H., J. S. McDonald, and G. Abbo (1967). *Lancet* 2:1066.

—— (1967). *Lancet,* 2:1306.

12 The Use of Indirect Indicators for Mutagenicity Testing

M. S. Legator

At the present time no practical screen exists for evaluating point mutations in mammals. There is no conclusive evidence of direct correlation between induction of point mutations and other practical measurable effects in animals such as the production of chromosome abnormalities. In the absence of a practical, direct procedure for the measurement of point mutation in mammals, a series of indirect indicators have been suggested or are currently used to detect mutagenic agents. Of the four procedures, all but one, that of employing ascites tumor cells, determine the induction of point mutations in the indicator system. In all of the procedures an attempt is made to include the metabolic detoxification or potentiation of the compound by the host prior to the assessment of mutagenic activity by a nonhost-related indicator. The cytogenetic analysis of ascites tumor cells in treated mice, the host-mediated assay, assessment by biological indicators of the presence of mutagenic substances in tissues or body fluid of experimental animals, and the use of microsomal enzymes to simulate the in vivo conversion of a nonmutagenic substance to an active mutagen, are examples of model systems that can be used for the indirect assessment of chemically induced mutations, or cytogenetic effects.

1. Ascites Tumor Cells

Adler [1970] recently reviewed and presented data on the cytogenetic analysis of ascites tumor cells in treated mice. In this procedure, tumor cells are injected into the intraperitoneal cavity of mice, and the animals are treated, usually by oral administration, with a suspected mutagenic substance during the growth phase of the tumor cells. One to two hours before harvesting the tumor cells, the mice are injected with colcemide. The ascites cells are then harvested and the cells are analyzed to determine chromosome abnormalities. Adler concluded that this method is a sensitive indicator of cytogenetic effects and can be conducted without great difficulty. The normal numerical chromosome distribution in these tumor cells is highly variable, and only an assessment of structural chromosome alterations can be made. This technique is simple and can be used to screen a large number of chemicals. The standardization and characterization of the cell inoculum and the use of different strains are advantages of this procedure. This technique could augment direct in vivo cytogenetic analysis, but it offers little advantage over direct conventional cytogenetic analysis in animals.

2. Cell-Free Systems Simulating *in vivo* Metabolism

The use of specific enzymes, or selective non-enzymatic preparations, or mixtures of hepatic microsomal enzymes, can be used to simulate the metabolic conversion of chemicals to either an active mutagenic agent, or the detoxification of a mutagen to a nonmutagenic compound. A model hydroxylating system has been used to convert inactive dimethyl and diethylnitrosamines to mutagenic compounds, using Neurospora as the biological indicator [Malling 1966; Mayer and Legator 1970; Udenfriend et al. 1954]. This conversion is presumably analogous to what occurs in animals where the dialkylnitrosamines are metabolized to yield an active alkylating agent presumably diazoalkane, an active alkene, or an alkyl carbonium ion. It is quite possible that this reaction could also be carried out by microsomal enzyme preparations.

The use of microsomal enzymes, and other similar procedures, can be used to evaluate drugs where there is a lack of suitable animal facilities, or as an adjunct to in vivo procedures for screening mutagenic agents. The possibility of isolating specific intermediary metabolic compounds under controlled conditions makes these procedures attractive.

3. Body Fluid or Tissues

Analysis of tissues or body fluids from mammals treated with suspected mutagenic agents is a technique that has yet to be exploited, but potentially it could be of great value in evaluating mutagenic substances in animal and man. A number of microbial indicators are presently available that are well characterized genetically, and these indicators have been or are being used in a routine manner for the in vitro evaluation of mutagenic agents. It should be possible, by the use of sensitive indicators, to detect mutagenic agents in blood, urine, or tissues of treated animals, including man. The feasibility of this approach was demonstrated by Gabridge et al. [1969a, b, c], where mutagenic activity was found in the blood and urine of rats following the administration of the antibiotic, streptozotocin. The requirements needed to determine mutagenic activity by this approach are quite stringent, requiring adequate amounts of the mutagen in either body fluid or tissue and a highly sensitive indicator. Although the sensitivity of this procedure is questionable, the ease with which it can be conducted, and the number of agents that can be screened, make this an attractive assay. In this procedure, urine or blood is analyzed periodically after the administration of the compound under study by using one or a number of suitable biological indicators. Plate tests can be run (see section 4.1), and the presence or absence of induced mutations can be determined with the same ease as obtains for the detection of inhibitory effects following the administration of antibiotics. The development of sensitive microbial indicators, such as the repair-lacking histidine auxotrophs of *Salmonella typhimurium*, should make this procedure extremely useful. Not only is it theoretically possible to sequentially evaluate mutagenic substances in various body fluids and tissue of animals, but one could also evaluate drugs administered to man for possible mutagenic activity. The drugs of abuse that on the basis of chemical structure are suspected of mutagenic activity could be quickly studied in a number of experimental animals, and possibly also in man, by this procedure. A negative result, at the present state of the art, would not be significant, but a positive result would be meaningful.

4. The Host-Mediated Assay

This assay is the method of choice for determining mutagenic activity by the use of an indirect indicator. It is sensitive and practical, and it has been used to screen a number of suspected mutagenic agents. The host-mediated assay is one of the three major procedures recommended by the Advisory Panel on Mutagenicity in the Report of the Secretary's Commission on Pesticides and Their Relationship to Environmental Health [1969]. Four papers on this procedure were published in 1969 [Gabridge et al. 1969a, b, c; Gabridge and Legator 1969].

In this assay, the mammal during treatment with a potential chemical mutagen is injected with an indicator microorganism in which mutation frequencies can be measured. It is important to note that mutagen and organism are always administered by different routes. After a sufficient time period, the microorganisms are withdrawn from the animal, and the induction of mutants is determined. The comparison between the mutagenic action of the compound on the microorganism directly, and in the host-mediated assay indirectly, indicates whether the host can detoxify the compound or whether mutagenic products can be formed as a result of host metabolism. The indicator organisms utilized in this technique include histidine auxotrophs of *Salmonella typhimurium* and the forward mutation system in *Neurospora crassa*.

Table 1. Classification and Derivation of *S. typhimurium* Mutants

Mutant	Class	Origin
G–46	Ochre	Spontaneous
C–117	Ochre	Spontaneous
C–120	Misserse	Spontaneous
C–203	Frame Shift	X-ray
C–207	Frame Shift	X-ray
C–340	Amber	Apparent
C–527	Amber	Spontaneous
TA–1530	Ochre Repair Deficient	

The histidine genes of *Salmonella typhimurium* are one of the best characterized operons. The structural genes for the enzymes of histidine operon, 10 enzymes that convert the 5-carbon chain of phosphoribosil pyrophosphate to histidine, are in a cluster on the Salmonella chromosome. Well over a thousand histidine-requiring mutants have been located in a fine structure map of the operon [Whitfield et al. 1966].

Frame-shift missense, ochre, and amber mutants were the indicators used. Table 1 indicates the mutants used and their classification and derivation. To illustrate this technique, the activity of selected compounds using G-46 as the indicator organism and the mouse as the host will be described.

4.1. Materials and Methods

4.1.1. Histidine Auxotrophs of *Salmonella typhimurium*

The G-46 (nonsense mutant), was maintained on tryptone agar slants. Swiss albino mice (Flander's strain), 18-23 g, were used throughout, and were treated in groups of three. Test compounds were dissolved in saline solution wherever possible. When necessary, dimethylsulfoxide or ethanol was used, along with appropriate controls. Final concentrations selected reflected factors including solubility, mouse toxicity, and organism toxicity.

For the host-mediated test, tryptone broth was inoculated from an agar slant culture of *S. typhimurium* and incubated in a reciprocating shaker for 2 hours at 37°C. This culture was diluted 1:4 with saline solution, yielding a final OD_{660}, and 2 ml of the resulting suspension was injected intraperitoneally into the mouse.

Each mouse was given the first of three intramuscular injections (0.1 ml) of the test compound; the remainder was administered at 1-hour intervals. All mice were sacrificed 30 minutes after the third injection. Each mouse then received 1 ml of saline solution intra-

peritoneally and as much fluid as possible was aseptically removed from the peritoneum.

Ten-fold serial dilutions, from 10^{-1} to 10^{-7}, of each peritoneal fluid sample were made in saline solution. The four highest dilutions were plated on minimal agar with a histidine overlay to give the total Salmonella cell count, and the three lowest dilutions were plated on minimal agar without histidine for mutant growth.

Plates (15 × 100-mm plastic petri dishes) containing a base layer of 20 ml minimal agar with 0.5 percent glucose were used. With standard pour plate techniques, 0.1 ml of the proper dilution and 2 ml of molten 0.6 percent agar were added to a sterile tube, mixed, and poured over the surface of a base plate. The histidine overlay contained 0.1 ml of 0.1 *M* L-histidine/40 ml of agar. Plates were incubated at 37°C for 48 hours, and the ratio of mutants:total cells (mutant frequency, MF) was determined.

A modification of the Szybalski [1958] method was used for the in vitro tests. Molten 0.6 percent agar (2 ml) was added to 0.1 ml of an overnight broth culture of Salmonella and the mixture was poured over the surface of a minimal agar base plate. Positive results consisted of mutant colonies in a ring formation around the sample of test compound after incubations.

4.1.2. *Neurospora crassa*

De Serres used this organism to develop a direct method for the recovery of forward mutations [De Serres and Osterbind 1962]. Mutants with genetic blocks in either one of two successive steps in adenine biosynthes (aminoimadazole ribonucleotide to 5-amino-4-imidazole-carboxylic acid ribonucleotide and continuing to 5-amino-4-imidazole-H-succinocarboximide ribonucleotide) will accumulate a reddish-purple pigment in the mycelium. In this system, both mutant conidia and the nonmutant conidia grow into colonies of the same size and morphology. The mutant conidia form reddish-purple colonies, and can be easily distinguished from the white nonmutant colonies.

This use of this system in the host-mediated assay was described by Malling [Malling and Cosgrove 1970]. The cultures are grown from single-colony isolates of heterokaryotic colonies after plating of conidial from silica gel stock culture. The conidia are harvested after 7 to 9 days at 25°C and a suspension prepared. The conidia are injected into the animal, and the chemical is administered 4-5 hours later. Twenty-four hours after the administration of the conidia, they are harvested from the animal and plated, and their mutation frequency is determined.

4.2. Results

This indirect method of assessing point mutations has been used to a greater degree than any of the other outlined procedures. This is especially true where *S. typhimurium* has been used as the indicator organism. A variety of laboratory animals have been used, including rats, mice, and hamsters. Theoretically it should be possible to utilize almost any experimental animal. Routes of administration of the drug can vary, and studies can be conducted on animals that are being treated with the drug for varying lengths of time. Most of the standard mutagenic agents, including EMS, MMS, EDB, MNG, and ICR-170, have been studied by this procedure. All of the tested standards were active in the host-mediated assay as well as in the in vitro test, with the exception of ICR-170. ICR-170 was positive in *in vitro* tests with both *Salmonella* and *Neurospora*, but was negative in animal studies with both these biological indicators. It is interesting to note that MNG and EDB, although active in *in vitro* tests with both *Neurospora* and *Salmonella*, was positive when administered to mice with *Salmonella* as the indicator organism, but not with *Neurospora*. Of special interest is the positive results obtained with the naturally occurring plant

Table 2. Comparison of Selected Mutagens in In Vitro Tests and in the Host-Mediated Assay

Chemical	Sal In Vitro	Salm. Host-Me-diated	Neur In Vitro	Neur Host-Me-diated
E.M.S.[a]	+	+	+	+
M.M.S.[b]	+	+	+	+
M.N.N.G.[c]	+	+	+	−
D.M.N.A.[d]	−	+		
Cycasin	−	+		
Streptoz	+	+		
ICR-170[e]	+	−		

[a] E.M.S. = Ethyl methane sulfonate
[b] M.M.S. = Methyl methane sulfonate
[c] M.N.N.G. = N-Methyl-N[1]-nitro-nitrosoguanidine
[d] D.M.N.A. = Dimethylnitrosamine
[e] ICR-170 = Acridine mustard (2-methoxy-6-chloro-9-(3-(ethyl-2-chloroethyl) amino propyl-amino)-acridine dihydrochloride)

toxin cycasin, and with the known animal carcinogen, dimethylnitrosamine. The investigations with cycasin in this assay indicated that the metabolite of cycasin, methylazoxymethanol (MAM), was responsible for the mutagenic activity, and the metabolite was formed by the action of the intestinal flora. The mutagenic activity could be correlated with the known carcinogenic activity. Dimethylnitrosamine, like cycasin, is not mutagenic in vitro. This compound is also active in ths host mediated assay, serving as an additional example of this procedure to detect mutagenic activity after the host has metabolized the administered chemical.

Table 2 summarizes the activity of a selected group of compound in this assay.

This technique, for the first time allows one to compare potential mutagenic activity and carcinogenicity in the same animal, as illustrated by cycasin and the nitrosamine.

5. Summary and Recommendations

A variety of methods exists where an indirect indicator is used in animals to determine potentiation or detoxification of a chemical by metabolic action of the host. None of these procedures have been used extensively for screening chemicals, including drugs of abuse. The host-mediated assay has been used more extensively than any of the other indicator procedures, and it seems well suited for routine screening. The discovery of new indicator organisms and the expanded use of existing procedures should establish the indirect indicator systems for detecting mutagenic activity as one of our better approaches to aid in the complex problem of characterizing chemically induced mutations.

References

Adler, I. D. (1970). In F. Vogel, ed., *Chemical mutagenesis,* New York: Springer-Verlag.

De Serres, F. J., and R. S. Osterbind (1962). *Genetics* 47:793.

Gabridge, M. G., A. Denunzio, and M. S. Legator (1969a). *Nature* 221:68.

——, A. Denunzio, and M. S. Legator (1969b). *Science* 163:689.

——, E. J. Oswald, and M. S. Legator (1969c). *Mutat. Res.* 7:117.

——, and M. S. Legator (1969). *Proc. Soc. Exp. Biol. Med.* 130:831.

Malling, H. V. (1966). *Mutat. Res.* 3:537.

——, and G. E. Cosgrove (1970). In *Chemische mutagenese bei sauger und mensch. Testysteme und ergebnisse.* Proceedings of a symposium held Mainz, Germany. In press.

Mayer, V., and M. S. Legator (1970). In press.

Report of the Advisory Panel on Mutagenicity (1969). Report of the Secretary's Commision on Pesticides and Their Relationship to Environmental Health. U.S. Dept. of Health, Education and Welfare. Washington D.C.:

Szybalski, W. (1958). *Ann. N.Y. Acad. Sci.* 76:475.

Udenfriend, S., C. Clark, J. Axelrod, and B B. Brodie (1954). *J. Biol. Chem.* 208:731.

Whitfield, H. J., R. Martin, and B. J. Ames (1966). *J. Mol. Biol.* 21:335.

13 The Dominant Lethal Assay for Mutagenicity Testing

S. S. Epstein

Requirements for a definitive test method for mutagens include speed, simplicity, sensitivity, and presumptive human relevance. The dominant lethal (DL) assay satisfies all these requirements. Its value as a convenient indicator of major genetic damage has already been demonstrated in studies with ionizing radiations [Russell et al. 1954; Bateman 1958a], and with chemical mutagens [Bateman 1960, 1966; Röhrborn 1965, 1968; Cattanach et al. 1968; Ehling et al. 1968; Epstein and Shafner 1968; Generoso 1969; Epstein et al. 1970a, 1970b]. With regard to human relevance, it is well known that mutagenic effects in different test systems may exhibit wide variations, *inter alia*, probably reflecting differences in metabolism of the chemical under test. The human relevance of data from any particular test system cannot therefore be guaranteed, but the probability of relevance is obviously much greater if mammals are used as test systems. Data on induction of DL mutants in mammals may be appropriately extrapolated to man, especially as most recognizable human mutations are due to dominant autosomal traits [Report of the U.N. Scientific Committee on the Effects of Atomic Radiation 1966]. Genetic hazards to man are not, however, particularly concerned with DL mutations, which will merely produce abortions, but rather with dominant viable mutations which are expressed in heterozygotes.

 The genetic basis for dominant lethality is the induction of chromosomal damage and rearrangements, such as translocations, resulting in nonviable zygotes; evidence for zygote lethality induced in mammals by x-rays and by chemical mutagens has been obtained embryologically [Snell et al. 1934; Snell and Picken 1935; Hertwig 1940], and cytogenetically [Bateman 1969 personal communication; Russell and Russell 1954; Generoso 1969; Epstein et al. 1970d; Joshi et al. 1970], respectively. Additional evidence for the genetic basis of dominant lethality is derived from the associated induction of sterility and heritable semisterility in F_1 progeny of males exposed to X-irradiation [Snell et al. 1934; Koller and Auerbach 1941], and to chemical mutagens [Falconer 1952; Cattanach 1964; Epstein et al. 1971b]; translocations have been cytologically demonstrated in such semisterile lines in mice [Koller 1944; Slizynski 1952; Cattanach et al. 1968] in hamsters [Lavappa and Yerganian 1970 personal communication], and more recently in fetal mice [Schleiermacher 1970 personal communication].

A DL mutation is one which kills an individual heterozygous for it, carrying it in single dose. It is not therefore possible in any particular case to confirm its genetic nature or to allocate it to a particular chromosome by breeding tests, such as applicable to other kinds of mutation. The mutation will have arisen in an egg or sperm prior to fertilization, and theoretically it could kill the zygote at any time during development, either prior to or after implantation. In practice, however, it is found that the deaths are restricted to a brief and early period of gestation. Preimplantation losses, early fetal deaths, and sterility and semisterility in F_1 offspring constitute a spectrum of adverse genetic effects, of which early fetal deaths clearly afford the most convenient and quantitatively unequivocal parameter of mutagenicity; hence, the utility of the DL assay.

1. Preimplantation losses due to Dominant Lethal Mutations

After parental exposure to mutagens and subsequent mating, adverse genetic effects may manifest sequentially by preimplantation losses of fertilized ova and zygotes, early fetal deaths, and sterility and semisterility in F_1 progeny [Cattanach, 1964; Epstein et al. 1971b]. Effects of ionizing irradiation of the male or of sperm in vitro on fertilization and subsequent development of the zygote have been extensively studied in the rabbit [Amoroso and Parkes 1947; Chang et al. 1957; Bedford and Hunter 1968], and in the mouse [Brenneke 1937; Bruce and Austin 1956; Edwards 1957]; such data are comparatively rare for chemical mutagens. Embryos with chromosomal damage have been demonstrated following artificial insemination of mice with spermatozoa treated with nitrogen mustard in vitro [Edwards 1958]. Administration of chemical mutagens to female mice prior to ovulation produced genetic damage, histologically recognizable as early as the 2-cell zygote stage [Generoso 1969].

In recent studies, based on recovery of ova from female mice following sequential mating with males treated with TEPA at 10 mg/kg, mating rates of treated and control males were generally similar, apart from the second mating week, when matings in treated groups and numbers of mated females with normal ova were reduced [Epstein et al. 1970d; Joshi et al. 1970]. Penetration and fertilization of ova by sperm of treated males were apparently normal, except in the sixth week following drug administration, when the majority of ova in mated females were not penetrated. Such striking premeiotic antifertility effects have been attributed to a brief inhibition of Type A spermatogonia [Steinberger 1962] and aspermia [Fox et al. 1963]. The increased incidence of polyspermy in treated groups was of particular interest, suggesting interference with blockage factors that normally prevent penetration of more than one sperm; polyspermy has been associated with embryonic triploidy [Carr 1965, 1969]. Micronuclei suggestive of chromosomal damage in sperm were observed in a high percentage of first cleavage blastomeres in the first 3 weeks following TEPA administration to male mice; this is consistent with previously described effects of x-rays and alkylating agents in rats and mice [Russell and Russell 1954; Edwards 1957, 1958]. Subsequently, retardation in rates of cleavage and morphological mal-formations in retarded and normally developing embryos were noted. Malformations were generally preceded by retarded cleavage as the ratio of malformed to retarded ova increased from 60 hours to 82 hours post-ovulation. These observations of retardation and malformation in fertilized ova accord with data indicating that reduced ability of sperm to form viable embryos is a more sensitive index of injury than reduced fertilization [Bishop and Walton 1960].

Administration of TEPA to male mice thus induced a biphasic effect on spermatogenesis [Epstein et al. 1970d; Joshi et al. 1970]. Postmeiotically, the effect on epididymal spermatozoa and spermatids manifested by normal fertilization followed by retardation in the cleavage and malformation of embryos. With severe embryopathies, zygotes died prior to implantation, resulting in reduction in the overall incidence of pregnancy or in the number of total implants per pregnant female. With less severe damage, the retarded and malformed embryos implanted and evoked a deciduoma reaction, but died shortly after. Such deciduomas or early fetal deaths are the basis for the dominant lethal assay [Bateman 1966; Epstein and Shafner 1968; Epstein et al. 1970a,b]. Premeiotically, infertility is probably due to aspermia, resulting from the high sensitivity of spermatogonial cells to the lethal effects of TEPA, besides certain other alkylating agents and x-rays. DL mutations induced in stem cells, which are generally resistant, are likely to be eliminated by germinal selection prior to maturation, so that apparently normal fertilization and embryonic development will ensue. It is, however, unlikely that point mutations would be subject to such selection [Bateman and Epstein 1971].

Enumeration of corpora lutea, which is relatively difficult in mice and relatively easy in rats, affords a good measure of total fertilized ova; the difference between total implants and corpora lutea counts thus is a measure of pre-implantation losses. In the absence of super-ovulation or systemic infection, corpora lutea counts are generally constant in controls. Thus, a simple alternative method of determining preimplantation losses in mice is to determine the differences between total implants in test and control females.

2. Sterility and Semisterility due to Dominant Lethal Mutations

Treatment of parental male rodents with x-irradiation or with various chemical mutagens induces dominant lethal mutations, as indicated indirectly by preimplantation losses of early zygotes and directly by early fetal deaths [Cattanach and Edwards 1957–1958; Cattanach 1959; Ehling et al. 1968; Epstein and Shafner 1968; Epstein et al. 1970a–d–1971b; Röhrborn and Vogel 1969]. Chromosomal translocations causing the heritable trait of semisterility have been demonstrated in progeny of irradiated males [Snell et al. 1934; Snell 1935, 1946; Gruneberg 1952; Carter et al. 1955; Ford and Clegg 1969; Ford et al. 1969]; more restrictedly, similar effects have been demonstrated with ethylmethane sulfonate [Cattanach et al. 1968], nitrogen mustard [Falconer et al. 1952], TEM [Cattanach 1966] and trenimone [Röhrborn and Vogel 1969]. Selection against translocation-bearing germ cells during sperm maturation has been demonstrated [Ford et al. 1969].

In a recent study, mutagenic effects of TEPA in mice, as manifested by heritable reduced fertility—sterility and semisterility—were observed in male progeny conceived within the first 3 mating weeks following treatment of parental males (Epstein et al. 1971b). Thus, in general accord with previous results of DL tests [Epstein and Shafner 1968; Epstein et al. 1970a], only postmeiotic stages of spermatogenesis were affected by this

Table 1. Recommended Protocol for Dominant Lethal Assay in Male Mice

Dosage	Number of Treated Males	Mating Procedure
Acute: $1 \times (LD_5-LD_{25})$	20	3 ♀/wk for 4 weeks
Subacute: $5 \times (LD_5-LD_{25})$	20	3 ♀/wk for 4 weeks
Chronic: Continuous for 3 months at maximum tolerated dose	20	2 ♀/wk for 3 months, commencing with third treatment month

mutagen. The genetic basis of the DL test is thus clearly confirmed by the associated occurrence of heritable reduced fertility. The DL test is clearly a more sensitive, and practical measure of mutagenic effects than are more laborious tests for reduced fertility. Semisterility in these studies was established in F_1 progeny by 3 criteria: increased incidence of early fetal deaths and/or reduced number of viable implants; reduced size of F_2 litters at birth; and reduced fertility in F_2 progeny. In F_2 male progeny, the same criteria were additionally confirmed by cytogenetic demonstration of translocations as the genetic basis for semisterility [Epstein et al. 1971b]. Sterility, in accordance with previous findings [Cattanach et al. 1968], can also be due to translocations. Of the 160 test F_1 male progeny from all 8 mating weeks, 12 induced a high incidence of early fetal deaths and/or a reduction in numbers of viable implants; litter size at birth confirmed reduced fertility in 4 of these males, 3 of which had subfertile F_2 progeny. The latter 3 F_1 males were conceived in the second and third weeks following TEPA treatment of paternal males, indicating the high sensitivity of postmeiotic germ cells. Of the treated males, 7 produced sterile and or semisterile male progeny. Thus, a single subtoxic dose of TEPA induced mutant progeny in 23 percent (7/30) of treated males [Epstein et al. 1971b].

3. Protocols for the Dominant Lethal Assay
Formal protocols for routine testing have been recently developed [Epstein and Shafner 1968; Epstein et al. 1970a; Epstein and Röhrborn 1971]. Chemicals should be tested for mutagenic effects following acute, subacute, and chronic administration to male mice (Table 1), and to male rats. Testing must reflect modes of human exposure and thus must include oral, parenteral, cutaneous, and respiratory routes. For chemicals to which man is exposed by aerosols, testing

should include oral and parenteral routes, in the absence of facilities for inhalation exposure. Subacute testing is recommended, in addition to acute, largely to anticipate and reflect the role of possible hepatic microsomal detoxification or activation. Chronic administration can be used to detect both cumulative and noncumulative spermatogonial mutations; however, evidence from acute studies reveals selection against DLs induced in spermatogonia.

Following acute or subacute drug administration to male mice or rats, they are mated sequentially with groups of untreated females over the duration of the spermatogenic cycle. For mice, the entire duration of spermatogenesis is approximately 42 days, comprising the following stages: spermatogonial mitoses —6 days, spermatocytes—14 days, spermatids—9 days, testicular sperm—5.5 days, and epididymal sperm—7.5 days [Bateman 1958b]. Thus, matings within 3 weeks after single drug administration represent samplings of sperm exposed during postmeiotic stages; and matings from 4 to 8 weeks later represent samplings of sperm exposed during premeiotic and stem cell stages.

The classical form of the DL assay involves autopsy of females approximately 13 days following timed matings, as determined by vaginal plugs in mice and vaginal cytology in rats, and enumeration of corpora lutea and of total implants, as comprised by living fetuses, late fetal deaths, and early fetal deaths. The test can be considerably modified and simplified and hence made more suitable for routine practice by sacrificing the females at a fixed time, e.g., 13 days in mice, following the midweek of their caging and presumptive mating; additionally, this procedure allows determination of effects of drugs on pregnancy rates. Similarly, corpora lutea counts, which afford a measure of total fertilized zygotes, but which are difficult and inaccurate in mice, can be omitted, and numbers of total implants in test animals can be related to those in controls, thus affording a simple measure of preimplantation losses. Additionally, matings may be restricted to 4 weeks following drug treatment of the males (Table 1). Using such modified procedures, together with computerized data handling, large numbers of test agents can be simply and rapidly tested for mutagenic activity [Epstein and Shafner 1968]. A modified form of the DL assay has been recently described in female mice, in which both premeiotic and postmeiotic germinal stages can be tested [Röhrborn 1968].

DL mutations are directly measured by enumeration of early fetal deaths and indirectly by preimplantation losses, as measured by reduction in the number of total implants in test compared with control females. Results are best expressed as early fetal deaths per pregnant female, rather than the more conventional mutagenic index—early fetal deaths × 100 per total implants, for the latter index can be markedly altered by variation in the number of total implants [Epstein et al. 1970a]. Preimplantation losses offer a presumptive index of mutagenic effects, but there is no precise parallelism between preimplantation losses and early fetal deaths. These should be regarded as concomitant and not alternate parameters. Furthermore, the use of the mutagenic index presupposes that the number of early deaths is proportional to the number of implants regardless of preimplantation losses; this would anticipate that absolute number of early deaths are lower in those animals with reduced numbers ot total implants. This has been shown experimentally not to be so [Epstein et al. 1970a]. Finally, an additional disadvantage of such ratios as measures of mutagenic effect is that their variability is high, as both numerator and denominator are contributory, and estimates of standard deviation hence are complex.

The justification for restricting testing of

Table 2. Chemicals Tested for Induction of Dominant Lethal Mutations in Mammals

Compound	Reference	Species (Sex)
Acriflavine	Epstein and Shafner 1968	Mouse (male)
Acrolein	Epstein and Shafner 1968	Mouse (male)
Aflatoxin	Epstein and Shafner 1968	Mouse (male)
Aminopterin	Epstein and Shafner 1968	Mouse (male)
Atmospheric Pollutants		
organic extract Boston 1966	Epstein and Shafner 1968	Mouse (male)
acid fraction New York 1967	Epstein and Shafner 1968	Mouse (male)
basic fraction New York 1967	Epstein and Shafner 1968	Mouse (male)
insoluble fraction New York 1967	Epstein and Shafner 1968	Mouse (male)
Azaribine	Epstein and Shafner 1968	Mouse (male)
Benzanthrone	Epstein and Shafner 1968	Mouse (male)
Benzo[a]pyrene	Epstein and Shafner 1968	Mouse (male)
5-Bromodeoxyuridine	Epstein and Shafner 1968	Mouse (male)
Butter yellow	Epstein and Shafner 1968	Mouse (male)
Butylated hydroxytoluene	Epstein and Shafner 1968	Mouse (male)
Caffeine	Lyon et al. 1962	Mouse (male)
	Cattanach 1964	Mouse (male)
	Kuhlmann et al. 1968	Mouse (male)
	Adler 1969	Mouse (male)
	Epstein et al. 1970c	Mouse (male)
	Epstein et al. 1970c	Mouse (male)

Dosage (route and duration)	Weeks of spermatogenesis sampled	Antifertility effects (weeks when maximal following administration of chemical)	Induction of dominant lethal mutants (weeks when maximal)	Comments
10.6 mg/kg (i.p. × 1)	3	0	0	
1.5 mg/kg (i.p. × 1)	8	0	0	
68 mg/kg (i.p. × 1)	8	+ (1–3)	+ (3–5)	
10 mg/kg (i.p. × 1)	8	± (1)	0	
333 mg/kg (i.p. × 1)	8	0	0	
333 mg/kg (i.p. × 1)	8	0	0	
333 mg/kg (i.p. × 1)	8	0	0	
333 mg/kg (i.p. × 1)	8	0	0	
1000 mg/kg (oral × 1)	8	0	0	
1000 mg/kg (i.p. × 1)	8	0	0	
750 mg/kg (i.p. × 1)	8	+	+ (3)	
500 mg/kg (i.p. × 1)	8	0	0	
216 mg/kg (i.p. × 1)	8	0	0	
1000 mg/kg (i.p. × 1)	8	±	0	
0.1% in drinking water (for 7 weeks)	4	0	0	
0.3% in drinking water (for 6 weeks)	3	+ (1–3)	0	
0.025–0.5% in drinking water (for 14–20 weeks)	NS	+	0	Mutagenic effects claimed on basis of preimplantation losses
0.25 g/kg (i.p. × 1)	8	+	0	
168–240 mg/kg (i.p. × 1)	3 or 8	+	0	
0.1% in drinking water (for 8 weeks)	8	+	0	

Table 2. Chemicals Tested for Induction of Dominant Lethal Mutations in Mammals (continued)

Compound	Reference	Species (Sex)
Caffeine + x-ray	Epstein et al. 1970c	Mouse (male)
	Epstein et al. 1970c	Mouse (male)
Caffeine + methyl methane sulfonate	Epstein et al. 1970c	Mouse (male)
Caffeine + TEPA	Epstein et al. 1970c	Mouse (male)
Captan	Epstein and Shafner 1968	Mouse (male)
	Epstein and Shafner 1968	Mouse (male)
Chloramphenicol	Epstein and Shafner 1968	Mouse (male)
Chloroethyl methane sulfonate	Cattanach 1964	Mouse (male)
Chlorpromazine	Epstein and Shafner 1968	Mouse (male)
Cumene hydroperoxide	Epstein and Shafner 1968	Mouse (male)
Cytoxan	Brittinger (1966)	Mouse (male)
D.D.T.	Epstein and Shafner 1968	Mouse (male)
	Palmer, Legator & Green	Rat (male)
1,2,3,4-Diepoxybutane	Cattanach 1964	Mouse (male)
	Epstein and Shafner 1968	Mouse (male)

Dosage (route and duration)	Weeks of spermatogenesis sampled	Antifertility effects (weeks when maximal following administration of chemical)	Induction of dominant lethal mutants (weeks when maximal)	Comments
168–200 mg/kg (i.p. × 1) + 50–250 r (acute)	8	+ (1–2)	+	Effect equivalent to x-ray alone
0.05–0.4% in drinking water (for 8 weeks) + 50 or 200 r (acute)	8	0	+	Effect equivalent to x-ray alone
168, 192 mg/kg caffeine (i.p. × 1) + 50 mg/kg MMS (i.p. × 1)	8	+ (1–2)	+	Effect equivalent to methyl methane sulfonate alone
200 mg/kg caffeine (i.p. × 1) + 0.312, 1.25 mg/kg TEPA (i.p. × 1)	8	+ (1–2)	+	Effect equivalent to TEPA alone
9 mg/kg (i.p. × 1)	8	0	0	
500 mg/kg (oral × 1)	8	0	0	
333 mg/kg (i.p. × 1)	8	0	0	
83 mg/kg (i.p. × 1)	NS	0	0	
8.3 mg/ka (i.p. × 1)	8	0	0	
34 mg/kg (i.p. × 1)	8	0	0	
60–240 mg/kg (i.p. × 1)	8	+ (4–8)	+ (1–3)	
105 mg/kg (i.p. × 1)	8	0	0	
50–70 mg/kg	8	NS	+ (2–3)	
27 mg/kg (i.p. × 1)	NS	NS	±	
17 mg/kg (i.p. × 1)	8	0	0	

Table 2. Chemicals Tested for Induction of Dominant Lethal Mutations in Mammals (continued)

Compound	Reference	Species (Sex)
Dimethyl hydrazide	Epstein and Shafner 1968	Mouse (male)
Dimethylnitrosamine	Epstein and Shafner 1968	Mouse (male)
Dimethyl sulfate	Epstein and Shafner 1968	Mouse (male)
Ethyl methane sulfonate	Ehling et al. 1968	Mouse (male)
	Generoso 1969	Mouse (female)
	Partington and Jackson 1963	Rat (male)
Formaldehyde	Epstein and Shafner 1968	Mouse (male)
Griseofulvin	Epstein and Shafner 1968	Mouse (male)
Hydrazine	Epstein and Shafner 1968	Mouse (male)
Hydroxyurea	Epstein and Shafner 1968	Mouse (male)
5-Iododeoxyuridine	Epstein and Shafner 1968	Mouse (male)
Isopropyl methane sulfonate	Partington and Jackson 1963	Rat (male)
Maleic hydrazide	Epstein and Shafner 1968	Mouse (male)
2-Methoxy-6-chloro-9-[3-(ethyl-2-chloroethyl) amino propyl-amino]acridine dihydrochloride (ICR-170)	Ehling et al. 1968	Mouse (male)
	Generoso 1969	Mouse (female)
Methyl cholanthrene	Epstein and Shafner 1968	Mouse (male)
Methyl ethane sulfonate	Partington and Jackson 1963	Rat (male)
Methyl hydroxylamine	Epstein and Shafner 1968	Mouse (male)
Methyl methane sulfonate	Partington and Bateman 1964	Mouse (male)
	Ehling et al. 1968	Mouse (male)
	Epstein and Shafner 1968	Mouse (male)
	Generoso 1969	Mouse

Dosage (route and duration)	Weeks of spermatogenesis sampled	Antifertility effects (weeks when maximal following administration chemical)	Induction of dominant lethal mutants (weeks when maximal)	Comments
25 mg/kg (i.p. × 1)	8	0	0	
8 mg/kg (i.p. × 1)	8	+ (5–8)	0	
23 mg/kg (i.p. × 1)	8	0	0	
100–250 mg/kg (i.p. × 1)	3	+ (1)	+ (2)	
325 mg/kg (i.p. × 1)	3	+ (1–2)	+ (1–2)	
100–200 mg/kg (i.p. × 1)	10	+ (1–4)	+ (1–4)	
20 mg/kg (i p × 1)	8	0	0	
750 mg/kg (i.p × 1)	8	+ (3–6)	0	
42 mg/kg (i.p. × 1)	8	0	0	
500 mg/kg (i.p. × 1)	8	0	0	
250 mg/kg (i.p. × 1)	8	±	0	
50 mg/kg (i.p. × 1)	12	+ (8)	0	Mutagenic effects claimed on indirect basis of preimplantation loss
500 mg/kg (i.p. × 1)	8	+ (1–2)	0	
4 mg/kg (i.p. × 1)	3	0	0	
4 mg/kg (i.p. × 1)	3	0	0	
100 mg/kg (i.p. × 1)	8	0	0	
50 mg/kg	12	+ (2–4)	+ (2–4)	
140 mg/kg (i.p. × 1)	8	0	0	
50–100 mg/kg (i.p. × 1)	5	+ (1–3)	+ (1–2)	
50–150 mg/kg (i.p. × 1)	3	+ (1–2)	+ (1–3)	
50 mg/kg (i.p. × 1)	8	0	+ (2)	
150 mg/kg (i.p. × 1)	3	+ (1–2)	+ (1)	

Table 2. Chemicals Tested for Induction of Dominant Lethal Mutations in Mammals (continued)

Compound	Reference	Species (Sex)
N-Methyl-N'-nitro-nitrosoguanidine	Ehlin et al. 1968	Mouse (male)
	Generoso 1969	Mouse (female)
Myleran (tetramethylene-1,4 dimethane-sulfonate	Partington and Jackson 1963	Rat (male)
Nicotine	Cattanach 1964	Mouse (male)
Nitrogen mustard	Cattanach 1964	Mouse (male)
	Falconer et al. 1952	Mouse (male)
4-Nitroquinoline-1-oxide	Epstein and Shafner 1968	Mouse (male)
Phosphorus[32]	Reddi and Vasuderan 1968	Mouse (male)
Strontium[90]	Lüning et al. 1963	Mouse (male)
Theobromine	Epstein and Shafner 1968	Mouse (male)
Theophylline	Epstein and Shafner 1968	Mouse (male)
Triethylmelamine	Bateman 1960	Mouse (male)
	Cattanach 1964	Mouse (male)
	Epstein and Shafner 1968	Mouse (male)
	Bateman 1960	Rat (male)
Trimethyl phosphate	Epstein et al. 1970b	Mouse (male)
	Epstein et al. 1970b	Mouse (male)
Tris (1-aziridinyl)-phosphine oxide (TEPA)	Epstein et al. 1970a	Mouse (male)
Tris (1-aziridinyl)-phosphine sulphide (THIOTEPA)	Epstein and Shafner 1968	Mouse (male)
Tris (2-methyl-1-aziridinyl)-phosphine oxide (METEPA)	Epstein et al. 1970a	Mouse (male)
2,3,5-Tris-ethylene-imino -p-benzoquionone (Trenimon)	Röhrborn 1965	Mouse (male)

Dosage (route and duration)	Weeks of spermatogenesis sampled	Antifertility effects (weeks when maximal following administration of chemical)	Induction of dominant lethal mutants (weeks when maximal)	Comments
50 mg/kg (i.p. × 1)	3	0	0	
70 mg/kg (i.p. × 1)	3	0	±(1)	
4–10 mg/kg (i.p. × 1)	10	+(7–9)	0	Mutagenic effects claimed on basis of preimplantation losses
0.2 mg (s.c. daily)	NS	0	0	
N.S.	NS	+	0	Mutagenic effects claimed on basis of fertility tests done
0.06–0.08 mg (i.p. × 1)	NS	+	±	
5 mg/kg (i.p. × 1)	8	0	0	
50–135 µCL (i.p. × 1)	4	+	+(2–3)	
18 µC (i.p. ± 1)	5	NS	+(1–3)	
380 mg/kg (i.p. × 1)	8	0	0	
380 mg/kg (i.p. × 1)	8	0	0	
0.2.–0.8 mg/kg (i.p. × 1)	4	+(2–3)	+(1–3)	
0.8 mg/kg (i.p. × 1)	4	+(1–2)	+(1–2)	
0.2 mg/kg (i.p. × 1)	8	+(1)	+(2–3)	
0.025–0.4 mg/kg (i.p. × 1)	6	+(1–4)	+(1–5)	
200–2000 mg/kg (i.p. × 1)	8	±	+(2)	
500–1000 mg/kg (orally on 5 successive days)	8	+	+(1–2)	
0.156–20.0 mg/kg (i.p. × 1)	8	+	+(1–3)	
5 mg/kg (i.p. × 1)	8	0	+	
0.782–100.0 mg/kg (i.p. × 1)	8	+	+(1–3)	
0.125–0.250 mg/kg (i.p. × 1)	8	+(1–6)	+(1–3)	

Table 2. Chemicals Tested for Induction of Dominant Lethal Mutations in Mammals (continued)

Compound	Reference	Species (Sex)
Tritiated thymidine	Bateman and Chandley 1962	Mouse (male)
Urethan	Epstein and Shafner 1968	Mouse (male)
Water pollutants		
Maine 1961	Epstein and Shafner 1968	Mouse (male)
Yonkers 1961	Epstein and Shafner 1968	Mouse (male)

NS = not specified; 0 = no effect; ± = equivocal effect; + = unequivocal effect; *commencing at 4th week following injection

Dosage (route and duration)	Weeks of spermatogenesis sampled	Antifertility effects (weeks when maximal following administration of chemical)	Induction of dominant lethal mutants (weeks when maximal)	Comments
300 µC (i.p., in 6 fractions over 2 days)	3*	NS	+(4–6)	
1000 mg/kg (i.p. × 1)	8	0	0	
333 mg/kg (i.p. × 1)	8	+	0	
699 mg/kg (i.p. × 1)	8	+	0	

acute and subacute regimes to meiotic and postmeiotic stages, i.e., to weeks 1–4 following drug administration to male mice (Table 1), is that no chemical has yet been shown exclusively to induce premeiotic DL mutations. A variety of agents, x-rays, Cytoxan, Trenimon, TEPA, METEPA, and aflatoxin, have been shown to induce premeiotic effects, as measured by early fetal deaths and/or by preimplantation losses, but these also produce more marked meiotic and/or postmeiotic effects. For chronic studies, test matings should extend over a period which will allow detection of effects of exposure on meiotic and postmeiotic, as well as premeiotic, stages. Thus chronic testing should also detect cumulative and noncumulative spermatogonial mutations.

4. Results of the Dominant Lethal Assay

Using these techniques, a wide range of chemicals to which man is exposed in the totality of the environment, including pesticides, food additives, drugs, and air and water pollutants, have been tested for mutagenicity in mice [Epstein and Shafner 1968; Epstein et al. 1971a]. Additionally, detailed dose-response studies with the aziridine alkylating agents, TEPA and METEPA, which have been used as chemosterilant pesticides, have revealed mutagenic thresholds in the region of 0.04 mg/kg and 1.4 mg/kg, respectively, following acute single parenteral administration in mice [Epstein et al. 1970a]. More recently, trimethylphosphate, a weak alkylating agent used till recently as a fuel additive, has been shown to be mutagenic in the DL assay [Epstein et al. 1970b].

Chemicals which have been tested for mutagenicity in male and female mice and rats by the DL assay are listed and reviewed in Table 2. As can be seen, of 58 agents tested, only 15 have been shown to be mutagenic. The overwhelming majority (13/15) of these mutagenic chemicals are alkylating agents. There are no published data on DL assays on drugs of abuse, except for phenothiazine

tranquilizers (see Chapter 13). Recent discrepancies between results in mice and rats for cyclohexylamine and for DDT have emphasized the need for dominant lethal testing in both these species [Epstein and Legator, 1971 unpublished data].

The DL assay has also been used to study problems of interactions, both synergistic and antagonistic, among known mutagens such as x-rays or alkylating agents, and among agents that modify DNA repair mechanisms. Such interactions have been extensively studied with reference to caffeine [Epstein et al. 1970c], in view of its effects in inhibiting DNA repair mechanisms [Witkin 1958; Rauth 1967; Wragg et al. 1967]. Caffeine was found to have no mutagenic effect itself, or any synergistic effect when combined with x-rays, MMS, or TEPA.

It must be emphasized that the DL assay should be applied together with other in vivo mammalian mutagenicity tests, notably in vivo cytogenetics, karyotype analysis of bone marrow, and the host-mediated assay, in addition to ancillary submammalian tests. Such mammalian systems can be simply and practically incorporated in the course of routine toxicity testing.

5. Integration of the Dominant Lethal Assay and Other Mutagenicity Tests into General Toxicological Practice

Hazards due to chemical pollutants may be classified by acute and chronic toxicity, teratogenicity, carcinogenicity, and mutagenicity. Historically, each has been studied and applied independently and by nonconverging disciplines; toxicity per se has largely been the province of classical pharmacologists, generally with little interest in carcinogenesis or mutagenesis. Mutagenesis has been even more isolated from other aspects of toxicology. Indeed, publications on mutagenic hazards are rarities in toxicological or public health journals; in general, they appear only in journals read by geneticists. Obviously, the present fragmentation of toxicological research is artificial and even wasteful. New organizational patterns and training programs are needed to coordinate toxicological approaches, and to have toxicology reflect current needs, especially at the laboratory level [Epstein 1969].

Mutagenicity tests in mammals, particularly the DL assay, the host-mediated assay, and in vivo cytogenetics, in addition to ancillary non-mammalian tests, should be incorporated into the armamentarium of routine toxicological practice.

Toxicological practice could be feasibly integrated by developing "catchall" screens for chronic toxicity, carcinogenicity, mutagenicity, teratogenicity, and reproductive effects in the same test animals [Epstein 1969]. For instance, in any type of chronic toxicity or carcinogenicity study, representative groups of males and females would periodically mate, the female would be allowed to go to term and the F_1 progeny would be retained; the parents then would be returned to the main body of the experiment. Effects would be scored in relation to incidence of pregnancies and malformations, and to litter sizes. Under these conditions, malformations would be teratologically or, less likely, genetically induced; reduction in litter size may be due to induction of DL mutations in parental males or females, manifesting as preimplantation losses of fertilized zygotes and as early fetal deaths, or due to other nongenetic factors. Reproductive tests on F_1 progeny, inter alia, would also indicate viable translocations manifesting as sterility or heritable semi-sterility. F_1 progeny would also provide a measure of carcinogenic effects, especially if test materials were administered continuously during maternal pregnancy, and during lifetime of the progeny commencing in infancy; enhanced sensitivity of infant rodents to a variety of carcinogens has been well documented. Cytogenetic tests could be performed serially on the marrow of parental animals and also on their progeny; single testes could also be sampled for the same reasons.

Positive effects of any kind in catchall screens would, of course, be subsequently further investigated by more specific standard test procedures. Both catchall screens and appropriate standard procedures would be simultaneously applied for test materials with high a priori reasons for anticipating particular toxic effects, e.g., congeners of known mutagens or their metabolic precursors. The validity and logistics of the catchall approach should be initially evaluated with a wide range of carcinogens, mutagens, and teratogens; such studies may also meaningfully reveal associations between these various effects in the same test system. Once established in principle, many variations in the catchall theme would be feasible; however, irrespective of the precise initial form, it should be flexible and dynamically reflect technical and conceptual advances in any aspect of toxicology.

The catchall screen is proposed not as a simple toxicological panacea, but as an integrated attempt to determine, though not necessarily completely characterize, any kind of deleterious effect by in-depth study of a group of animals over more than one generation. It should be further appreciated that this holistic approach, oriented toward a multiplicity of end points, is closer to the human situation than standard approaches in which single toxic agents are singly tested on model systems designed to demonstrate single hazards only.

6. Summary

A number of in vivo procedures are presently available in mammals, the majority of recent origin, that can be used to determine the mutagenic activity of drugs of abuse. Our ability to characterize mutagenic agents no longer depends exclusively on nonmammalian systems, such as Drosophila, bacteriophage, microorganisms, and cell culture, although these procedures should be considered as ancillary to available mammalian tests. Mammalian tests, which should be considered as the definitive basis for evaluating potentially mutagenic agents, are in vivo cytogenetics, the host-mediated assay, and the DL assay. These procedures are as relevant to man as any other procedure presently used in the field of toxicology; they are also practical. The DL test can be concluded in less than three months; similarly, the host-mediated assay can be carried out in a few weeks. The cost of these tests is considerably less than that of many procedures currently used in chronic toxicity testing. It is anticipated that a protocol, relying on both the in vivo mammalian tests and on nonmammalian ancillary procedures, should detect the majority of mutagenic psychotropic drugs. At the present time, none of these drugs has been adequately, if at all, tested for mutagenic activity.

The phenothiazine tranquilizers represent one of the most widely used classes of drugs in our society, with over a dozen formulations in commerce. Recent studies in the dominant lethal assay, using both rats and mice, and using both oral and parenteral routes of administration, indicate that trifluoropromazine and chlorpromazine produce dose-dependent mutagenic effects over a dose range of 27-75 mg/kg [Petersen and Legator, 1971, personal communication]. In addition, these two drugs increase the number of mitotic recombinants in the host-mediated assay, using *Saccharomyces cerevisiae* as the indicator organism [Brusick and Legator, 1971, personal communication]. The phenothiazine tranquilizers thus may represent the first class of apparently noncytotoxic drugs that are active mutagens in mammals, and thus they pose potential genetic hazards to man.

References

Amoroso, E. C., and A. S. Parkes (1947). *Proc. Royal Soc.* B. 134 : 57.

Bateman, A. J. (1958a). *Heredity* 12 : 213.

——— (1958b). *Heredity* 12 : 467.

——— (1960). *Genet. Res. Camb.* 1 : 381.

——— (1966). *Nature* 210 : 205.

—(1969) Personal communication.

———, and S. S. Epstein (1971). In A. Hollaender, ed., *Chemical Mutagens—Principles and Methods for Their Detection*, New York: Plenum Press.

Bedford, J. M., and R. H. F. Hunter (1968). *J. Reprod. Fertil.* 17 : 49.

Bishop, M. W. H., and A. Walton (1960). In A. S. Parkes, ed., *Marshall's Physiology of Reproduction,* London: Longmans, Green, vol. I, part 2, 98 pp.

Brenneke, H. (1937). *Strahlentherapie* 60 : 214.

Bruce, H. M., and C. R. Austin (1956). *Proc. Soc. for the Study of Fertility* 8 : 121.

Cattanach, B. M. (1959). *Zeitschrift fur Vererbungslehre* 90 : 1.

——— (1964) In W. D. Carlson and F. X. Gassner, eds., *Effects of Ionizing Radiation on the Reproductive System*, New York: Macmillan, 415 pp.

——— (1966) *Mutat. Res.* 3 : 346.

———, and R. G. Edwards (1957–1958). *Proc. Royal Soc.* (Edinburgh) B67 : 54.

———, C. E. Pollard, and J. H. Isaacson (1968). *Mutat. Res.* 6 : 297.

Carr, D. H. (1965). *Obstet. Gynec.* 26 : 308.

——— (1969). *Am. J. Obstet. Gynec.* 104 : 327.

Carter, T. C., M. F. Lyon, and R. J. S. Phillips (1955). *J. Genetics* 53 : 154.

Chang, M. C., D. M. Hunt, and E. B. Romanoff (1957). *Anat. Rec.* 129 : 211.

Edwards, R. G. (1957). *Proc. Royal Soc. B.* 146 : 469.

——— (1958) *Proc. Royal Soc. B.* 149 : 117.

Ehling, U. H., R. B. Cumming, and H. V. Malling (1968). *Mutat. Res.* 5 : 417.

Epstein, S. S. (1969). *Experientia* 25 : 617.

———, E. Arnold, and G. Bishop (1971a). In preparation.

———, E. Arnold, K. Steinberg, D. Mackintosh, H. Shafner, and Y. Bishop (1970a). *Toxicol. Appl. Pharmacol.* 17 : 230.

————, W. Bass, E. Arnold, and Y. Bishop (1970b). *Science* 168 : 584.

————, W. Bass, E. Arnold, and Y. Bishop (1970c). *Food Cosmet. Toxicol.* 8 : 381.

————, W. Bass, E. Arnold, Y. Bishop, S. Joshi, and I. D. Adler (1971b). *Toxicol. Appl. Pharmacol.*, in press.

————, S. R. Joshi, E. Arnold, E. C. Page, and Y. Bishop (1970d). *Nature* 225 : 1260.

————, and M. Legator (1971). Unpublished data.

————, and G. Röhrborn (1971). *Nature,* 230 : 459

————, and H. Shafner (1968). *Nature* 219 : 385.

Falconer, D. S., B. M. Slizynski, and C. Auerbach (1952). *J. Genetics* 51 : 81.

Ford, C. E., and H. M. Clegg (1969). *Brit. Med. Bull.* 25 : 110.

————, A. G. Searle, E. P. Evans, and B. J. West (1969). *Cytogenetics* 8 : 447.

Fox, B. W., H. Jackson, A. W. Craig, and T. D. Glover (1963). *J. Reprod. Fertil.* 5 : 13.

Generoso, W. M. (1969). *Genetics* 61 : 461.

Gruneberg, H. (1952). In Martinus Mijhoff, ed., *The Genetics of the Mouse*, The Hague.

Hertwig, P. (1940) *Z. Indukt. Abstamm. Vererb. L.* 79 : 1.

Joshi, S. R., E. C. Page, E. Arnold, Y. Bishop, and S. S. Epstein (1970). *Genetics* 65 : 483.

Koller, P. C. (1944). *Genetics* 29 : 247.

————, and C. A. Auerbach (1941). *Nature* 148 : 501.

Lavappa, K., and G. Yerganian (1970). Personal communication.

Palmer, K., M. Legator and S. Green (1971). Unpublished data.

Rauth, A. M. (1967). *Radiat. Res.* 31 : 121.

Report of the United Nations Scientific Committee on the Effects of Atomic Radiation, New York : United Nations, 1966, 99 pp.

Röhrborn, G. (1965). *Humangenetik* 1 : 576.

———— (1968), *Humangenetik* 6 : 345.

————, and F. Vogel (1969) *Humangenetik* 7 : 43.

Russell, L. B., and W. L. Russell (1954). *Cold Spring Harbor Symp. Quant. Biol.* 19 : 50.

Russell, W. L., L. B. Russell, and A. W. Kimball (1954). *Amer. Naturalist* 88 : 269

Schleiermacher, E. (1970). Personal communication.

Slizynski, B. M. (1952). *J. Genetics* 50 : 507.

Snell, G. D. (1935). *Genetics* 20 : 545.

————, E. Bodemann, and W. Hollander (1934). *J. Exp. Zool.* 67 : 93.

————, and D. I. Picken (1935). *J. Genetics* 31 : 213.

———— (1946). *Genetics* 31 : 157.

Steinberger, E. (1962). *J. Reprod. Fertil.* 3 : 250.

Witkin, E. M. (1958). *Proc. X. Int. Kongr. Genet.* 1 : 280.

Wragg, J. B., J. V. Carr, and V. Ross (1967). *J. Cell. Biol.* 35 : 146A.

14   Epidemiological Surveillance of Human Populations for Mutational Hazards

J. F. Crow

Other discussions on monitoring the human population have assumed that the environmental mutagen in question was completely unknown and probably widespread. The monitoring system, it is hoped, would discover a rise in the mutation rate, whereupon the detective work could begin and the culprit be discovered. For preliminary discussions of the ways that such a "genetic emergency" might be detected, see Neel and Bloom [1970], Sanders [1969], and Crow [1968, 1970]. The strategy would be to monitor a large sample of the population, chosen to be representative of the population at risk.

With drugs of abuse the problem is different, and, at least in one way, much simpler. The high risk population is already identifiable, at least to a large extent. In fact, the method is already in use, as evidenced by the numerous reports of association and nonassociation of LSD and chromosome breakage.

It is clear at the outset that the best time to study the mutagenic properties of a drug, or anything else, is before it is used. Many efficient test systems for screening at the source are described in previous chapters. It is equally clear that such study has rarely been done and that means are needed for discovering if, among the drugs now being used and abused, some are mutagenic. If this mutagenicity is to be discovered efficiently and promptly, before more harm is done, there must be effective ways of monitoring the human population. This is in addition to, and not a replacement for, mutagenicity tests on the drugs, using experimental organisms.

The possible methods of population monitoring that have been discussed include cytogenetic screening, monitoring for particular phenotypes whose incidence is closely correlated with the mutation rate, monitoring for changes in proteins or metabolic pathways, and looking for more general changes such as congenital anomalies, as well as systems based on detection of somatic mutations. Not all of these methods are practical, and we need to consider those which are likely to be the most promising.

1. Criteria for Selecting Monitoring Systems

A desirable monitoring system should be *relevant,* in that it is based on indicators that are strongly correlated with the human genetic damage that is feared; *prompt,* so that the increased mutation rate is discovered before further harm is done; *sensitive,* so that a small or moderate change in the mutation rate can can be detected; *broad* enough so that all of the kinds of genetic damage that are anticipated—from single nucleotide changes to gross aneuploidy—can be found; *organized* so that the cause of the increased genetic damage can be identified; and *economically feasible* and *available soon.*

It is clear that any system based on detecting germinal changes will have to be carried out on an enormous scale if it is to be sensitive to small percentage increases in rare events. This should prompt us to look for somatic cell indicators where the individual cell, rather than the person, is the unit of observation. This could increase the sensitivity of the test by several orders of magnitude.

2. Cytogenetic Screening

This subject is discussed in considerable detail in Chapter 11, and I shall make only a few remarks here.

We badly need, I think, better ways of identifying in somatic cells those kinds of chromosomal events that indicate transmissible genetic damage. Chromosome breaks often restitute on the one hand, or lead to cell death on the other. In either event, there is no damage to descendant cells, either because they are normal or because there are not any left. The kinds of change that lead to abnormality and disease in the next generation need to be identified. To some extent these changes are already known. Structural rearrangements, such as translocations, can lead to partial sterility and abnormalities that persist for several generations. Errors in chromosome distribution can also lead to congenital anomalies if they lead to the transmission of aneuploid gametes.

One possibility is to concentrate specifically on chromosome breaks of particular kinds, such as the characteristic figure X that is produced by a reciprocal translocation. Such a configuration is very conspicuous, and it might be possible to get more relevant information by searching many cells for highly diagnostic configurations than by a more careful study of a smaller number of cells. This would appear to be an area where automation and computerization could increase the feasibility. This assumes, reasonably I think, a high correlation between somatic and germinal effects.

A high research priority should, I think, go to a systematic study of the correlation among particular kinds of cytological configurations in somatic cells of the parents and genetic damage in the descendants. This can be done very effectively in mice, where leukocytes can be examined in the parents and the progeny could be scored for dominant lethal mutations or other kinds of evidence of genetic change. The dominant lethal study is relatively cheap and a number of mutagens could be tested this way, as a test of the reproducibility of the correlation (Chapter 13). The specific locus mutation test is also available in mice for correlation with somatic cytogenetic changes, although this test is much more expensive and time-consuming.

3. Somatic Mutation-Detecting Systems

There are now several systems that use animal or human cells and where biochemical mutants have been studied. According to Krooth [1968], over 25 biochemical mutants are known in human cell lines. For three of the mutants there are selective media that permit the growth of normal, but not mutant, cells, so reverse mutation studies are feasible. What is needed is the adaptation of such methods to *in vivo* tests for somatic point mutations, to complement those now possible for cytogenetic changes.

Although, as far as I know, there are no tested methods of measuring mutation rates in somatic cells *in vivo*, they would not appear to be beyond present techniques. For mutation monitoring they are badly needed.

Early work foreshadowing this possibility was done by Atwood with human red blood cell antigens. There are numerous other possibilities using selective growth media, selective killing by antibiotics, and cell strains specific for particular enzymes. It should be possible to find systems that detect both forward and reverse mutations. I suggest that one of the most important kinds of research, if not the most important, is the finding of such systems and refining them for large-scale testing.

4. Screening for Genetic Changes in Children of Drug-Exposed Parents

Various indicators have been suggested for identifying an overall increase in human mutation rate—an increase in specific traits, such as achondroplasia, that are known to be caused by dominant mutants, an increase in novel types of proteins such as hemoglobin detected by chemical procedures, and possibly such doubtful indicators as changes in the sex ratio. None of these seems appropriate for drug studies. They all require monitoring an enormous number of persons, more than are likely to be available.

On the other hand, the possibility of using less direct evidence for genetic change should not be overlooked. Newborn infants of drug-using parents could possibly provide evidence, particularly if there were a very large increase in the mutation rate—the situation most to be feared.

Perhaps the best procedure would be the straightforward one: an examination of each newborn infant of drug-using parents for any signs of congenital defect. At the same time, cord blood is readily available, and a cytogenetic examination could be included. The data could be compared with a control group, or with standard risk data for the same age, income, racial, and economic group. I realize that such data are "dirty." The criteria for different phenotypes are not uniform, the acuity of the observer is a factor, hospital and birth clinic standards vary, and so on. Moreover, if a change is detected, it is not necessarily caused by mutation; it may be caused by a prenatal teratogen. But, on the other hand, we are just as interested in discovering teratogenic effects of drugs as mutagenic effects. Furthermore, even heterogeneous data may be sensitive to a change in the trend.

A large program to examine newborn children for congenital anomalies may not be worth the expenditure if the sole purpose is to detect mutations, but combined with a similar program for detection of teratogens, it may well be economically feasible. The cost of caring for one child with severe mental retardation can be enormous, and the saving from preventing only a small number may pay off even in the crassest economic terms, humanitarian considerations aside.

To the extent that the thalidomide incident can serve as a guide, the discovery of any phenotype that was previously rare or absent is a danger signal, not so much for mutation as for teratogenesis. If the normal incidence is zero, even one case is statistically significant! Much more likely, especially if mutation is the cause, is an increase in types that already exist and where a much larger number is needed for statistical validity.

One advantage of a nonspecific search for deviant phenotypes, an advantage of all such dirty systems, is that the system is responsive to several different kinds of causes, including those that are unknown or unforeseen. A sophisticated system of protein analysis depending on the discovery of amino acid substitutions would probably fail to detect a change in chromosome rearrangements. The cruder system would be sensitive to changes of all kinds, including nongenetic changes; of course, if suffers not only from lack of resolving power but from ambiguity of interpretation if a trend is found.

In addition to prospective studies such as I have just been discussing, there is also a chance of getting useful information from retrospective studies. Retrospective research has obvious pitfalls, and many that are not so obvious. There are considerations of reliability of response to questions and invasion of privacy in studies of a socially sensitive area such as drug abuse. Despite all this, I think it could still be of value to examine the history of children with congenital anomalies and mental retardation. The sample could be considerably enriched from the standpoint of detecting possible drug effects by choosing children whose parents belong to age groups, economic and education classes, races, and cultural groups where drug usage is greatest.

There is the additional possibility of trying to measure effects caused by the cumulative effects of several minor mutant genes. I do not know how promising this method is, but perhaps it deserves a try. We could try to identify those phenotypes that are particularly sensitive to small insults, whether these are genetic or environmental.

Among the various body measurements that might be used, Lederberg has suggested that minor asymmetries between right and left sides might be sensitive indicators of the kind of developmental imbalance that could be caused by mutation. He suggests that dermatoglyphics might be particularly easy to quantify for such use.

It is abundantly clear from such diverse lines of evidence as cytogenetic anomalies, children of consanguineous parents, and twins in comparison to singletons, to say nothing of a host of environmental studies, that a lowered intelligence score is a particularly sensitive indicator that something has gone wrong. Perhaps it could be used in monitoring. Downward deviations from the IQ expected for this group might be a useful signal that something is happening, though it is not likely to give any hint as to what it is that is wrong.

5. Indirect Monitoring, using Laboratory Test Systems

Assuming that there is extensive testing of drugs in microbial, mouse, and cell culture systems, there is still the possibility that drug effects in man are different because of the way the drug is metabolized, or because people who use drugs have other habits that lead to mutagenesis.

Another monitoring system that might perhaps offer promise is to see if the blood serum of drug users contains substances that are mutagenic in other test systems. If a highly efficient microbial test system is used, it may be discovered that there are mutagenic influences not explained by the drug itself. Such influences might be detected in this way, even if their concentration were so low that any direct test on the person or his descendants would not be powerful enough to detect the effect. This may be a promising second line of defense, between screening of chemicals at the source and human monitoring, that permits the detection of effects, such as synergistic interactions, that might not be otherwise foreseen.

6. Summary and Recommendations

The best time to determine whether a drug produces genetic damage is before it comes into general use. However, since a number of drugs are already in use, it is necessary to study the effects that they are actually having in addition to the laboratory screening methods discussed elsewhere in this chapter.

Since there is only one zygote per individual compared with the enormous number of somatic cells, it follows that systems based on somatic cells are enormously more efficient in detecting genetic changes. Somatic cyto-genetic studies are now being done, but we need better criteria for distinguishing those types of aberrations that are correlated with genetic damage that is transmitted to future generations. Effective means for detecting somatic gene mutations in man are not now ready for use, but such methods do not appear to be beyond present technology.

Tests for geminal mutations are much more difficult, because of the numbers needed to demonstrate an increased mutation rate even in the most favorable conditions. However, it might be feasible to search for phenotypic abnormalities in the newborn children of parents who had been exposed to drugs. If combined with a search for teratogenic effects, this might be more feasible economically. It is not likely that the results would be easily interpretable, but it is important to detect an increase whether the drug is acting as a mutagen or teratogen.

References

Crow, J. F. (1968). *Scientist and Citizen* 10:113.

Crow, J. F. (1971). In A. Hollaender, ed., *Environmental Chemical Mutagens*, New York: Plenum Press.

Krooth, R. S. (1968). *Somatic Cell Genetics*, Symposium on Human Cytogenetics. Tallahassee: University of Tennessee, pp. 21–26.

Neel, J. V., and A. D. Bloom (1969). The detection of environmental mutagens. *Med. Clin. North Amer.* 53:1243–1250.

Sanders, H. J. (1969). *Chem. Eng. News* 47:51 (May 19) and 54 (June 2).

15 Mutations in Human Populations—Estimation of Mutation Rates

K. C. Atwood III

This chapter reviews the methods employed at the population level for the estimation of human mutation rates, and examines the question whether any of these can be adapted to monitor changes in mutation frequency that may be brought about by such environmental factors as drug abuse. Any useful means of recognizing environmentally induced genetic effects in populations would be subject to two constraints that do not apply to ordinary mutation studies: first, the method must be capable of detecting changes in mutation frequency within a reasonable time of their inception; second, the method must be feasible in limited subpopulations of special interest from the standpoint of environmental risk.

When available methods are measured against these requirements it will be seen that, with the possible exception of one new and untried method, none of the current approaches to the study of mutation in human populations can be turned to practical use for the purpose of genetic surveillance. The first three methods to be mentioned do not estimate the present mutation rate, but rather the rate prevailing in past generations, while the fourth method requires a population so large that the gathering of reliable information on the degree of exposure to a specific agent—particularly an illegal one—seems impracticable. These procedures and results are relevant, however, from the heuristic standpoint, and because they are instructive in regard to the nature of the problem posed by the introduction of mutagens to the environment: its seriousness as a menace to public health, and the deceptively delayed onset of its consequences.

1. Regression of Sex Ratio on Age Difference of Mother and Maternal Grandfather (Method 1)

The presence of carriers of sex-linked recessive lethal mutations among the mothers of any given generation accounts, in part, for the difference between the primary and secondary sex ratios in the progeny; that is, for some of the males lost during development. The age difference between mother and maternal grandfather represents the time during which lethal mutations in the male germ line may accumulate before being transmitted to a carrier. The greater this age difference, the greater is the probability that the given female carries a lethal mutation. Therefore, the secondary sex ratio is expected to decline with increasing age difference between mothers and maternal grandfathers. With sufficient data, this effect can be isolated from other factors such as birth order and paternal age that have been correlated with the sex ratio in some populations.

The method, introduced by Cavalli-Sforza [1961], estimates the sum of the mutation rates of all sex-linked recessive lethals that act during antenatal development. A modification given by Krehbiel [1966] uses the sex ratio in spontaneous abortions, which *increases* with the mother-grandfather age difference. Results with both of these approaches indicate that sex-linked recessive lethal mutations arising spontaneously in the male germ line are being added to the human population at the rate of about 2.5 per thousand X chromosomes per generation. If we assume a per locus mutation rate consistent with other evidence, say 10^{-5} per generation, it would suggest that about 250 of the genes on the human X chromosome are capable of mutating to recessive lethal alleles. Since the total genome is about twenty times larger than the X chromosome, the further assumption that the genetic content of most chromosomes is roughly proportional to their size leads to the speculation that the total number of genes capable of mutating to recessive lethals in man is of the order of 5,000, and the expected overall

recessive lethal mutation rate per gamete is around 5 per cent.

2. Deleterious Effects of Inbreeding (Method 2)

In a randomly mating population each homozygote frequency would be the square of the corresponding gene frequency, but inbreeding increases the frequency of homozygosis by a factor that can be calculated for each type of consanguineous mating. Therefore, the incidence of anomalies, defects, and mortality as a function of the degree of consanguinity may provide an estimate of the frequency of recessive deleterious genes in the population. By means of a reduction of such data to lethal equivalents per gamete, Morton, Crow, and Muller [1956] estimated the mutation rate per gamete required to equal the observed rate of elimination of deleterious and lethal recessives; it ranged from 6 to 15 per cent. These estimates were based on limited available data, and other investigators have found somewhat smaller effects of consanguinity in different populations [Neel 1962].

Differences are to be expected because the outcome of consanguineous matings at a given epoch depends not only on the overall gene frequencies, but also on the previous history of inbreeding patterns tending to produce a more or less nonuniform distribution of gene frequencies in different segments of the population. Perhaps the most that can be said is that the reported effects of inbreeding do not run contrary to expectations based on reasonable assumptions concerning the mutation rate per locus and the number of loci involved.

3. Inference from the Relative Fertility of Specific Phenotypes (Method 3)

Haldane [1935] estimated the mutation frequency for hemophilia (about 2×10^{-5}, now known to comprise two loci) on the reasonable assumption that the genes arising by mutation are in equilibrium with those eliminated because of the low relative fertility of affected males. In principle, specific locus mutation rates are given by $m = (1 - f)q/2$ for autosomal dominants, $m = (1 - f)q/3$ for sex-linked recessives, and $m = (1 - f)$ $\times [Fq + (1 - F)q^2]$ for autosomal recessives, where f is the relative fertility of affected persons, F is the inbreeding coefficient, and q is the mutant gene frequency. In practice, it is often uncertain what degree of confidence should be attached to estimates of f and F. Departures from equilibrium must have resulted from recent changes in F, but it is not feasible to reconstruct these events accurately enough to apply a correction. Finally, selection for or against heterozygotes, even if sufficient to have a much greater effect on the gene frequency than mutation, would in most cases be undetectable.

In view of these limitations, the method is of interest only because none other is available for specific recessives in which the heterozygotes cannot be efficiently detected. Some of the ostensible mutation rates obtained in this way are probably correct, but we cannot be certain which ones they are. Unusually high rates, e.g. 10^{-3} for cystic fibrosis of the pancreas, are best interpreted as balanced polymorphisms maintained by heterozygote advantage, as has been proved for sickle cell anemia and glucose-6-phosphate dehydrogenase deficiency. Examples [Lenz 1963] of mutation rates for autosomal recessives are infantile amaurotic idiocy, 10^{-5}; ichthyosis congenita, 10^{-5}; albinism, 3×10^{-5}; epidermolysis bullosa, 5×10^{-5}. Afflictions that are lethal in childhood, such as ichthyosis congenita and amaurotic idiocy, at least present no problem of estimating the value of f.

4. Direct Ascertainment of New Dominant Mutants (Method 4)

This method makes use of distinctive phenotypes known from pedigrees to be inherited as simple dominants. It consists in exhaustive enumeration of the population under study and of the affected persons. Familial cases are identified and excluded; isolated cases represent the new mutations. The estimate of mutation rate per gene per generation is one half the relative frequency of isolated cases. Some mutation rates obtained in this manner are shown in Table 1.

In contrast to the previous methods with inherent delays of two or more generations, this method has at least the potential of detecting increased mutant frequency in the immediate progeny of persons exposed to mutagens. Sources of error (discussed in detail by Neel [1962]) can be classified according to whether they would interfere with the early detection of induced mutations. Uncertainty concerning the number of loci that can mutate to the dominant phenotype is no hindrance, since it is not necessary that the mutation rate per locus be known; indeed, the sensitivity of the method would increase with the number of participating loci. On the other hand, misleading results would be obtained if recessive genes or nongenetic causes contributed significantly to the number of affected persons, for in that case the induced incidence of the phenotype would be diluted by an irrelevant background incidence which, in turn, might differ in the control and exposed populations because of genetic and environmental factors other than those under study. Phenotypes with late onset, such as Huntington's chorea, polycystic kidney, and intestinal polyposis, could not be used.

Human mutation studies are probably somewhat biased toward a disproportionate representation of loci with exceptionally high

Table 1. Estimate of the Rate of Appearance of Certain Mutant Phenotypes Based on the Direct Method (Method 4).

Trait	Locale	Author	Mutant phenotypes per 10^5
Epiloia	England	Gunter and Penrose 1935 Penrose 1936	0.8–1.6
Retinoblastoma	England U.S.A., Michigan U.S.A., Ohio Germany Switzerland Japan	Philip and Sorsby 1944 Neel and Falls 1951 Macklin 1959, 1960 Vogel 1954 Bohringer 1956 Matsunaga and Ogyu 1959	2.4 4.6 3.6 3.4 4.2 4.2
Aniridia	Denmark U.S.A., Michigan	Mollenbach 1947 Shaw, Falls, and Neel 1960	1.0 1.0
Achondroplasia	Denmark North Ireland Sweden Japan	March 1941 Stevenson 1957 Book 1952 Neel, Schull, and Takeshima 1959	8.4 28.6 14.0 24.5
Partial albinism with deafness	Holland	Waardenburg 1951	.7
Pelger's nuclear anomaly	Germany Japan	Nachtsheim 1954 Handa 1959	5.4 3.4
Neurofibromatosis	U.S.A., Michigan	Crowe, Schull, and Neel 1956	26.0–50.0
Microphthalmos-anophthalmos without mental defect	Sweden	Sjogren and Larsson 1949	1.0
Huntington's chorea	U.S.A., Michigan	Reed and Neel 1959	1.0

Source: From J. V. Neel (1962), in W. J. Burdette, ed., *Methodology in Human Genetics*, San Francisco: Holden-Day. Reprinted with permission of the publisher. Details of references cited in Neel.

spontaneous rates. Experience with animal, plant, and microbial systems indicates that loci with high spontaneous rates are often quite ordinary in their response to mutagenic agents; hence the use of relatively frequent phenotypes, such as achondroplasia or neurofibromatosis, would not necessarily ensure a gain in sensitivity; it might even be misleading. Finally, the various difficulties involved in ascertainment become more serious in subpopulations that are, of necessity, chosen without regard for the convenience of the investigator.

The most serious limitation, however, is the low frequency of occurrence of the specific phenotypes that can be used. Even with the assumption that phenotypes of high incidence would provide a trustworthy measure of induced mutation, the incidence is not high enough for a reasonable expectation of success. Suppose, for instance, that we would be satisfied with being able to detect a doubling of the mutation rate by means of a five-year study. By combining the usable phenotypes one might expect to observe an overall spontaneous rate of perhaps 3×10^{-4}. For an observed doubling of this rate to be significant at the 5 percent level, the size of the exposed population would have to be such as to yield about 30 affected individuals during the five-year period; that is, about 5×10^4 births with the doubled mutation rate. At the crude birth rate of about 25 per thousand per year, the parent population would have to comprise some 4×10^5 persons. Despite a more favorable age distribution than that of the general population, the birth rate in the drug subculture is probably lower than the crude rate. It appears that a rather insensitive test with this method would require a formidable—perhaps impossible—effort in order to engage a sufficient number of persons who would both reproduce and provide reliable histories of significant drug use.

5. The Pseudohemizygote Frequency (Method 5)

It has long been recognized that heterozygotes for X-linked recessives occasionally manifest the recessive character. These exceptions, previously explained as "variable dominance," are now commonly ascribed to chance variation in the proportion of cells in which a given X homologue is active. A different interpretation emerges, however, if we consider the consequences of the Lyon phenomenon of X chromosome inactivation in the presence of a cell lethal mutation on one of the X chromosomes. Clearly, the only viable cells would be those in which the active X chromosome carried the normal allele of the cell lethal. If the same X chromosome happened to carry the recessive allele of a heterozygous marker, the individual would manifest the recessive character. Such cases will be called *pseudohemizygotes*.

The combined mutation rate of all X-linked loci that mutate to cell lethals, or to alleles that confer a very strong selective disadvantage at the cell level, can be estimated from the pseudohemizygote frequency if three assumptions are correct: first, X-linked cell lethals survive despite random inactivation of the X chromosomes; second, the numbers of founder cells for most tissues are large enough so that chance variations in the proportion of cells in which a given X homologue is active cannot account for a significant fraction of the pseudohemizygotes; third, somatic crossing over is negligible. Although these assumptions are not conclusively proved, they are consistent with many different lines of evidence, to be presented elsewhere.

The foregoing combined mutation rate per X chromosome in males could be obtained by means of a marker gene for which the recessive allele has a reasonably high frequency, Xg^a, for instance. The estimate is then $m = n/Ng$, where n is the number of — females with + fathers, i.e., pseudohemizygotes; N is the total number of females with $+$ fathers, and q is the gene frequency of the $-$ allele.

The pseudohemizygote frequency obtained by means of ascertainment of affected females with normal fathers appears—although data are still insufficient—to be well in excess of 10^{-3}, suggesting that a large number of loci are involved, and that this method may turn out to be sensitive enough for induced mutation studies.

6. Summary

Established methods utilizing human population data are entirely unsuited to rapid, sensitive testing for mutagenic effects. They have shown, however, that the human genome already sustains sufficient spontaneous mutational injury so that at least several percent of human zygotes per generation are eliminated. These represent the aggregate of some very large number of different kinds of genetic defects. It is likely that other, less severe, defects are even more frequent. These are important considerations in judging the potential hazard of further increase in mutation frequency that could be brought about by exposure to mutagenic agents.

References

Cavalli-Sforza, L. L. (1961). *Atti Ass. Genetica Ital.* 6:151.

———, (1962). In *Seminar on Vital and Health Statistics for Genetic and Radiation Studies*, New York: United Nations World Health Organization, 221 pp.

Haldane, J. B. S. (1935). *J. Genetics* 31 : 317.

Krehbiel, E. L. (1966). *Amer. J. Human Genetics* 18 : 127.

Lenz, W. (1963). *Medical Genetics*, Chicago: University of Chicago Press.

Morton, N. E., J. F. Crow and H. J. Muller (1956). *Proc. Nat. Acad. Sci.* 42 : 855.

Neel, J. V. (1962). In W. J. Burdette, ed., *Methodology in Human Genetics*, San Francisco: Holden-Day, pp. 203–224.

Appendixes

A. Psychiatric Perspectives on Drugs of Abuse

H. Brill and J. Willis

Psychiatry plays a central role in drug abuse.[1] For the drug taker the subjective experience is basically what drug abuse or addiction is all about, and for society the induced psychiatric aberrations and their behavioral consequences constitute a problem of national and international dimensions. However, the operation of psychic factors in drug dependence is not limited to the subjective experiences of the drug user or to his behavioral aberrations. Psychic contagions accounts for the spread of the problem. Psychiatric disorders are either mimicked, initiated, or precipitated by the abuse of drugs, and psychiatric considerations govern the propensity to relapse long after the demonstrable somatic elements have disappeared.

Finally, the process of recovery is never completely independent of psychotherapeutic considerations and is often entirely dependent on them. This is not to minimize the role of somatic factors in drug dependence; it must be assumed that they underlie all psychic level events. The somatic effects set in motion by these drugs undoubtedly appear first in the temporal sequence, but an unbridged gap still lies between them and the observed psychic responses. For the present the two responses can be described only as irregularly parallel, the mechanism by which somatic events are translated into psychic experience being unknown. As a result, it is possible to describe either response independently of the other, but a complete picture of the present state of knowledge in this field requires some consideration of both aspects.

With these facts in mind, it will be our purpose to present here in general terms a brief account of the psychiatric aspects of drug dependence and abuse which might seem appropriate as background for this

[1] The W.H.O. term *drug dependence* includes drug addiction and drug abuse. It is further subdivided by drug type, i.e., drug dependence of the opiate type, the alcohol-barbiturate type, cannabis type, etc.

monograph, which centers on the non-psychiatric hazards of drug abuse. We shall include some specific data for illustrative purposes, but for a more complete account of the technical side of this problem we refer the reader to various standard works in the field [Nyswander 1956; Connell 1958; Chopra and Chopra 1965; Kalant 1966; Freedman and Kaplan 1967; Hollister 1968].

1. A Philosophical Note

In a review of this type it is difficult to avoid becoming entangled with questions about the relation of psyche to soma—classical problems that have produced much fine philosophy but no rigorous scientific answers as yet. The dilemma of mind-body relations is not limited to drug dependence; it pervades all of psychiatry. For the most part these are academic issues because most psychiatric phenomena occur in the absence of demonstrable specific somatic correlates. The issue is much more difficult to avoid in the case of mental disorder associated with demonstrable organic lesions, although even here one finds a striking lack of correlation between the apparent extent of organic damage and the amount of mental disturbance. Severe organic psychoses are associated with almost trivial demonstrable organic change, while relatively extensive damage appears to be compatible with only minor psychic disturbances.

In the case of drug dependence the mind-body issue is particularly hard to avoid because only here among all the organic conditions the agent is known, quantifiable, and subject to chemical manipulation of chemical structure and investigation in vitro and in vivo. In addition, many psychic level experiences are relatively specific for a given drug and are dose related if not fully dose dependent. Thus, in drug dependence psychiatry deals with the most clear-cut of somatic factors on the one hand and the most abstract of mental phenomena on the other. The gap which separates our understanding of events between somatic and psychic levels seems narrowed, perhaps to a tantalizing degree, but a gap still remains. One can only choose from several alternative formulations as to the nature of the relationship between the two series; these formulations are neither new nor derived from rigorous scientific data. We may accept some variant of the hierarchical monism of Aristotle and Aquinas [Jaspers 1963], which assumes a unity of mind and body; or we may select the dualism of Descartes, which sees events in the two spheres as incommensurate; or finally we may accept some form of existentialism which gives primacy to the psychic events. No matter which way we turn, we still cannot escape the fact that in the last analysis a dilemma of a philosophical nature underlies all interpretations of data from this field.

This chapter, because it is confined to the psychic aspects of drug dependence, may easily give the impression that a primacy of the psychic events is assumed; this is particularly true when only the psychic aspects of such demonstrably somatic syndromes as those of drug withdrawal are described. The authors wish to emphasize that any such impression is a result of the nature of our assignment and not an expression of a covert vitalism or even an undercurrent of existentialism; it is merely a recognition of the fact that a gap still divides our knowledge of somatic aspects from the psychic, and that our task lies on the psychic side. The two sets of events remain only essentially parallel and not translatable into each other at this time, although it is to be hoped that the results of future investigations will change this situation. Such progress will inevitably cast important light on mental illness generally. Indeed it is this hope that has led psychiatrists to be involved with studies of drug dependence almost since psychiatry emerged as a medical speciality.

2. Some Definitions

The subject of drug dependence generally has become so emotionally charged that the terms of discussion must be carefully defined if one is to avoid problems of communication and even complete misunderstanding. For example "drug abuse" has been generally defined as any improper use of drugs, more particularly improper use outside of medical practice. This would include drug suicides or attempted suicides as well as overmedication, especially chronic overmedication, with almost any pharmaceutical agent. While these forms of drug abuse are all of obvious medical importance, they are not the forms which have led to the current public concern about drugs; and many of these forms are not at all new.

Man has always been a drug-taking animal, and his excesses in the name of therapy have long been the subject of satire and condemnation in plays, essays, and cartoons. This therapeutic problem, still the subject of vigorous discussion [Mintz 1965; Johnson 1967] and posing an important public health issue, is clearly distinct from the problem of "street" or social drug dependence, which is the real focus of current concern. This problem has taken on massive proportions within the last few years. It has spread rapidly and the population involved is young, often immature, and predominantly male. These individuals take drugs for hedonic and social purposes, and their habit, which spreads by psychic contagion, has reached within less than a decade many hundreds of thousands of young persons in the pursuit of pleasure through drugs. This problem is clearly different from that of medical abuse, even though many of the same drugs are used. The medical cases are middle-aged and older, they are predominantly women, and

most of all they do not behave in such a way as to transmit their habit to others, nor do they interfere with the general public in any significant fashion. Theirs is essentially a personal problem, and a problem for their immediate families.

Both the medical and nonmedical forms of drug dependence have important psychiatric aspects, but they are essentially different [Brill 1966; Bejerot 1969]. This discussion will be confined to the psychiatry of the non-medical type, which in its present manifestations and extent represents a new problem of contagion in our society.

3. Psychic Contagion in the Spread of Drug Dependence

The epidemiology of drug dependence is the subject of another chapter in this volume, but a brief comment on the element of psychic contagion appears warranted here to illustrate the operation of this factor in historical perspective. The term *epidemic* is only now being generally applied to episodes of spread of drug dependence, but the phenomenon itself is probably quite old. It can be assumed that psychic contagion accounted for the rapid proliferation of opium addiction in China [Livingston 1958] from about the seventeenth century onward; and such contagion led to the transitory ether-sniffing vogue among American students in the early 1800s, as well as to the more serious outbreak of ether drinking in Ireland in the latter part of the nineteenth century. A most convincing example of epidemic spread was the ten-year methamphetamine epidemic which swept Japan at the close of World War II [Brill 1969], producing an estimated 2,000,000 abusers and 300,000 addicts.

The present situation in the United States cannot be viewed in isolation from events elsewhere in the world and is undoubtedly related through psychosocial mechanisms to the recent spread of stimulant abuse in

Sweden [Sjoquist and Tottie 1969], and to the less extensive but well-studied simultaneous drug episodes in Britain [Glatt 1967; de Alarcon 1969]. The course of events in the United States has been reasonably well defined, and it is clearly related to other events on the social scene. The current situation began in the early 1960s, apparently in connection with an academic interest in psylocibin and mescaline. Interest then rapidly shifted to LSD–25, which caught the fancy of a considerable number of young intellectuals; and finally marijuana, long a ghetto drug, suddenly emerged on the national scene and far outstripped all other substances of abuse. Within the space of about five years marijuana has become the most widely used illicit drug in the country and has been adopted by students and young liberals alike as a symbol and a basis for confrontation with the establishment.

4. Psychiatric Factors in the Predisposition to Drug Dependence

As Willis [1969] has pointed out,

The majority of psychiatric evidence supports the view that addiction to narcotics, heroin particularly, is usually associated with major personality disorders. For instance, large-scale surveys of addicts such as those carried out by Hill et al. [1962] provide convincing evidence in support of this general statement. This was a study carried out on three groups of institutionalized narcotic addicts, alcoholics and criminals—each group containing 200 subjects. Using the Minnesota Multiphasic Personality Inventory (MMPI) ... the scores obtained could be shown to demonstrate the presence of ... personality configurations of an abnormal sort. The predominant finding in this and similar studies is the elevation of the psychopathic deviate scale in the MMPI.
Clinical psychiatric evidence linking psychopathy with addiction is also well documented. But the relationship between personality disorder and addiction, however, is not a simple one. The very diagnosis of personality disorder can too easily become a process of labelling in which pejorative epithets are applied to patients and may reveal the observer's prejudices as well as his psychiatric orientation... . It is a factor which should

not be ignored. It is all too easy to label as "psychopathic" someone whose behavioral standards offend against one's own. A further problem is ... that the majority of addicts who have been studied have been studied after their addiction has been established so that it may be thought hard strictly to exclude the effects of the drug on their personality. However, there have been studies ... on addicts or rather ex-addicts in prison after a period of abstinence of sufficient length to exclude any drug effect. Also, there is no experimental evidence to back up the idea that drugs such as opiates alter personality. [Thus] ... there is no evidence that any of the personality disorders in drug addiction can be attributed to changes in personality caused by the drug.

A very contrary point of view is maintained by some observers, for example as Willis [1969] points out:

Lindesmith [1947] postulates a theory of addiction which does not acknowledge the role of personality disorder. His theory is that addiction is developed and maintained by the development of withdrawal distress—providing that the user is fully aware of its significance. He takes the view that addiction may just as easily develop in "normal" personalities provided they take the drug for long enough. In this way an individual who identifies himself as an addict accepts the idea that he is one and that he needs to take opiates to prevent withdrawal distress ...

Willis [1969] however concludes that

The bulk of personality studies confirm the general statement that heroin addiction is most likely to occur in highly deviant individuals whose abnormalities are manifest in persistent antisocial or asocial acts or attitudes; people with severe disorders of emotional development, such as immaturity and hypersensitivity. They are likely too to be passive individuals with major defects in their abilities to sustain stable interpersonal relationships. These are handicaps and deficiencies of which they are often only too painfully aware.

These principles are usually considered to apply to drug-dependent youth generally, and thus psychiatric findings appear to constitute an element of predisposition to drug dependence. Although studies on this question are necessarily retrospective there is good agreement that the predisposed individuals are predominantly young males who suffer from character disorder which often has already manifested itself in truancy and delinquency and other asocial or antisocial behavior which preceded the drug dependence.

5. Psychic Experience as a Reinforcer

The addicted are in part driven by demonstrable physical needs, as manifest in withdrawal phenomena, which are reproducible in animals. However, withdrawal hunger alone falls far short of a complete explanation of the drug-seeking compulsion which is the hallmark of drug dependence. Withdrawal hunger fails to explain why addicts tend to relapse years after complete withdrawal; for the most part addicts must resist a life-long drive to return to drugs. Furthermore, physical dependence seems either lacking or minimal in drugs of dependence other than the opiates and the alcohol-barbiturate group. Yet, stimulants such as cocaine are powerful dependence producers in animals as well as man, an effect subsumed under the term *reinforcement potential.*

From the point of view of the drug-dependent person, the subjective effects constitute the primary motive for drug taking. These subjective effects are obviously a reflection of somatic events which however remain unidentified, and as a result this important aspect of the problem can be studied on a descriptive level only, although much of it can be reduced to objective terms by double blind techniques. The drug-dependent person can identify the reinforcing quality in the drug experience far more easily than he can describe it, especially to the naive and uninitiated. This is not surprising since it is also true of other subjective experiences; pain and pleasure are real enough, but they are not understood by words alone.

Some understanding of the subjective aspects of drug dependence can be gained from the accounts of such writers as DeQuincey [1822 (1932)], Baudelaire [1860 (1964)], and Huxley [1954] to mention but a few. These must, of course, be read with the reservation that the drug experience is dependent in part on the innate capacity of the person as well as the drug itself. Baudelaire long ago emphasized that one must have poetically imaginative capacity to have poetically imaginative experiences, and that a pedestrian imagination produces only pedestrian experiences.

The psychiatry of drugs of dependence is largely concerned with the negative or adverse psychic reactions or, more poetically, the pains of drug dependence. In addition, psychiatry has an interest in all of the experiences produced by these substances, because the study of their acute effects is an approach to the pharmacology of pleasure, pain, and motivation. Besides their powerful motivational effects, many of these drugs are powerful analgesics capable of alleviating physical as well as psychological pain, while the hallucinogen LSD has been shown to relieve the anxiety of patients with intractable pain, leaving them comfortable even though the somatic pain itself appears to continue unabated [Kast and Collins 1964].

The motivation-producing power of these drugs is so great as to reach the level of an artifically induced compulsion. Intense drug-seeking behavior can be demonstrated in animal experiments with opiates, sedatives, and stimulants, although it has not as yet been done with hallucinogens. Reinforcement is strongest when a drug is taken intravenously; in man the experience is then described as a *rush* or a *bang* and likened to a sexual orgasm.

The traditional classification of drugs of dependence is pharmacological—sedatives, stimulants, hallucinogens, opiates, and others—but this classification can be misleading because it leaves the impression that the effect sought is simply pharmacological—

sedation, stimulation—or hallucinogenic. However, something more is obviously involved since not all drugs which produce such effects are abused. Atropine, for example, produces hallucinations, but it is a deterrent rather than an attractive drug. Stramonium also produces hallucinations, but it is rarely used for this purpose more than once or twice. Ephedrine is a stimulant, but is not favored for abuse. Finally, bromides, which are powerful sedatives if used in sufficient dose and which have been abused medically, are not taken for pleasure and do not produce abuse of the contagious type.

A further indication of the incompleteness of a purely pharmacological classification of drugs of dependence is that drugs of opposing pharmacological action are regularly taken in combination; sedatives, in particular, are combined with the stimulants, apparently to cancel out excessive sedation and stimulation and to leave an experience which is preferred to either alone. Cocaine, for example, is mixed with heroin, and amphetamines with barbiturates. Especially in the case of the hallucinogens, the classical pharmacological action is not the one usually sought, and the user often attempts to hold the dose below the level of hallucinations in order to experience only the rest of the drug effect, which is described as essentially one of euphoria [Solomon 1966]. Finally, individual drugs appear to have mixed actions; for example the toluene-containing glues are described as being hallucinogens for about 50 percent of the exposed population and simple euphoric anesthetics for the rest. There is no indication that the degree of dependence is related to the occurrence or lack of occurrence of hallucinatory experiences [Press and Done 1967a, b].

In general the acute drug effects may be divided into those which are dose dependent and those which are not. The dose-dependent group are relatively simple and predictable and include progressive sedation to the point of narcosis or progressive stimulation to mania and the hallucinogen effects which progress to active acute psychotic episodes; but the nondose-dependent effects partake of the qualities of pathological intoxication and are quite unpredictable, although these effects as well as the dose-related ones are subject to modification by a very large number of "psychic" factors.

6. Acute Psychiatric Reactions

Among the acute psychiatric complications, the best known are the so-called "bad trips" with hallucinogens, conduct disorders and paranoid reactions with stimulants, and states of pathological intoxication with the barbiturate-alcohol group, all of which may result in suicidal or aggressive acts. However, the adverse reactions associated with virtually all drugs of dependence have been known to mimic a variety of psychiatric disorders. Usually these are of a transitory nature, but in some cases they become protracted and develop into subacute or chronic forms, similar to those not associated with drugs. While the "bad trip" and acute reactions are highly variable, a certain degree of specificity does attach to reactions with individual drugs. These include the visual and combined hallucinations of cannabis and LSD, the delerioid barbiturate reactions, and the aggressive behavior with stimulant drugs, which have also been reported as producing paranoid hallucinatory reactions after brief exposure, although such reactions are more typical of chronic abuse.

As mentioned above, there is room for academic debate as to whether the drugs actually produce the nondose-dependent pathological mental states, or whether they merely release a pre-existing pattern. It is also possible to reason that the drugs create a new balance of mental forces, by diminishing or reinforcing various components of the mental life, and this imbalance creates a new and disordered outcome which is neither a simple release of a previously performed pattern nor yet the creation of a new psychiatric illness. Regardless of the explanation, the fact is that for various drugs of dependence, outbreaks of mental disorder have been recorded with sufficient regularity to indicate that such episodes constitute a hazard for some of those exposed to drugs.

7. Subacute Psychiatric Reactions

The most consistent subacute effect in drug dependence of all types is the induced compulsive drug taking which can replace other drives; in well-marked cases of drug dependence, this condition can become the overriding motivation of the individual's life. As already mentioned, this can be attributed only in part to withdrawal or fear of withdrawal symptoms. It is now generally recognized that the maintenance of drug dependence involves a purely psychic state. This state long outlasts any withdrawal symptoms and accounts for relapse years after the last withdrawal, and also explains the fact that dependence on nonaddictive drugs like cocaine or methamphetamine may be no easier to control than dependence on opiates or other physically addicting drugs.

It may also be that the underlying psychic dependence is less specific than might be thought from observation of active opiate addiction alone. This fact may account for the nonspecific way in which one drug may be substituted for another, even though the two are of very different pharmacological groups. Illustratively, it was noted in the London methamphetamine epidemic of 1968 that this stimulant, taken intravenously, was being substituted by preference for the opiate heroin which had become unobtainable except in special clinics. The addicts appeared to prefer to switch to methamphetamine, then readily available, rather than go to the trouble of reporting to a clinic. The important fact is that the effect which was sought was not totally specific for heroin but could be produced to a satisfactory degree by methamphetamine.

8. Psychiatric Aspects of Long-Term Drug Dependence

The chronic adverse effects of drug dependence vary with many factors. Common to virtually all forms of fully developed chronic drug dependence, however, is a degree of social and economic disability and a moral deterioration which is easier to recognize than to measure or reduce to objective terms. It is seen as a falling off of consideration for others and a narrowing of interest to the self and particularly to those activities which relate to drugs; such a constriction is similar to that which occurs in persons suffering from chronic somatic disease.

A significant proportion of drug-dependent persons become an economic and social burden, and when they become sufficiently numerous in any society their existence stimulates social responses which include legislation for control. This occurred long ago in China, the Near East, and North Africa, with respect to opium and cannabis, and more recently in Japan with respect to methamphetamine and in North America, Sweden, and to a lesser extent in Britain [Glatt et al. 1967; Brill and Hirose 1969; Sjoquist and Tottie 1969].

The frank psychiatric complications of chronic drug dependence include the psychoses associated with stimulant use. These complications are of particular interest because certain paranoid types are often quite indistinguishable from ordinary paranoid schizophrenia, although a wide variety of other psychoses have been described, especially with cocaine, where episodes of delirium with haptic hallucinations are prominent. Delirium and convulsions are a frequent complication of withdrawal from the barbiturate-alcohol group, and less well defined psychotic states also occur. As already mentioned, the hallucinogens and particularly LSD have been noted to precipitate "bad trips" which may lose their acute character and turn into typical schizophrenia where the drug experience plays only a historical role. The opiates appear to be singularly free from active and positive psychiatric symptoms, such as psychosis, delirium, or drug-induced aggression.

When we come to a discussion of the negative symptoms or loss of capacity, we find much in common among the chronic effects of various drugs of dependence. Such negative symptoms affect only a minority of drug-dependent persons, and when they do occur it is always possible to point to other factors as the real explanation of the pathology. Such factors obviously contribute to the total picture, but at present there is no data to indicate just how large this contribution may be. Some observers are inclined to feel that factors such as poor nutrition, chronic infection, social deprivation, stress, and pre-existing psychopathology account for all defect symptons, and for all chronic and acute psychiatric disorders as well, except for obvious dose-dependent acute drug reactions. Other observers are more inclined to stress chronic drug abuse as the primary and decisive factor in the production of defect symptoms. For the present we can do no more than rely on clinical judgment, which generally favors the view that severe drug dependence is in most instances the decisive factor, and it is on this assumption that most therapy is founded.

9. Psychiatry, Conduct Disorders, and the Legal Basis of Compulsion

The rapid spread of drug dependence has roused serious public concern and has led to widespread demands for proof as to the adverse effects of this practice. Such demands, whether from those who favor or from those who oppose legal controls, are for incontrovertible data—tangible, measurable, and fully demonstrable under controlled conditions. Those who favor legal controls expect further support for their views from such proof, and those opposed to control are equally certain that the evidence will provide constitutional grounds for decontrol of one or more drugs, at least with respect to personal use.

In such discussions, the psychiatry of drug dependence and its behaviroal correlates finds relatively little favor from either side of the debate. Adverse psychiatric reactions associated with drug dependence and abuse are easy to identify clinically, but they are not tangible like evidence of somatic damage; in the psychiatric reactions, the use of drugs is but one of a bewildering variety of other elements of potentially pathogenic nature. The timing of the reaction and its specific pattern may convince the clinician that the drug is the cause, but post hoc reasoning is always open to debate; in any given instance of drug-related psychotic reaction, the abuse of drugs can also be interpreted either as a symptom of the oncoming disorder rather than its cause, or merely as a trigger which releases an underlying predisposition to such disorder.

In the past, society readily accepted the consensus of clinical judgment, and drug dependence was generally thought to lead to a variety of social ills through the behavioral and psychiatric disorder induced by such abuse [Lewin 1924; Adams 1937]. As we have seen, however, the debate was reopened some years ago, first with demands for rigorous scientific proof as to the damage from LSD and the more potent hallucinogens, and later with respect to cannabis and even the opiates. The specifications of these demands are such that they are not likely to be satisfied by field and clinical data, where the nature of the agent is often in doubt, its amount a matter of conjecture, and the variables of personality and of environment essentially uncontrolled. McIver [1964] has written a clear account of the problem of evaluating social factors alone.

What the current debate seems to demand is a set of tangible, objective, and controlled proofs which can fulfil a series of postulates analogous to those Koch developed for tuberculosis, an isolation of factors to be achieved only in a laboratory setting and at the present not foreseeable for chronic dependence in humans. In view of these considerations, it might seem pointless to dwell on the psychiatry of drug dependence or its psychic aspects as a consideration relevant to the current debate about drugs and their adverse effects; one might be led to believe that for purposes of public policy only irrefutable proofs of somatic damage would be relevant.

Unfortunately the reverse tends to be true. As has been vigorously maintained by Solomon [1966] and by most legal authorities, society has only limited rights to interfere with what the individual does with his own body, except insofar as that activity impinges on the welfare of others. This position was long ago enunciated in a very different context by John Stuart Mill, and it appears to be one of the basic elements in both English and American law. The proponents of decontrol argue that demonstration of purely personal harm to the drug user provides no basis for laws which control his taking such drugs, any more than obesity statistics justify legislation against overeating. These proponents also make an equally strong case against control of personal use if such control is based purely on the ground of dependence. Only when an individual's conduct interferes with society to a significant degree may society in turn interfere by law with that conduct and with the person's civil liberty. Some liberals go so far as to include suicide in this concept of personal freedom [Szasz 1968]. One does not need to invoke such extreme positions to arrive at the conclusion that in the last analysis the case for legal controls which go so far as to interfere with possession of a drug for personal use must be based on conduct of the drug taker as it affects others; and this position in turn springs directly from the psychiatric effects of drug dependence.

10. Psychiatry in Therapy of Drug Dependence

Just as group influences have a powerful effect in spreading drug habits, so also they play a large role in treatment. This is most clearly evident in such organizations as Synanon and Daytop Village, which derived their initial impulse from Alcoholics Anonymous and which have since added elements from a wide variety of psychotherapeutic modalities, such as behavior therapy, the therapeutic community, and formal group therapy. Regardless of the specific mix of any given program, the effort still centers on change at the psychic level. Even where the basis of the treatment is a chemical modality, such as methadone, the psychotherapeutic element is still significant.

Some addicts recover spontaneously by a process which resembles religious conversion through an abrupt experience of revelation somewhat like that described for religious conversion [James 1929]. Other addicts are able to overcome an inveterate addiction as a result of a happy marriage or some other psychic experience of equally positive value. All this is not to be taken as proof that the process must be entirely or even fundamentally on a psychic level; it is cited merely as a description of the data as they are now available, and these indicate that for the healing of drug dependence, psychic factors are as significant as they are for its inception and its maintenance.

11. Relation of the Psychiatry of Drug Dependence to Broader Issues

The psychiatry of drugs of dependence and abuse is unique perhaps in that it provides a situation in which a range of known agents act on persons in such a way as to produce a variety of observable psychic changes at the highest levels—including stimulation, sedation, and changes of content of thought —as well as states which resemble all of the known mental disorders. The agents are quantifiable and suitable for investigation and chemical manipulation to a high degree, and this fact promises to bring some of the basic problems of psychiatry within reach of the experimental laboratory.

References

Adams, E. W. (1937). *Drug Addiction,* London : Oxford Medical Publications.

de Alarcon, R. (1969). *Bull. Narcotics* 21 : 17.

Baudelaire, C. (1964). *Les Paradis Artificiels,* Paris : Editions Gallimard et Librarie Generale Francaise Livre de Poche 1326. Originally published in French in 1860.

Bejerot, N. (1969). *Internat. J. Addictions* 4 : 391.

Brill, H. (1966). *Proc. Vth Internat. Congr. CINP.,* pp. 267–270.

——, and Hirose T. (1969). *Seminars in Psychiatry* 1 : 179.

Chopra, R. N., and I. C. Chopra (1965). *Drug Addiction with Special Reference to India,* Council of Scientific and Industrial Research New Delhi : Delhi Press.

Connell, P. H. (1958). *Amphetamine Psychosis,* London : Maudsley Monographs, Chapman and Hall.

DeQuincy, T. (1932). *The Confessions of an English Opium Eater,* New York : Three Sirens Press. Originally published, ca 1822.

Fraigneau, A. (1957). *Cocteau par Lui-Meme,* Paris : Editions du Seuil.

Freedman, A. M., and H. I. Kaplan (1967). *Comprehensive Textbook of Psychiatry,* Baltimore : Williams and Wilkins.

Glatt, M. M., D. J. Pittman, D. G. Gillespie, and D. R. Hills (1967). *The Drug Scene in Great Britain,* London : Edward Arnold.

Hill, H. E. (1962). *Quart. J. Stud. Alc.* 23 : 18.

——, C. A. Haertzen, and M. Davis (1962). *Quart. J. Stud. Alc.* 23 : 411.

——, C. A. Haertzen and Glaser (1960). *J. Gen. Psychol.* 6 : 127.

Hollister, L. E. (1968). *Chemical Psychoses* Springfield, 111. Thomas.

Huxley, A. (1954). *The Doors of Perception* New York : Harper.

James, W. (1929). *The Varieties of Religious Experience,* New York : Modern Library.

Jaspers, K. (1963). *General Psychopathology* Chicago : University of Chicago Press. Translated from the German by J. Hoenig and Marian W. Hamilton.

Johnson, G. (1967). *The Pill Conspiracy,* Los Angeles : Sherbourne.

Kalant, O. J. (1966). *The Amphetamines,* Toronto : University of Toronto Press.

Kast, E. C., and V. J. Collins (1964). *Anesth-Anal.* (Cleveland) 43 : 285.

Lewin, L. (1964). *Phantastica,* New York : Dutton. First published in German in 1924.

Livingston, R. B. (1958). *Narcotic Drug Addiction Problems,* Washington, D.C. : U.S. Dept of Health, Education and Welfare, Health Service Publication No. 1050.

McIver, R. M. (1964). *Social Causation,* New York, Evanston, and London : Harper Torchbooks, Harper and Row.

Mintz, M. (1965). *The Therapeutic Nightmare,* Cambridge Mass : Houghton Mifflin.

Nyswander, M. (1956). *The Drug Addict as Patient,* New York : Grune and Stratton.

Press, E., and A. K. Done (1967a). *Pediatrics* 29 : 611.

——, (1967b). *Pediatrics* 39 : 451.

Sjoquist, F., and M. Tottie (1969). *Abuse of Central Stimulants,* Stockholm : Almqvist and Wiksell.

Solomon, D. (1966). *The Marijuana Papers,* New York : Bobbs Merrill.

Szasz, T. S. (1968). *Law Liberty and Psychiatry,* New York : Collier Books 07477.

Willis, J. H. (1969). *Drug Dependence,* London : Faber.

B. The National Institute of Mental Health

B. S. Brown

The National Institute of Mental Health administers the federal government's major program of support for the nation's work in mental health. From a fairly modest beginning in 1949 with an overall budget of $3 million and a staff of 192, the Institute has moved to a current budget of over $450,000,000 and more than 6,000 employees. Due to its growth and expansion, NIMH was separated from the original nine Institutes of Health in 1967, and became a Bureau of the Public Health Service. In 1968, as part of the reorganization of the Public Health Service, NIMH became part of the newly established Health Services and Mental Health Administration, Public Health Service, Department of Health, Education, and Welfare.

The Institute, in addition to its central intramural and extramural research, training, and service offices, operates the Fort Worth and Lexington Clinical Research Centers for the treatment of drug addicts; St. Elizabeth's Hospital for psychiatric patients in Washington, D.C.; the Mental Health Study Center in Adelphi, Maryland; the Epidemiological Study Center in Kansas City, Missouri; and animal research laboratories in Poolesville, Maryland. NIMH employees also serve in ten Regional Health Offices.

The Institute's programs fall into three major categories—research, training, and services; and about one-third of the budget is appropriated to each category. There are nine administrative Divisions, one Center, and four Offices listed on the administrative chart.

The Divisions are Division of Extramural Research Programs, Division of Manpower and Training Programs, Division of Mental Health Service Programs, Division of Special Mental Health Programs, Division of Narcotic Addiction and Drug Abuse, Division of Alcoholism (newly established), Division of Clinical and Behavioral Research, Division of Biological and Biochemical Research, Division of Special Mental Health Research, and National Center for Mental Health Services, Training, and Research. The Divisions of Clinical and Behavioral Research, of Biological and Biochemical Research, and of Special Mental Health Research are all segments of the National Institute of Mental Health intramural research program. The other Divisions are concerned with extramural research, training, and delivery of services. The National Center for Mental Health Services, Training, and Research at St. Elizabeth's Hospital offers inpatient treatment, training, and a special division devoted to clinical research.

The National Institute of Mental Health is devoted to the eradication of mental and emotional disorders, by finding a delicate balance between genetic and physical factors and the psychological, social, and environmental influences which can either help to preserve and enhance the mental health and spiritual well being of man, or conversely, to threaten or undermine that mental health. Dr. Stanley Yolles, Director of the Institute from 1964 until June 1970, put the matter very well when he said, "The interests of the Institute cover an awesome spectrum—from the most molecular of the biological sciences to the broadest of the social sciences, from a single brain cell to the total culture."

The single theme which runs throughout research in mental health today is the essential unity of man's nature. It is an absolute composite of biological, psychological, social, and cultural factors of human behavior.

C. The Division of Narcotic Addiction and Drug Abuse and the Center for Studies of Narcotic and Drug Abuse, NIMH

E. Carroll, R. C. Petersen, and J. D. Blaine

The Division of Narcotic Addiction and Drug Abuse, formed in November 1968, includes the Clinical Research Centers in Lexington and Forth Worth, the Addiction Research Center in Lexington, the Narcotic Addict Rehabilitation Branch, and the Center for Studies of Narcotic and Drug Abuse, the extramural research arm of the Division. Within the National Institute of Mental Health, the Division of Narcotic Addiction and Drug Abuse bears primary responsibility for prevention, education, research, training, and treatment in the entire area of drug abuse.

The Lexington and Fort Worth Clinical Centers plan and conduct a broad program of studies on the management, treatment, rehabilitation, and aftercare of drug-dependent persons and serve as model treatment, training, and demonstration centers for professionals and other persons concerned with the problems of drug dependence. Both centers provide vocational rehabilitation services. The Lexington Center admits both male and female patients from east of the Mississippi River, while the Fort Worth Center admits only males from west of the Mississippi.

Both centers use a variety of treatment modalities, in an attempt to tailor treatment to the particular presenting needs of the addict patient. At present the two centers both offer examination and evaluation services for addicts under the civil commitment programs of Titles I and III of the Narcotic Addict Rehabilitation Act (PL 89–793). It is expected that the number of patients served under the commitment procedures will decline as communities develop their own examination and evaluation facilities. Staff from both centers have participated in a variety of educational programs for both professional and lay persons.

The Addiction Research Center, the intramural basic research arm of the Division, conducts a wide variety of investigations on the nature of the addictive process, the addiction potential of new drugs, and the therapeutic potential of various drugs to be used in the treatment of narcotic addiction. For example, during the past year a pilot study was completed to determine if post-addicts would perform a moderate amount of work to obtain a single dose of dilaudid, and would refuse to work for a placebo. Data indicated that addicts would work to obtain dilaudid, but not a placebo. The investigators feel that the methods they employed might be useful in studying the effects of various treatments of addiction on drug-seeking behavior as well as for the study of the absolute and relative abuse potential of drugs.

The Narcotic Addict Rehabilitation Branch is responsible for the development and admini-stration of the narcotic addict civil commit-ment program authorized under Title I and III of the Narcotic Addict Rehabilitation Act of 1966 (PL 89–793). This Act was a land-mark in that narcotic addiction was viewed as an illness and not as a criminal activity, and the federal government assumed re-sponsibility for addicts committed under Titles I and III for a maximum period of thirty-six months. The Branch, through approxi-mately 130 contracts, provided for the delivery of a wide range of treatment and re-habilitation services to narcotic addicts in 118 cities in 42 states. Approximately 950 patients are now receiving aftercare services. Civil commitments for examination and evaluation (the suitability of the addict for treatment) totaled more than 3,000 in the past year.

In addition to aftercare contracts, the Branch is responsible for the development and administration of narcotic addiction treatment center grants, under Title IV of the original NARA Act and its legislative successors, PL 90–574, and PL 91–211. All applicants for these grants must agree to furnish, either themselves or through contract, five essential services, which include inpatient, outpatient,

partial hospitalization (including half-way houses), twenty-four-hour emergency care, and community consultation and education.

The federal government provides funds, on a matching basis, for both the construction and staffing of these treatment centers. All these centers provide a variety of treatment modalities, on the general premise that not all addicts are the same, and that any one addict, depending on the stage of his addiction, might respond better to one treatment modality, or combination of modalities, rather than another. There are approximately 3,000 patients now in treatment at the 17 treatment centers. All of the grantee agencies are re-quired to use uniform admission and evalua-tion data collection forms, so that meaningful comparisons, with adequate numbers, might be made of the relative efficacy of various treatment modalities.

The Center for Studies of Narcotic and Drug Abuse, the extramural research arm of the Division, was established in 1967 as one of the special sections of the Division of Mental Health Programs. It became part of the Division of Narcotic Addiction and Drug Abuse in 1968.

The term *drug abuse* covers an extremely broad range of problems which, in turn, demand a wide range of activities to cope with them. These activities include focused investigation of the underlying causes and consequences of the various kinds of drug abuse ; pharmacological isolation and pro-duction of dangerous drugs to permit re-plicable research ; development of innovative and effective treatment methods as well as their evaluation ; and dissemination of authoritative information to the general public as well as to the scientific community for the purpose of education, prevention, treatment, and stimulation of expanded research.

The creation of narcotic addiction treatment centers and the expanded program of treatment offered for drug users through staffing grants in the community mental health centers, as well as the need for more health personnel to serve in preventive and treatment capacities, have led to the establishment of three training centers, one each on the East and West Coasts, and one in a continuing education department of a university in Oklahoma. In addition, the Center is underwriting the production of training films.

Significant aspects of the training grant program include the training of youths from 14 ethnic groups at high risk of addiction, to work as case finders and treatment personnel for members of their peer groups in San Francisco, as well as an exchange program between the Hunter College School of Social Work and the School of Social Work of the University of Puerto Rico to increase awareness of the cultural factors in addiction of Puerto Ricans on the island and in New York City. Workers trained in this program will be able to serve in the narcotic addiction treatment center funded by the Narcotic Addict Rehabilitation Branch in San Juan.

The Center, in active collaboration with the Office of Communications, participates in the development of a wide range of public information and educational materials related to drug abuse. This includes the preparation and revision of descriptive brochures describing the various drugs of abuse, materials for educators and others, and a wide range of audiovisual materials.

Since its inception, the Center has had the responsibility for the development and administration of a program for obtaining necessary supplies of research drugs and their orderly distribution to qualified investigators. Originally, the program began with the distribution of LSD through the joint FDA–NIMH Psychotomimetic Agents Advisory Committee. With the increasing use of marihuana and related drugs, the program has come to include a considerably wider spectrum of drugs, including LSD, psilocybin, radioactively tagged and untagged THC (delta 8 and 9), a uniform grade of natural marihuana, and most recently, heroin.

The Center embarked in 1968 on a program to make available to the research community supplies of natural marihuana of known potency, as well as supplies of THC in synthetic form. In addition to supporting an expanded contract program in these areas, the Center has underwritten a wide variety of research grants which include investigations of the basic chemistry of cannabis and cannabis products; studies of the pharmacology of the drug; the mutagenic, carcinogenic, and teratogenic implications of its use; as well as applied research.

Two overseas studies are currently underway to investigate the possible psychological and physiological concomitants of chronic cannabis use. One study, in Greece, is concentrated on hashish users; the other, in Jamaica, will study users of ganja, marihuana much more similar to the potency of that used in the United States.

Evaluation of currently promising addiction treatment approaches, particularly chemotherapeutic methods, is probably the single most important applied aspect of the Center's research program. Research has expanded in the area of methadone maintenance particularly, since this treatment modality has secured such a wide degree of acceptance. The clinical desirability of having long-acting chemotherapeutic agents to control addiction has led to the development of support to develop new and longer acting materials.

Emphasis on the development and evaluation of chemotherapeutic treatments for addiction is paralleled by studies having to do with the neuropharmacological and biochemical aspects of opiate dependence.

Studies of the amphetamines and the barbiturates include investigation of the neurophysiological effects of amphetamine abuse, the neurochemical correlates of such abuse, and the relative role of enzyme induction in tolerance to barbiturate use.

Studies on LSD and other hallucinogenic drugs include investigation of the pharmacology and biochemistry of these drugs, as well as genetic studies and studies of mutagenicity and teratogenicity.

More accurate knowledge of the epidemiology of drug use is essential for devising more effective means of prevention, early intervention, and treatment. The illicit character of much of this use makes the collection of accurate figures even more difficult than is the case, for example, in psychiatric epidemiology.

The Center underwrites the Narcotic Addiction Register in New York City, the only one of its kind in the country. In addition, in the field of heroin addiction, the Center currently supports one epidemiology study in New Orleans and another in Chicago which looks at "copping areas"—places where buyers and sellers of heroin meet. Another investigator in an East Coast city is looking at the natural history of addiction careers by examining one group of lower-class whites in an ethnic enclave.

Two nationwide studies of student drug use—one concerned with high school students, and the other with college students —are currently underway. In addition, the Center supports studies of specialized drug-using populations on both the East and West Coasts.

In sum, drug abuse and narcotic addiction are still growing public health problems in the United States and in most of the highly industrialized nations of the world. The tasks of understanding the many facets of this problem, of devising prevention, education, treatment, and research strategies to cope with it, are ones which challenge the best scientific efforts of the research community.

Index

See also individual tables for further listing of drugs of abuse